Mi Chelle
Rhus tox
Calcare Carb
Sulphur
Nitric Acid
Conium
Urticaria U.

Kent Rep

DISEASES OF THE SKIN INCLUDING THE EXANTHEMATA

FAROKH J. MASTER

B. JAIN PUBLISHERS PVT. LTD.

Printed in India

Price : Rs. 150.00

First Edition 1993

Reprint Edition 1994,**1995**, 1996,1998

Published by:
B. Jain Publishers (P) Ltd.
1921, Street No. 10th Chuna Mandi,
Paharganj, New Delhi-110055 (INDIA)

Printed in India by :
J.J. Offset Printers
7, Wazirpur, Delhi

ISBN 81-7021-136-0
BOOK CODE B-3424

CONTENTS

Chapter		Page
1.	Introduction	1
2.	Anatomy, Physiology, Embryology, Bacteriology and Pathology	4
3	Case - taking and Symptom Analysis	26
4.	Laboratory and other Aids in Dermatological Practice	50
5.	The Principles of Dermatological Treatment	62
6.	Aids to a Healthy Skin	67
7.	Affections due to Physical Agents	81
8.	Virus Infection	126
9.	Dermatitis & Eczema	214
10.	Erythematous Rashes	289
11.	Psoriasis	315
12	Napkin Rash	338
13	Acne Vulgaris	349
14	Pyoderma	380
15	Angular stomatitis	396
16	Furunculosis	399
17	Syphilis	419
18	Chancroid	452
19	Tinea or Ringworm	480
20	Lichen Planus	492
21	Pemphigus Vulgaris	503
22	Hair Loss (Alopeçia)	513
23	Nail Diseases	525
24.	Pruritus	539
25	Diseases of the Sweat Glands	563

Preface

It is now over eighty-six years since the first edition of the text book "Diseases of the Skin Including the Exanthemata" by Dr. Frederick M. Dearborn was conceived and published. During these eight long decades the vistas of dermatology have spread far and wide, and vast experience has been gained in the field of homoeopathic therapeutics of dermatology. Results are obvious. Ideas have crystallised. Practice can be separated from theoretical hypothesis and investigative tools, as chaff from grain.

It is sad to mention that during these eighty-six long years not a single book was published of such a kind on homoeopathic therapeutics of dermatology. Also what interests me the most is that to-day about twenty to twenty-five per cent of total cases that come for homoeoapthic consultation have dermatological disease and still we have no reference book on homoeopathic therapeutic of dermatology which presents clearly and concisely the subject of dermatology. It has been my aim in the succeeding pages to present the subject matter in a comprehensive manner with stress on etiology, symptomatology, pathology, diagnostic aids, differential diagnosis, miasmatic interpretation, homoeopathic approach, clinical cases and cases from old homoeopathic journals. In the preparation of the text, I have heavily relied on experience, suggestions and assistance of my colleagues all over India and abroad.

I hope this first edition of homoeopathic therapeutics of dermatology will help the students, homoeopathic practitioners and dermatologists who are interested in practising homoeopathy to understand the vast subject of skin diseases and thereby render skilled, efficient and yeoman service to the suffering humanity.

I take this opportunity of expressing my gratitude to the following persons.

Staff of my clinic

Dr. Afshan Deshmukh
Dr. Zubin Marolia
Dr. Kamal Kodia
Dr. Meena Shebet (Rowhani)
Dr. Meherzin Turel (Dubash)
Dr. Benaz Mistry
Dr. Bhavna Trivedi
Dr. Sejal Shah
Dr. Shahrukh Pavri
Dr. Nilufer Panthaky
Dr. Bamji Niloufer
Dr. Farhana Shaida
Dr. Sharmila Lulla
Dr. Swati Kanakia
Dr. Vincent Castelleno
Dr. Diana Minbattiwala
Dr. Kehkashan Deshmukh
Dr. Renuka Naik
Dr. Zenobia Colabawalla
Dr. Ronak Shah
Dr. Pratik Maniar

They have helped me throughout the preparation of this book. Also Dr. Shailen Petigara and Sangeeta Pooran who have been pillars of support.

Contributors

Dr. B.N. Chakravarty
Dr. K.N. Kasad
Dr. B.H. Dastur
Dr. D.P. Rastogi
Dr. R.P. Patel
Late Dr. Kirpal Singh Bakshi
Dr. Satinder Pal Bakshi
Dr. A. Salam Pathan (London)
Dr. R.S. Bakshi (London)

Secretarial Help

Mrs. Yogita Gurunath, Miss Roda Bandrawalla and Mrs. Mridula T. Bedi gave their unstinted co-operation in maintaining the records and in typing. I regret very much the printer's devil, if any, inspite of my best endeavours. Finally I wish to acknowledge my gratefulness to Dr. Premnath Jain and Mr. Kuldeep Jain for publishing this edition and thereby assisting me to accomplish the task with satisfaction.

24.02.1993 **FAROKH JAMSHED MASTER**

Vatcha Gandhi Memorial
Building No.1
Hughes Road
Bombay - 400007

CHAPTER 1

Introduction

Dermatology is an essential part of general medicine since the skin is not, by any means, foreign to the body which it covers. Diseases of the skin are a common occurrence. There are not many statistics to prove the exact frequency of skin diseases in this country, but my experience in Bombay Hospital tells me that of the patients attending the hospitals about 10 per cent suffer from skin diseases. While infections are more common in the tropics, chemical and psychogenic dermatoses are common in western countries.

Diseases of the skin account for a great deal of misery, suffering, incapacity and economic loss. Besides this, they are a great handicap in society because they show. Fortunately however, due to recent advances, cutaneous scars can be successfully removed by plastic planing and skin grafting.

There is a popular adage that skin patients are never cured and never die. Like all generalisations, this is quite untrue. Admittedly, skin diseases are seldom fatal; but I assure you, the cure rate in skin diseases compares quite favourably with that in any other speciality, and cases which cannot be cured outright are often favourably influenced by the control of troublesome complaints. Contrary to popular belief, only a few skin diseases are really contagious. Our task in this country is made more difficult by the illiteracy and economic backwardness of the people and by the superstitions prevalent amonst them. Many diseases are attributed either to visitations by evil spirits or to the anger of the gods, with the result that they are worshipped in temples. A good example of this is smallpox or *Mata.* We medical people will have to root out these ideas before we can succeed in controlling, and then eradicating such diseases. Besides the presence of ubiquitous and the tropical diseases, and the problems created by poverty and illiteracy in tropical countries, climatic factors too create special problems in the treatment of skin diseases. A homoeopath practising in the tropics, therefore, must take them into account.

Since the subject matter of dermatology is superficial, and so available for observation, the practice of dermatology pertinently requires an acute observation with an ability to pay attention to details; it requires recognition of trifles from which deduction can often be made. It has been appropriately said, especially in the diagnosis of contact dermatitis and eczema, that the homoeopath should be a good detective with power of observation and deduction almost like Sherlock Holmes. The diagnosis of cutaneous diseases is essentially objective, and attention to details of eruptions, occupational stigmas, bearing of the patient and clothing is important. Laboratory tests and instrumental aids do not afford any short-cuts to diagnosis.

In chalking out a practical line of treatment, one must never omit reassurance and explanation. Reassurance is the stock-in-trade of faith-healers and quacks. It goes a long way towards the ultimate recovery of the patient and it is a pity that qualified doctors often lose sight of it. A mysterious approach produces anxiety; an explanation of the diseases helps to prevent this unhealthy reaction. The practice of dermatology demands a good background of general medicine which, far from being alien, is closely allied to dermatology. However superficial its subject matter, dermatology is not merely skin-deep. Its scope includes the whole range of life from the human mind to the various micro-organisms, vast external environments and complex endocrine and metabolic transactions within the body. In the practice of dermatology, undue stress should not be laid on giving diagnostic labels; time would be more usefully spent if emphasis were given to establishing the cause/causes of the malady in question.

A skin disease, as seen in practice, is often a reaction pattern resulting from the effects of different etiological stresses on a particular diathesis.

Last of all, the line of treatment should be simple but sure; one should not play with potent, powerful drugs without knowing their specific side-effects. It is a strange fact of modern practice that a large percentage of diseases are man-made; undoubtedly, there should be a strong plea for the prevention of such man-made dermatoses. This could be achieved to a great extent by the timely realization of the dangers involved in the use of potent drugs and the promotion of healthy team work in medical practice.

Sincerity, charity and skill are the bases of practice of medicine; loving tender care is essential for winning the patient's co-operation and confidence essential for his ultimate recovery. Economy is important, more so in these days of rising cost of medical practice. It involves austerity in the use of drugs, cheaper effective drugs and medicaments, only essential laboratory investigations, cutting down the period of morbidity and quicker return to work, so that the least working time is lost.

CHAPTER 2

Anatomy, Physiology, Embryology, Bacteriology And Pathology

The skin is a protective covering of the body. It, with all its specialized derivatives, makes up what is called the integument (Latin = a covering) which covers the entire surface of the human body.

The human skin shows wide regional variations in structure like scalp, face, ear lobes, back, palms, soles, etc. Thickness varies; the number of sebaceous glands, collagen fibre and vasculature differ in different parts of the integument.

ANATOMY

The skin is composed of a superficial epithelial layer — the epidermis, and an underlying connective tissue layer, the dermis or corium. Beneath the corium is another connective tissue layer, rather loose in texture — the hypodermis or subcutaneous layer.

Structure of Epidermis

The epidermis is formed of non-vascular stratified epithelium. Its usual thickness is between 0.07 to 0.12 mm. But in certain parts, like the soles of the feet and the palms of the hands it is very thick, ranging from 0.8 to 1.4 mm. Squamous epithelium is ten to twelve cells thick in the palms and soles and 3 to 4 cells over the eyelids and forearms.

The epidermis is mainly divisible into two main systems, viz., Keratinizing or Malpighian system (Keratinocytes) which forms the bulk and the pigmentary system (Melanocytes) which produces the pigment Melanin is transferred to keratinocytes through the dendrites of melanocytes (Cytocrine secretion).

The following are the main layers of the epidermis which can be made out microscopically in a section perpendicular to the skin surface :

1. Stratum Germinativum : This is the deepest portion of the epidermis and is composed of columnar cells placed perpendicular to the skin surface. The whole of the epidermis germinates from this stratum and hence the name "stratum germinativum". Any trauma to this layer would result in scarring; traumata above the level of this layer heal without scarring. The basal layer contains many mitotic figures signifying the occurrence of cellular multiplication. More and more cells are formed and pushed off to the superficial layers.

2. Stratum Malpighii or Prickle Cell Layer: It is superficial to the basal cell layer, and is composed of several layers of polyhedral cells connected to each other by intercellular bridges. Electron microscopic studies have revealed that adjacent epidermal cells have at their point of contact areas of thickened membranes. These are called desmosomes. Between the desmosomes of two cells there appears to be structureless cement like substance, giving an appearance of bridges. All keratinocytes adhere together by desmosomes. Half size desmosomes occur on the under surface of basal cells which play an important part in anchoring the epidermis to dermis.

3. Stratum Granulosum: It is superficial to the stratum Malpighii. It is composed of flat, fusiform cells which are one to three layers thick. These cells contain irregular granules of keratohyalin.

4. Stratum Lucidum: Superficial to the stratum granulosum is the pale, wavy-looking layer known as stratum lucidum. It is formed by many layers of flattened and closely packed cell whose outlines have become quite indistinct and the nuclei have disappeared.

5. Stratum Corneum: This is the most superficial layer, the outer surface of which is exposed to the atmosphere. It consists of many layers of non-nucleated, flattened, cornified cells. Almost all the cellular structure is lost. It is this layer which becomes thicker with the application of intermittent pressure. This layer is thickest on the palms of the hands and soles of the feet, but thinnest on the outer aspect of the lips, on the glans penis and the eyes. When interior of the keratinocytes are studied with the help of electron microscope, they reveal cytoplasmic filaments in the cytoplasm (tonofilaments), forming bundles (tonofibrils) which are inserted in the cell membrane at the desmosomes. In the stratum Malpighii cytoplasmic organelles are diminished, the centrioles absent and tonofibrils increased whereas in the basal layer (stratum germinativum) a full complement of cytoplasmic organelles and centrioles is present. At the level of the stratum granulosum most of the organelles have disappeared, tonofibrils have increased and dense keratohyalin granules are seen surrounding the tonofibrils. Then there is an abrupt change to the cells of the stratum corneum, no organelles, no nuclei but tonofibrils are seen embedded in a dense structureless matrix. These tonofibrils at the final stage are considered as mature fibrous protein keratin; early prickle (spinous/Malpighii) cells with tonofibrils which contain sulphahydril and disulphide bonds are precursors of keratin. Keratohyalin granules do not contain sulphahydril groups. Epidermal horny layer because of content of keratohyalin cement is referred to as soft keratin. Hard keratin is present in nails and hair.

6. Dendritic Cells of Epidermis: These are melanocytes, Langerhan's cells and indeterminate cells. The melanocytes are the pigment producing cells and are derived in foetal life from the neural crest; their numbers are subject to regional variation. They are normally present in the ratio of 1:5 to 1:10 to the epidermal basal cells.

The cells of Langerhan are found about the middle of epidermis; they can be identified by histochemical methods and electron microscopy. These cells are dopa negative and contain the hydrolytic enzyme, adenosine triphosphatase. These cells are also stained by gold chloride method.

7. Basal Lamina (Basement membrane): The basement membrane as it was known before is now called basal lamina to conform to the terminology of other epithelial surfaces. P. A. S.

stain reveals a condensed zone of mucopolysaccharides in between the epidermis and dermis. Dermal side of the basal lamina contains a few scattered collagen fibres.

Time of Maturation of Epidermal Cells

Basal germinal cells are continuously producing daughter cells by normal mitotic division. The mitotic activity may be increased during stress, inflammation and psoriasis. Normally basal cells to the final maturation stage of horny cells take 4 to 5 weeks. It may be as short as 72 hours to 7 days. Time varies according to the stimulus.

Structure of Dermis (Cutis Vera or Corium)

This layer consists of bundles of collagen and elastic fibres arranged in a reticular fashion. It is profusely supplied with blood vessels. Superficially the dermis is condensed into a dense fibrous network — the basement membrane — to which are attached the epidermal cells. Its deeper parts merge imperceptibly into the hypodermis. Beneath the basement membrane are distributed many blood vessels forming a capillary network.

The connective tissue cells in the dermis are spindle-shaped and are more numerous in the superficial layers than in the deeper ones. Thickness of dermis is 1 to 3 mm.

In a microscopic section passing through the dermis, besides the structures mentioned above, are also seen hair follicles, various types of sebaceous and sweat glands, plain muscle fibres, sensory end-organs like Pacinian and Meissner's corpuscles and adipose tissue. There are a few round cells, an occasional fibrocyte and a few pigment-carrying histocytes called melanophores.

Within the skin the blood supply and drainage lie along well-determined pathways. There are rich capillary beds in the papillae and round appendages and in sub-papillary plexus; deep reticular plexus is much less rich. In the deeper layer of dermis, there is arterio-venous anastomosis surrounded by sphincter like group of smooth muscles under autonomic control. Skin is richly innervated by myelinated and non-myelinated sensory fibres and via non-myelinated autonomic fibres supplying blood vessels and appendages. Conspicuous nerve supply consists of plexuses in the papillae, Meissner's corpuscles, Pacinian cor-

Percentage Pattern of Dermatology

50% Infection	25% Miscellaneous	10% Allergy	15% Climate
•Pyoderma	•Acne	•Eczema	•Intertrigo
•Scabies	•Alopecia	•Drug eruption	•Miliaria
•Mycoses	•Vitiligo	•Urticaria	
•Warts	•Psoriasis		
•Herpes	•Pemphigus		
•Leprosy	•Lichenplanus		
•Tuberculosis			
•Syphilis			

puscles, Merkel's discs and nerve endings in the basal layer of the epidermis.

Sebaceous Glands

They are scattered all over the integument in association with the hair follicles. They are absent from the hairless portion of the body like the palms of the hands, the soles and sides of the feet. These glands, however, occur independently of hair follicles at certain places like the eyelids, margins of lips, external auditory meatus, nipples, anus and around the external genitalia, and at these sites the glands are more superficial. The sebaceous glands are numerous and large on the scalp, forehead, ears, face, the sternal and interscapular regions. In the hairy portions of the skin, the ducts of these glands open into the hair follicles, while in the non-hairy portions, they open directly on the surface of the skin. One or more sebaceous glands may be attached to one hair follicle. Meibomian glands, mammary glands and smegma glands of the penis are modified sebaceous glands. Perspiration in the hot climate and in hot weather stimulates the production

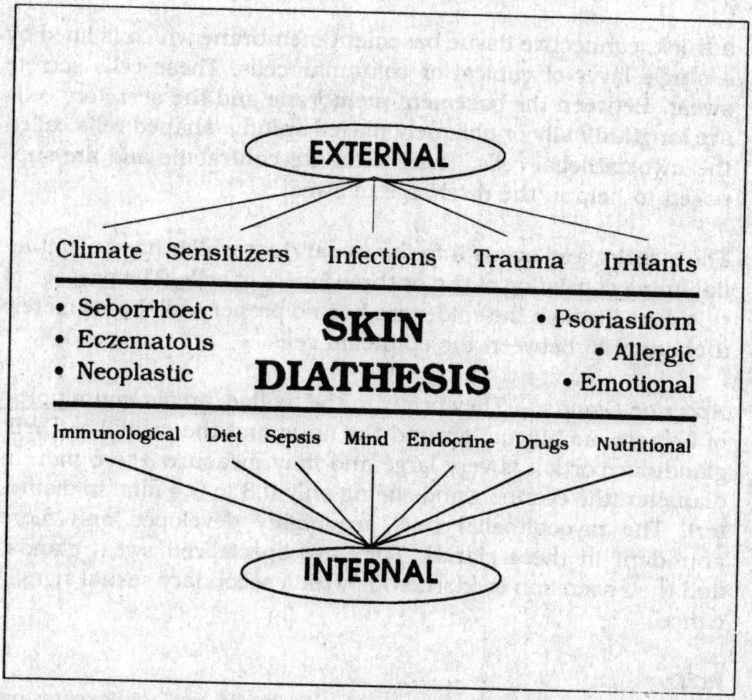

of sebum. Further, the sebaceous glands are active at and after puberty, during menstruation and pregnancy.

Structurally, these are small glands composed of a number of rounded sacs, the alveoli. Adjacent alveoli form a mass like a bunch of grapes. The ducts of the sebaceous glands are lined by stratified squamous epithelium which is continuous with the external root sheath of the hair, and with the Malpighian layer of the epidermis.

Sweat Glands

These are of two types :

Eccrine Glands–They are the ordinary, small-sized sweat glands which are distributed all over the skin except on the beds of nails, margins of lips and the glans penis.

The glandular portion is a simple tube folded by a number of unequal twists into the shape of a ball. This tube is composed of a thick, connective tissue basement membrane which is lined by a single layer of cubical or columnar cells. These cells secrete sweat. Between the basement membrane and the secretory cells are longitudinally or obliquely placed spindle-shaped cells called the myoepithelial cells. These cells are contractile and are supposed to help in the discharge of sweat.

The sweat gland opens into the sweat duct which has an epithelial lining consisting of two or three layers of cells. The passage of this duct through the epidermis has no proper wall, but is merely a channel in between the epithelial cells.

Apocrine Glands — They occur in the axillae, areola and nipples of breasts, umbilicus, around the anus and the genitalia. Their glandular portion is very large and may measure 3 to 5 mm. in diameter (the eccrine glands being only 0.3 to 0.4 mm. in diameter). The myoepithelial cells are highly developed and more abundant in these glands. They are specialized sweat glands, and their secretion is odoriferous with a secondary sexual significance.

Hair

Hair is found on every part of the body surface except on the palms and the soles, the dorsal surface of the terminal phalanges, the inner surface of the labia, the inner surface of the prepuce and the glans penis. Hair differ in length (short or long), thickness (thick or thin) and colour (black, brown or blonde) in different parts of the body and in different races (curly or straight). There are three types of hair :

1. Long, medullated, pigmented hair seen on the scalp.

2. Short, fine, non-medullated and non-pigmented 'lanugo' hair seen in women, children, and on the faces and trunks of adults (Vellus hair).

   Even in bald persons vellus hair may be present.

3. Thick bristles seen in the nose and ears.

   Hair grows about 1-2 cm. per month. The growth varies in different people, races and also on the different parts of the body.

Hair growth and development is under endocrine control. Fine balance of oestrogens, androgens and gonadotrophins determines the pattern in an individual.

Hair follicle and its hair can be anatomically divided into three segments :

1. *Infundibulum* : Extends from pilar orifice above to the entrance of sebaceous gland below.

2. *Isthmus* : The short midsection of the follicle bounded superiorly by the sebaceous duct and inferiorly by the insertion of arrector pilorum muscle.

3. *Inferior* : This extends from the insertion of muscle to the base of the follicle. The upper segments of the isthmus and infundibulum are permanent. The entire follicle beneath the isthmus disappears during the involutionary stages of the hair cycle and again re-forms during the growth cycle.

The hair follicle and its hair are fundamentally one structure derived partly from undifferentiated cells of the foetal epidermis. It is better to combine hair follicle, hair and sebaceous glands as one functional unit. In post-foetal life following the establishment of hair germ, growth occurs upwards as well as down the dermis. Hair follicles are found at different levels in the dermis. Coarse terminal hair extend up into the subcutaneous fat, fine body hair up to the mid-dermis, and fine vellus hair to superficial dermis.

The lower part of the hair is the site of growth. About half way up the follicle it becomes the keratinized structure devoid of living cells. The junction of these two zones (Adamson's fringe) is the level up to which keratinophilic fungi infect the hair. Actually living cells are not infected and so no permanent hair loss occurs following ringworm infection of the scalp.

A hair is composed of a root — the part embedded in the skin, and a shaft — the portion projecting from the surface. The root of the hair at its lower end forms a bulbous enlargement which is called the root bulb. The hair is contained in the skin in a series of invaginations called the hair follicle. If the hair root is of considerable length, the follicle may extend even into the hypodermis. The hair follicle extends inwards from the surface of the epidermis, where it is funnel-shaped either perpendicularly or in a curved fashion — the latter in curly hair. It is dilated at its inner end and is known here as the hairpit. The hair bulb, i.e. the innermost portion of the hair root, fits into this pit. The hair shaft is a dead cornified structure that extends from the follicle to above the surface of the skin. It has three components — an outer cuticle, a cortex and inner medulla.

The hair follicle consists of two coats — the inner one corresponding to the epidermis and the outer one to the dermis. The outer one, therefore, consists of a hyaline basement membrane, external to which is a compact layer of connective tissue fibres and spindle cells, arranged circularly around the follicles. The inner coat, initimately attached to the root of the hair, further consists of an internal and an external root sheat'. The internal root sheath is made up of 3 layers : (*1*) a fine cuticle composed of a single layer of imbricated scales with indistinct or no nuclei, (2) Huxley's layer consisting of one or two layers of horny and flattened nucleated cells, and (3) Henle's layer consisting of a single layer of cubical cells with flattened nuclei. The external root sheath corresponds to the polyhedral cells of the stratum Malpighii. At the bottom of the hair follicle, these cells become continuous with those of the hair bulb.

The hair bulb lies over the vascular papilla and consists of epithelial cells of polyhedral shape. In the hair root, the cells are elongated, at the periphery, spindle-shaped, and in the centre, polyhedral. One or more sebaceous glands pour their secretion into the upper third of the follicular canal through a short duct.

The growth of the hair is cyclical. There are three phases in the life cycle of hair. Growing (anagen), involutionary (catagen) and resting (telogen).

Anagen begins between the papillae and the undifferentiated cell. As anagen begins, matrix cells generate a new hair which pushes upward and dislodges the old bulb of hair.

Mature anagen hair follicle consists of infundibulum, isthmus and inferior segments.

During catagen, entire inferior segment of follicle shrivels upward as a thin cord of epithelial cells and is followed upward by the papillae. During telogen — the club-shaped hair rests in its cornified sac at the level of the hair arrector muscle.

During telogen phase the hair melanocytes cease to synthesize melanin. This function of melanin formation begins again with anagen phase. Therefore, the root of the anagen hair is pigmented, whereas the tip of the telogen hair is unpigmented.

Arrector pili muscles are the small bundles of plain muscle fibres which extend from the connective tissue sheath of the hair follicles (below the level of the opening of the duct of the sebaceous gland) to the epidermodermal junction. When these contract under the effect of cold or emotions, they move the hair into a more vertical position. They also pull on the epidermis in the adjoining region, thus producing an effect whereby the skin in the region around the follicle appears to be raised, while in the adjoining region, it appears to be depressed. This gives the so-called appearance of "goose flesh". The contractions of these muscle fibres is also thought to squeeze out sebum from the duct of the sebaceous gland.

Nails

These are semi-transparent, plate-like horny structures, covering the dorsal surfaces of the distal phalanges of the fingers and toes.

The proximal edge of the nail is known as the root of the nail. The visible portion of the nail is called the nail plate. It is semi-transparent and looks red due to the abundant vascular supply in the nail bed. The more opaque and rather whitish semi-lunar portion of the nail plate near its root is known as the lunula.

The surface of the skin on which the nail rests is known as the nail bed. The fold of the skin surrounding the lateral and proximal borders of the nail are known as the lateral and posterior nail folds.

Nails may be objects of admiration and beauty; nevertheless they are homologous to the claws and hooves of lower animals. The material of the true nail develops from the matrix, which is the deeper portion of the proximal or posterior nail fold and the epithelium of the proximal part of the nail bed. The nail plate and the proximal nail fold are joined by a thin cuticle called the eponychium which makes the exterior groove waterproof. Its rupture by enthusiastic manicuring or dissolving of the eponychium, as in case of washermen results in disease.

There are definite differences between the skin and mucous membranes. In the latter, stratum corneum, lucidum and granulosum are absent. Stratum Malpighii has less number of layers. Dermal appendages like hair, sweat and sebaceous glands are absent; on the other hand, mucous glands are present. Pigmentation is minimal. On the lips, transition from skin to mucous membrane is typically seen. The outer vermilion border has more pigment and is somewhat thicker than the inner part. For this reason and also because of the absence of hair follicles, the chances of repigmentation are least in depigmentary disorders.

Lines of Langer denote lines of normal tension of the integument. These patterns are caused by the peculiar arrangement of elastic tissue in the corium which throws the papillary layer into definite folds. The main significance of these lines is surgical. Incisions along these lines close smoothly, while those across these lines tend to gape and cause wide scars. The pattern of these lines is fairly uniform in all persons.

PHYSIOLOGY

The skin performs a multitude of functions. These are :

1. Protective Function: As an organ of protection, the skin exhibits a wide range of modifications in the various species of animals. For instance, the skin of the alligator has horny plates, and that of the toad has poisonous glands located in it. In human beings, the tough, horny, and keratinized waterproof epidermis, and appendages like hair and nails, provide a sufficiently strong barrier against injury, epidermal penetration of harmful substances and bacterial invasions; they also protect the underlying structures.

Another protective function of skin is to protect against sunlight by synthesis of melanin pigment.

The stratum corneum has been held as a major barrier to penetration. External substances not only are unable to pass through this barrier, but water loss to outside by insensible perspiration is also restrained. There is about 70% of water in the epidermis and about 15% in the horny layer. The horny layer becomes hard and brittle when the water content falls below 10%. The skin looks dry and brittle. It is now appreciated that dry skin is due to lack of water and not due to lack of greasy lipids or fatty substances. Permeable properties of this cornified layer maintain the body's water content and electrolyte concentration. If the injury to the cornified layer is severe and widespread, death may result from dehydration or toxicity.

2. Sense Organ: The skin is richly supplied with nerves and various types of specialized sensory end-organs which provide information regarding environmental changes; the body can then adjust its activities accordingly.

3. Secretion and Excretion: The skin possesses various types of glands which pour secretions on the surface. The more important ones are the sweat and the sebaceous glands.

Sweat in its composition consists of 1.2 per cent solids (organic 0.4 per cent and inorganic 0.8 per cent) and 98.8 per cent water. The important substances excreted in it are : sodium chloride, sodium phosphate, sodium bicarbonate, keratin and a small amount of urea. Water and chlorides are by far the most important constituents. In the hot tropical summers, when sweating is profuse, one can lose a large amount of water and this can give rise to heat cramps and dehydration which can be rectified by the administration of salts and water.

Man perspires very little at low and moderate temperature, but his perspiration sharply increases at high temperature. Direct studies on the amount of sweat secreted on the surface of the human skin show that sweat glands react very strongly to changes in atmospheric temperature. This is known as thermal sweating. In places like the palms of the hands and soles of the feet sweating does not increase with the rise of temperature alone. It can also show an increase in different emotional conditions of fear, anxiety or mental stress. This is called cold sweating or mental sweating, and is under direct cerebral control. This forms one basis of LIE detection. It should be understood, however, that in exercise, sweating is both mental and thermal.

Eating of hot spicy food, causes facial sweating known as "Gustatory sweating". Emotional stress, pain, fear or anger causes generalized or localised sweating on the palms, soles, axillae and forehead.

The sweat glands are innervated by cholinergic fibres belonging to the sympathetic nervous system. These nerve fibres are axons of cells located in the sympathetic ganglia. The central efferent mechanisms of perspiration are located segmentally along the entire spinal cord corresponding to the distribution of the neurons from whose axons the sympathetic fibres are formed. Regional disorders in perspiration can, therefore, prove quite important in diagnosing the diseases in the corresponding divisions of the spinal cord.

Besides the substances excreted in sweat in the normal way (water, salts, lactic acid and products of nitrogen metabolism), the skin can also excrete certain drugs administered to the individual, for example mercury, arsenic, iodine,etc. In certain diseases of disturbed metabolism, a variety of substances have been found in sweat, i.e., cystine in cystineurea, and glucose in diabetes. Elimination of urea and other compounds through the skin, to some extent, can compensate for kidney failure.

The sebaceous glands of the skin secrete sebum which is composed of fatty acids, cholesterol, alcohols, etc. Fatty acids have a mild fungistatic activity. The sebum acts as a lubricant for the drying effects of the atmosphere. Another advantage of sebum and sweat is that they have a destructive action on streptococci and other organisms through certain fatty acids and enzymes.

Excessive production of sebum is called seborrhoea. Sebaceous glands undergo marked hypertrophy during puberty indicating hormonal control of these glands. Sebaceous gland is an androgen target organ. Sebum may evoke inflammation by action of free fatty acids leading to formation of comedones in acne. Sebaceous gland secretion being androgen dependent, excess or deficiency will cause dermatological disorders.

4. Body Heat Regulation: The vital activity of warm blooded species like human beings is,in a large measure, independent of the temperature conditions of external environments because of their constant internal temperature. This constancy is achieved by the existence of a heat regulating mechanism which adjusts the body heat loss to the heat generated in it.

The skin plays the most important roles in the regulation of heat loss. It loses heat to the external environment in three ways : by conduction, by radiation and by evaporation. Heat loss by the first two mechanisms takes place when the environmental temperature is lower than that of the skin. Heat loss by evaporation mainly means the amount of heat spent by the body to evaporate the sweat from the surface of the skin. Even when no perspiration is visible, a certain amount of fluid continues to evaporate through the skin. This is known as insensible or invisible perspiration. About 90 per cent of the total heat loss of the body is regulated by the skin.

The heat loss through the skin is regulated by various physiological mechanisms which include (1) the reaction of the cutaneous vessels, (2) perspiration and (3) the reaction of the smooth muscle fibres of the skin.

The temperature of the skin depends upon the amount of blood flowing through the vessels in the dermis. Therefore, for all practical purposes, the amount of heat loss by physical means is determined by the condition of these vessels. The most important way of reducing the loss of heat is to reduce the flow of blood through the skin. Thus, in the cold, when we want to conserve heat it is accomplished by the constriction of the arterioles in the dermal vascular plexuses. Flushing of the skin occurs when the environmental temperature rises and when one takes exercise, thus ensuring greater amount of heat loss.

Perspiration which adjusts the heat loss through evaporation also depends upon, *firstly*, the blood flow through the skin, and *secondly*, the stimulation of the sweat glands through the autonomic nervous system. Insensible perspiration depends mostly upon blood flow through the skin.

The sensory end-organs for heat (Organs of Ruffini) and cold (End Bulbs of Krause) are present in the dermis. These, when stimulated, send impulses to the heat regulating centres situated in the hypothalamus, which through its connections with the vasomotor mechanisms brings about vascular adjustments in the dermis by constricting or dilating the vessels, thus regulating the heat loss. It also regulates sweating through the autonomic nerves.

5. Storage Function of Skin: The dermis in conjunction with the hypodermis has a considerable capacity for storing various materials; of these the best known are fat and blood.

(a) Fat is laid down in fat cells as a permanent store of subcutaneous adipose tissue. This provides the reserve stores of body energy. Incidentally, it also prevents heat loss, and is a good shock absorber.

(b) Blood is stored in the rich subpapillary plexuses of the dermis. A rough estimate of its capacity in a normal adult comes to near about one litre. Whenever there is a greater requirement of blood by the muscles or other organs, blood is directed from this storehouse to those regions.

(c) The skin is also a good storehouse of ergosterol — the provitamin for vitamin D. This ergosterol is irradiated by the ultraviolet light of the sun and converted into vitamin D (calciferol).

(d) The other type of storage which occurs in the skin is what has been called by Cannon as storage by inundation. This in fact, is the storage of extracellular fluid in the interstitial spaces. This fluid represents an escape from the blood capillaries whenever the hydrostatic pressure in the capillaries increases. The extra fluid is thus held in the dermal and hypodermal layers. In pathological states, this may lead to oedema. Conversely, in dehydration or decrease of plasma volume, the water from such places can be drawn back to the blood.

Certain substances like glucose and chloride may also be stored in the skin temporarily, when their level in the blood registers a sudden rise.

6. Absorption: It is almost an established fact that the uninjured skin is impermeable to watery solution of salts or other substances. Ions can, however, be made to permeate with the application of an electric current by a process known as iontophoresis. In some measure, the skin can absorb substances dissolved in fatty solvents like vitamins and hormones. This is the principle behind the local application and massaging of various ointments, salves and creams dissolved in animal fats. Inflammation greatly increases the skin permeability. Substances that are completely insoluble in water and lipids do not penetrate. Percutaneous absorption mainly occurs via the pilo-sebaceous apparatus. Very little penetration occurs through the cornified cells via the intercellular spaces.

Skin without an epidermis, in extensive ulcers, erosions, etc., becomes freely permeable and absorbs substances easily.

7. Gaseous Exchange through Skin: A small amount of gaseous exchange occurs through the skin. In man the amount of CO_2 exchanged through the skin is negligible compared to the amount exhaled from the lungs (near about 1/150 to 1/200 of that exhaled by the lungs). But in a thin skinned animal like the frog the absorption of O_2 and the excretion of CO_2 through the skin may be sufficient for the proper oxygenation of its blood, so that it may continue to live even after the removal of its lungs.

EMBRYOLOGY

The whole of the skin, epidermis and dermis, is a unified integrated organ system but it develops from two different primitive embryonic layers — epidermis from the ectoderm and dermis from the mesoderm.

The general ectoderm of the early human embryo, except for the part that specializes as the neural ectoderm, consists of the single layer of cuboidal cells. By the fifth week of intra-uterine life, this becomes double layered. The most superficial layer of flattened cells is called periderm or epitrichium because the hair that grows later from the deeper layers is said not to penetrate through it, but to push it up and cast it off. During the third month of foetal life, three layers of cells are recognizable, the periderm, the intermediate and the basal layer which is close to the derma. The basal cells multiply rapidly and keep pushing the older cells towards the periderm, and thus, by the fifth month a stratum of these cells (prickle cells) superficial to the basal cells forms a definite stratum Malpighii.

The cells in the zone overlying the stratum Malpighii show keratohyalin granules and form the stratum granulosum. As the cells keep moving outwards owing to new cells being added from the basal layer, the most superficial ones culminate in cornification forming the stratum corneum nearer the surface. Next to the stratum corneum a thin clear zone containing homogeneous semi-fluid eleidin is evident, particularly on the palms and soles, giving rise to the stratum lucidum. The early intermediate layer of cells becomes a part of the stratum germinativum and the periderm by the end of the fourth month of foetal life is cast off as a part of the vernix caseosa.

The embryonic stratum germinativum, besides giving rise to the surface epidermis, forms the primary epithelial germ which later develops, by downward prolongations into the mesoderm into the hair, sebaceous glands and apocrine glands and also forms the eccrine sweat glands. Soon after birth, the cells of the stratum germinativum acquire pigment granules from the melanoblasts which migrate from the primitive neural crest and specialize in melanin pigment formation.

The dermis is derived mostly from the mesenchyme, though probably some cells from the ventro-lateral part of the somite (dermomyotome) may contribute to deeper layers of the corium. Until the end of the second month of intra-uterine life, the derma consists of closely packed, spindle-shaped mesenchymal cells, and by the third month of intra-uterine life, fine reticulum fibres are demonstrable, which later increase in number and thickness and form the collagenous fibres. The mesenchymal cells by now develop into fibroblasts. The elastic fibres appear later usually during the sixth month of foetal life. It is only during the later months of intra-uterine life that the distinction between the compact derma and subcutaneous tissue becomes evident. The subcutaneous fat is apparent by the end of the third month of intra-uterine life, but becomes abundant only during the later months of foetal life.

The nail starts as an epidermal specialization on the dorsum of the tips of the digits by the third month of foetal life.

The earliest hair appears on the eyebrows, upper lip and chin at the end of the second months of intra-uterine life. By the fourth month, hair appears over the general body surface. This hair is fine, silky, down-like, termed lanugo hair and is cast off before birth as a component of the vernix caseosa. The replacing hair develops to some extent from the new hair follicle and is shed thereafter and replaced periodically throughout life. The hair on the face, neck and trunk of the female and on the face, except for the beard, the flexor aspect of the upper arms and the trunk, in the male, remains apparently of the lanugo type throughout life. Under the influence of sex hormones at puberty, coarser and darker hair appear on the pubis and axillae of both the sexes and on the face and certain regions of the trunk of the male.

Most of the sebaceous glands in the body develop in connection with hair follicles during the fifth month of foetal life, as solid epidermal buds, which later become lobulated. In certain regions like the upper eyelids, hairless deeper parts of the vestibule of the nose, prepuce, vulva and the anal canal, these glands arise from the general epidermis, independent of the hair follicles.

Most of the eccrine sweat glands develop independently as solid down-growths from the epidermis. They first appear on the finger tips, the palms and the soles during the fourth month of intra-uterine life. By the sixth month of foetal life, they become simple cords, which later coil and acquire lumina.

Congenital Anomalies of the Integumentary System

As will be seen from the process of development of the integument, congenital anomalies could involve only a local area or the general body surface. They could also affect all the components of the integument or only the appendages of the skin. There are, however, other anomalies which occur at the regions where the ectodermal lines normally fuse in the early embryo. Here only a short description of a few anomalies is included.

Dermatoid cysts occur as a result of epidermal inclusions along the lines of fusionof embryonic structures, e.g., bronchial cysts and cysts along the mid-dorsal and mid-ventral body wall. The contents of the cyst will naturally show all the derivatives of integument.

Pilonidal (Latin = pilus — hair, and nidus — nest). Cyst. : A variety of the dermoid cyst, due to the persistent foveola coccygea near the tip of the coccyx at the embryonic site of the terminal attachment of the neural tube to the embryonic skin.

Congenital Ectodermal Defect : There is an absence of eye-brows, deformed nails and teeth which may be entirely absent; and sometimes accompanied by the absence of sweat glands. Scalp hair is sparse, the eyes have an upward slant and the nose is saddle-shaped.

BACTERIOLOGY

Normally, the integument harbours several resident organisms like staphylococcus albus and corynebacterium acnes on its surface and crevices. Pityrosporon ovale, a saprophytic fungus is frequently found on the scalp and face. Bacteria like streptococcus pyogenes and staphylococcus aureus, may occasionally be found on the skin as transient flora though they can often be demonstrated in the nose, mouth and throat. These pathogenic bacteria are also frequently found in the body folds particularly the perineum. Occasionally, candida albicans and intestinal bacteria may be seen on the skin particularly near the anus.

Despite the presence of these organisms, normally no harm is done to the skin, because the latter protects itself with its auto-disinfecting defence mechanism, viz. : the acidic pH mantie, the fatty acids of the sebum, the continuous desquamation of the stratum corneum and the enzymes of sweat. Daily washing and the sun's rays also inhibit the growth of bacteria. The normal resistance of the skin is reduced in debilitating diseases like diabetes; xerodermic skin lacks the defence mechanism and is, therefore, more prone to pyoderma. In the body folds, particularly in obese patients where sweating is increased, pH is high, maceration is more, local temperature is raised, hence the infection is frequent. Seborrhoeic individuals are supposed to have altered sebaceous secretion; hence they are also prone to infections. Resident bacterial flora like staphylococcus albus which is normally non-pathogenic, may become pathogenic in person with defective defence mechanism.

PATHOLOGY

The pathological processes in the skin may involve one or more of its constituents,viz.,epidermis, dermis or subcutaneous tissue or their component parts or layers. The changes are hypertrophic, atrophic, inflammatory or dystrophic. The student should be familiar with the meaning of these pathological changes and the terminology used to describe them.

Epidermis

Hyperkeratosis implies hypertrophy of the stratum corneum. In localized form it is seen in corns, warts and keratoses. In diffuse form, it is seen in ichthyosis, keratodermas and pityriasis rubra pilaris.

Parakeratosis implies incompletely cornified but abnormally increased horny layer. The latter is seen as swollen horny cells with oedema and retention of nuclei. Cells are loosely attached. Parakeratosis signifies oedema of prickle cell layer, usually due to an inflammatory process, e.g., psoriasis, eczema, seborrhoeic dermatitis.

Dyskeratosis implies imperfect and premature keratinization taking on various shapes. It may be benign as it is seen in Darier's disease Corps ronds and grains of Darier, and chronic benign pemphigus of Hailey and Hailey or it may be malignant as in epitheliomas (Bowen's disease, Paget's disease and squamous cell carcinoma).

Acanthosis implies hyperplasia of the prickle cell layer. It is usually a benign process and is seen typically in chronic eczema, psoriasis, lichen planus and warts. In tuberculosis cutis verrucosus and pyoderma vegetans, acanthosis and hyperkeratosis are secondary to the disease process in the corium. Special type of acanthosis is seen in condyloma acuminatum and molluscum contagiosum; the latter exhibits molluscum bodies.

If there is a typical proliferation of prickle cells with hyperchromatic nuclei and mitotic figures (anaplasia) accompanied by loss of intercellular fibrils malignancy must be suspected.

Spongiosis implies spongy appearance of the epidermis (mainly prickle cell layer) caused by intercellular oedema. With the increase of oedema, collections of fluid result in intra-epidermal vesicles or bullae e.g. eczema. Viral affections also produce intra-epidermal bullae.

Acantholysis is typically seen in pemphigus. Due to lysis of intercellular fibrils of basal and prickle cell layer degenerated epidermal cells become detached, shrunken and rounded with swollen, compact, hyperchromatic nuclei (Tzanck cells). Acantholytic bulla is seen in pemphigus.

Atrophy implies thinning of the epidermis and straightened epidermodermal junction with loss of rete ridges, e.g., senile atrophy, scleroderma, acrodermatitis atrophicans, lichen sclerosus et atrophicus, leprosy, etc. Basal cell degeneration is seen in discoid lupus erythematosus.

Corium

Infiltration: Polymorphonuclear cell infiltration is seen in acute inflammations, while in chronic inflammations, lymphocytes predominate. Infiltration is mainly around blood vessels (perivascular), pilo-sebaceous apparatus and sweat glands. Epitheloid cells are seen in infective granulomata, mainly tuberculosis, leprosy, sarcoid, etc. A granuloma, histologically speaking, implies circumscribed dermal infiltration which is usually persistent and slowly progressive. Granulomas are composed of histiocytes, epitheloid cells, giant cells (Langerhan's, foreign body) and plasma cells.

It is important to establish the different cells of the infiltration process, their location, number and distribution. Since these are differently affected in different disease processes, correct histological reading helps in conformation of diagnosis.

Bullae : Dermal bullae are seen typically in dermatitis herpetiformis, erythema, multiforme and epidermolysis bullosa. In filiaria profunda, sweat is imprisoned in the upper part of the corium.

Collagen tissue is increased in fibrosis. Increase accompanied by hyalinization and oedema is seen in scleroderma. Elastic tissue is affected in elastosis, cutis laxa and pseudo-xanthoma elasticum.

Neoplasms in the corium may arise from any of its constituents, viz., fibroma from fibrous tissue, a leiomyoma from smooth muscle of arrector pili, neuromas from nerve fibres, lipomas from fatty tissue,etc. Then there are different types of naevi, malignant melanomas, sarcomas and reticuloses particularly mucosis fungoides, etc. Tumours related to hair follicles are seen in trichoepitheliomas; and syringomas arise from sweat glands.

Cysts : Sebaceous, sweat,etc., may be seen in the corium. Degenerative changes may effect corium-collagen or elastic tissue or both. In stained sections, these tissues become basophilic, degenerated lumps or granules. Elastic tissue is more resistant than collagen, hence the latter shows degenerative changes first. Necrobiosis means partial destruction of tissues — nuclei are disintegrated but the cellular structure is preserved. It is typically seen in necrobiosis lipoidica diabeticorum.

Blood vessels of the corium are typically affected in syphilis (Panarteritis with perivascular cuffing of plasma cells.), Schamberg's disease, nodular vasculitis, angioma, angiokeratoma,etc. Extravasation of red cells is seen in purpura and Schamberg's disease; proliferation of capillaries in angioma, angiokeratoma; vaso-dilatation, in inflammations, etc.

Subcutaneous tissue is affected in panniculitis, erythema nodosum, erythema induratum and Milroy's disease.

CHAPTER 3

Case Taking And Symptom Analysis

SYMPTOMS

The common symptoms of skin diseases are itching, pain and disturbed sensations in the nature of crawling, sense of heat, stinging, anaesthesia or hyperaesthesia. These subjective symptoms, as much as the apparent rash, are responsible for bringing the patient to the doctor for consultation.

1. Itching (pruritus) : It is an annoying complaint. Its intensity varies according to the disease and the sensitivity of the individual. It may be continuous or spasmodic, localized or generalized, accompanied or unaccompanied by a rash. The objective evidence of itching is a scratch mark in the form of a linear excoriation. The common causes of itching are :

Scabies	Urticaria
Pediculoses	Dermatitis herpetiformis
Ringworm	Neurodermatitis
Eczema	Insect bite

Itching is typically absent in syphilitic rashes.

2. Pain : It may be localized to the skin, as in boils, abscesses, or radiate along a nerve, as in leprotic neuritis and herpes zoster.

3. Crawling sensation (formication) as if insects are crawling under the skin. It is a variety of itching,e.g.,acarophobia.

4. Sense of Heat (SOH) : In dermatological practice "Heat in the blood" or Sense of Heat is not an uncommon complaint. It is seen as the first sign or symptom of drug eruption, in urticaria and allergy. Lay patients even call venereal diseases as 'Heat-Garm' (syphilis in Arabic means heat). Ayurveda, Hippocrates and Galen have laid stress on constitution, temperament and elementary qualities like heat, cold dryness and moisture.

It is experienced as warm sensation to feeling of burning heat, warm to hot hands and feet, uncomfortable to burning sensation in the sun, and keeping feet and hands outside the covering while sleeping. Almost every case of urticaria, drug rash and disseminated eczema is preceded or accompanied by SOH. This is more in cholinergic, physical urticarias; SOH, as a matter of fact, is a more useful guide than leucocyte count or allergy tests in urticaria and endogenous eczema. Further, according to my experience, persons with SOH are more prone to skin disease. May be change in eating and living habits (vegetarian diet, no spices, chillies, tea, alcohol, etc.) help to reduce the SOH and hence the predisposition to allergic dermatoses.

5. Stinging sensation is characteristic of stinging of insect bites.

6. Hyperaesthesia signifies increased sensitivity, e.g. post-herpetic neuralgia.

7. Anaesthesia signifies loss of sensations. It is noticed in leprosy, syringomyelia,etc. The patient may notice the anaesthesia himself, but usually it is found on physical examination. The sensations tested, pertaining to skin diseases are : pain sensation (pin prick),touch and temperature (hot and cold).

SIGNS

Objective signs are more important in cutaneous diseases than subjective ones since cutaneous lesions are at once noticeable. Quite a few skin diseases are symptomless. Clinical lesions are basically of two types:

1. Primary
2. Secondary

In case-taking, primary lesions are the most important. The differential diagnosis centres mostly around them. The clinician must look for the primary lesion in the most recently developed eruption or at the periphery of the rash. The history and observation of an intelligent patient will be helpful. With the passage of time, primary lesions either involute or transform or get modified into secondary lesions.

Primary Lesions

1. **Macule** : A macule is a small-sized, not raised, circumscribed lesion with alteration in colour. There are two types of macules :

(a) Erythematous
(b) Pigmentary

When of large size, this alteration in colour is called a patch or a plaque or sheet of erythema or pigmentation. A macule must be palpated for infiltration or induration which is typical of granulomatous diseases and reticuloses. Further erythematous macules must be differentiated from purpuric macules. In the former, erythema disappears under pressure, while in the latter, the redness is brighter, and does not fade under pressure. Pigmentary macules are further differentiated into hyperpigmented, hypopigmented or depigmented types. The common causes of macular eruptions are :

Erythematous Macules

Dermatitis
Exanthemata
Drug eruption
Macular syphilide
Erythema multiforme
Tinea circinata
Psoriasis
Pityriasis rosea
Leprosy

Hyperpigmentary Macules

Chloasma
Fixed drug eruption
Melanodermas
Addison's disease
Freckles
Naevi
Lentigines

Hypopigmentation

Leprosy
Tinea versicolor
Pityriasis alba

Depigmentation

Leucoderma
Vitiligo

2. **Papule**: It is a solid, raised lesion about the size of split pea or smaller. A similar lesion, but larger in size, is called a nodule (a big as a hazel but, or smaller), or tumour (bigger than a hazel nut). A papule may be a static lesion or a transition to other lesions; hence in practice, a homoeopath may come across papulo-vesicular, papulo-pustular and erythemato-papular lesions. When dealing with papules, the points to be studied are : their size, shape, colour; whether they be discrete or grouped; whether they be follicular or interfollicular; inflammatory or non-inflammatory in nature. Further, an attempt should be made to distinguish epidermic from dermic and mixed papules. An epidermic papule is usually superficial, dry, solid and flesh coloured; a dermic papule is deeper, elastic and reddish. The common causes of papules are :

Warts
Epidermal and dermal naevi
Drug eruptions
Syphilis
Chickenpox and smallpox
Psoriasis
Lichen planus
Lichen scrofulosorum
Lichen spinulosum
Eczema and eczematides
Acne vulgaris
Rosacea
Prickly heat
Tumours

Papules in Lines

Warts
Insect bites
Psoriasis
Lichen planus

Examples of Nodules

Naevi
Neurofibromatosis
Skin cancer
Dermal leishmaniasis
Tuberculosis cutis
Sarcoid
Erythema nodosum
Xanthomatosis

Leprosy
Syphilis
Mycosis fungoides

Examples of Tumours

Epithelioma
Lymphosarcoma
Mycosis fungoides
Gumma
Keloid
Xanthoma
Naevi
Lipomas
Neurofibromas
Secondary carcinomatosis
Sarcoid

3. **Vesicle** : It is a circumscribed, serum or plasma containing elevation of the integument. When ruptured, the contents ooze out. The size of a vesicle varies from the size of a pin-head to that of a small pea. A similar lesion, but larger in size, is called a bulla. The following characters of vesicles must be studied: their shape, size — is there uniformity or irregularity of shape or size? Are they tense or flaccid, grouped or discrete? What is the mode of evolution? As a rule, vesicles are transitory and of short duration; they either rupture and ooze, or their contents coagulate to form crusts, or enlarge to form bullae, or transform into pustules, or their roofs get rubbed off to leave behind a moist, raw surface. On the palms of the hands, they are situated rather deeply, hence, their contents are discharged with difficulty. On the mucous membranes, their roofs get rubbed off very easily producing erosions. The common causes of vesicles are :

Herpes simplex
Impetigo
Scabies
Smallpox
Chickenpox
Dermatitis herpetiformis
Herpes zoster
Miliaria crystallina and rubra
Tinea
Drug eruptions
Insect bites
Eczema

The common causes of bullae are :

Impetigo contagiosa
Erythema multiforme
Pemphigus
Drug eruptions
Insect bites
Epidermolyss bullosa
Dermatitis herpetiformis

4. **Weal** : It is a flat, evanescent swelling of the skin caused by the local dilatation of blood vessels and increased permeability resulting in localized oedema. The temporary, evanescent nature of a weal and its duration (from a few hours to a maximum of 24 hours or so) is characteristic; it helps to distinguish a weal from a persistent granulomatous lesion. Weals disappear without leaving any trace of stains, scars or atrophy. A weal is usually pale in the centre and red at the periphery, but it may be uniformly whitish or reddish. Common examples of weals are :

Urticaria	Trauma
Insect bites	Urticaria pigmentosa
Drug rashes	

Occasionally, a weal may be surmounted by a vesicle, e.g.,papular urticaria of childhood, or accompanied by bulla formation, e.g.,urticaria bullosa.

5. **Pustule** : It differs from a vesicle or a bulla in the nature of its contents. It is a purulent, fluid-containing elevation. It may arise as such, or it may be a transformation from a papule or more so, a vesicle. The following characters should be studied : the size, shape, number. Is the pustule discrete or confluent, epidermal or follicular, superficial or deep?

An example of a superficial, epidermal pustule is impetigo and of a deep epidermal pustule is ecthyma. When a pustule is in the upper part of a hair follicle, it is called folliculitis. When it is in the deeper part of a hair follicle and involves the root of the hair which comes out as the core, it is called furunculosis (boil). When a conglomeration of boils forms a deep, dermic abscess with multiple holes on the skin through which pus is discharged, it is called a carbuncle. Pustules terminate by rupture, or desiccate to form irregular yellow crusts. Common examples of pustules are :

Impetigo	Bacterides
Sycosis barbae	Furunculosis
Carbuncle	Scabies
Drug eruptions (iodides and bromides)	Anthrax
	Tuberculides
Acne vulgaris	Smallpox and Chickenpox

Secondary Lesions

1.. Scale or Squama : It is a dry exfoliation of the skin due to increased or abnormal formation of stratum corneum (hyper or parakeratosis). It results from erythema or inflammation of the skin or increased dryness. Study the following characters : the colour, shape; whether the scale is dry or greasy; whether it is thin or thick, loose or adherent, whether powdery or squamous, etc.

In certain cutaneous diseases they are very characteristic, hence, of diagnostic value, e.g., the silvery layer-upon-layer scales of psoriasis, the greasy scales of seborrhoeic dermatitis the cigarette-paper-like centripetal scaling of pityriasis rosea, the furfuraceous (powdery) scaling of pityriasis versicolor and the adhesive scale, with its nutmeg-like under-surface of lupus erythematosus. In other disorders, the diagnosis is based upon the primary lesion to which the secondary feature of scaling has been added. The important causes of scaling are :

Dermatitis and eczema
Psoriasis
Exfoliative dermatitis
Pityriasis rubra pilaris
Tinea capitis
Syphilis
Lupus erythematosus
Exanthemata — following scarlet fever
Seborrhoeic dermatitis
Pityriasis versicolor
Tinea corporis
Drug eruptions
Ichthyosis
Lichen planus
Malnutrition-pellagra
Pityriasis rosea.

2. Crust or Scab : It represents a dried-up mass of oozing and other products of inflammatory tissues particularly epithelial debris. Scabs form on vesicles, pustules, bullae, ulcers, erosions and excoriations. The colour, thickness, adhesiveness, consistency and odour of a crust should be studied, also its underlying surface, visible only after the crust has been removed. These characters of the crust, its underlying surface and the primary lesion which the crust has supplemented, are all helpful in the making of an accurate diagnosis. The common causes of crusts are:

Impetigo contagiosa, ecthyma
Sycosis
Ulcers
Kaposi's varicelliform eruption

NON HEALING ULCER TREATED WITH SULPHUR

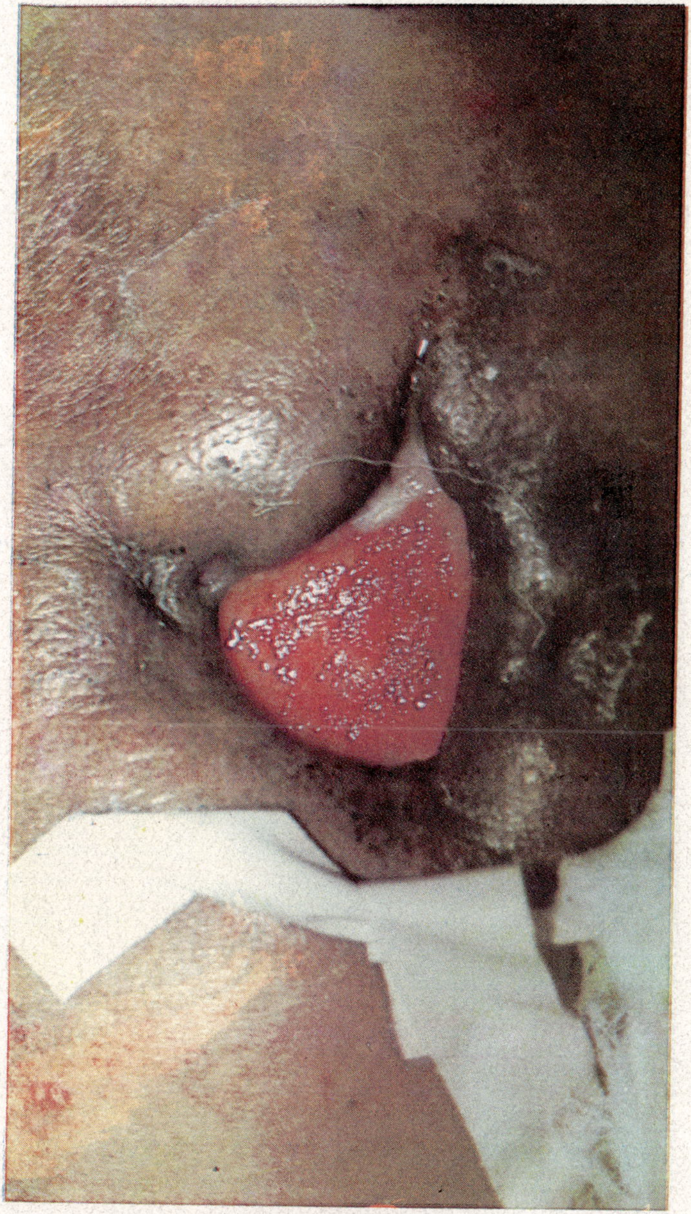

AFTER

NON HEALING ULCER TREATED WITH SULPHUR

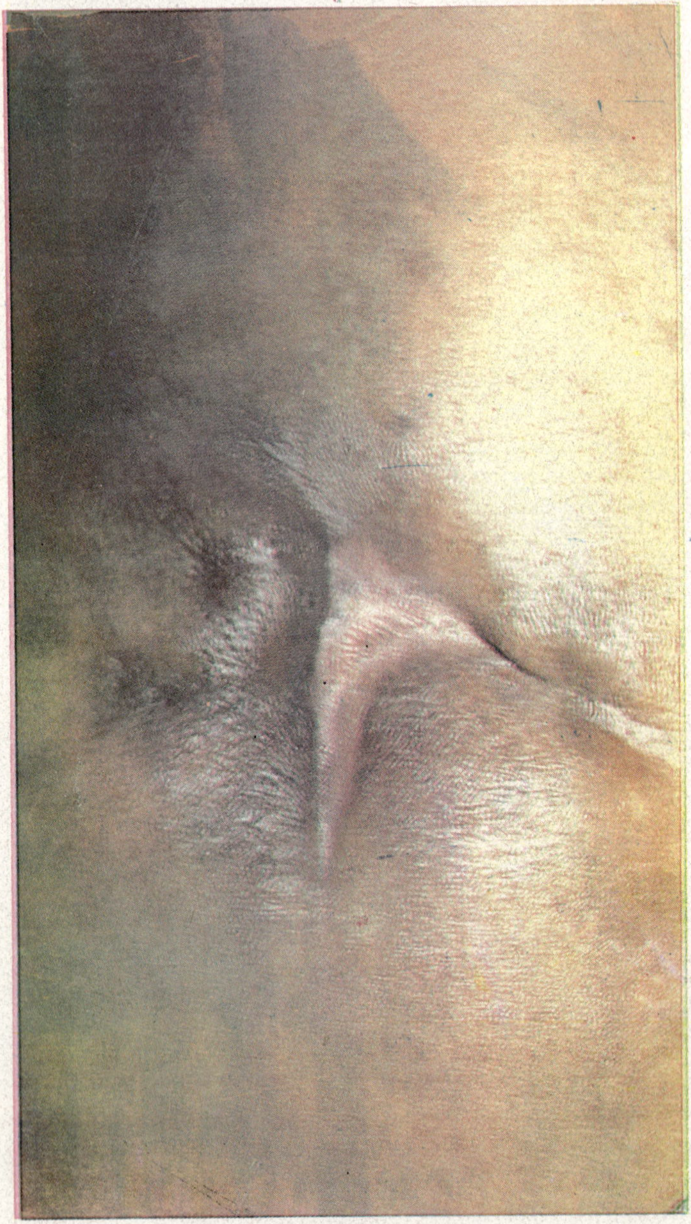

BEFORE

Seborrhoeic dermatitis
Pemphigus
Eczema and dermatitis
Exanthemata—Chickenpox and Smallpox
Herpes zoster
Drugs—iodides, bromides and heavy metals
Syphilis—rupial and nodulo—ulcerative
Scratch marks (blood crusts)

3. **Excoriations** : They are superficial, linear lesions characterized by the removal of the epidermis by scratching or by abrasion. An excoriation may be superficial or deep. It gets covered by a crust — simple, blood or impetiginous.

It is produced by trauma; an excoriation is an evidence of pruritus; a search should be made for its cause.

4. **Fissure** : It is a linear crack in the integrity of the skin reaching down to the papillary layer of the dermis or deeper. It has length but unlike an ulcer, no breadth. A fissure is usually accompanied by pain which interferes with the use of the affected part. Because of the loss in integrity, there is risk of secondary infection. Common examples of fissures are :

Chapping of hands as in extreme dryness
Chronic eczema of the palms and soles
Menopausal keratoderma
Syphilitic fissures
Fissure-in-ano
Intertrigo
Angular stomatitis

5. **Ulcer** : It is a circumscribed lesion starting from a break in the skin, reaching upto the level of the dermis. It has definite length, also breadth as opposed to a fissure. A homoeopath should study its size, contour, depth, edge, covering crust, contents, odour and the surrounding area of skin. The common causes of ulcers are :

Traumatic
Pyogenic
Tuberculosis
Syphilis
Actinomycosis
Neoplastic ulcers
Varicose ulcer
Trophic ulcers

Dermal leishmaniasis
Leprosy
Tropical ulcer
Frost-bite
Peripheral vascular disorders
Metabolic disorders
Syringomyelia and Tabes

Causes of ulcers in the mouth

Stomatitis
Dental irritation
Pemphigus
Tuberculosis
Syphilis
Epithelioma

6. **Scar** : It represents a healed destructive lesion of the dermis and deeper parts. Whenever any inflammatory or traumatic lesion destroys the basal layer of the epidermis and underlying corium, a scar is formed. Superficial epidermal lesions heal without scarring; these are important points to be remembered in surgery and in the treatment of cutaneous lesions. In people with dark skins — Indians and Negroes — scars have a tendency to be keloidal. So, due precautions should be taken in surgery and in the treatment of burns. Certain scars are very characteristic, viz. the tissue-paper like scars of lupus vulgaris, the wrinkled, achromic scars of leprosy, the depressed pigmented scars of cutaneous leishmaniasis, pock marks of smallpox. The clinician should study — the size, shape, colour, texture, depression or elevation of the scar whether it is attached or free, whether there is any accompanying deformity and loss of sensations, hair, sebaceous or sweat secretion. The common causes of scars are:

Traumatic
Ecthyma, acne necrotica and conglobata
Exanthemata — Smallpox and chickenpox
Herpes zoster
Granulomata — Tuberculosis, syphilis, leprosy, leishmaniasis, yaws and fungi
Varicose ulcer
Neoplasms

Certain Dermatological terms (Special Lesions)

Alopecia : It implies loss of hair resulting in a bald patch. Defluvium capillorum means fall or thinning of hair without areas of complete baldness. It must be remembered that hair occur in three states : Growing, stationary and falling. The last state comprises a very small percentage for causes of baldness.

Atrophy : It means wasting away of skin, which appears thin. There is loss of elasticity, wrinkling with diminished or complete loss of hair, sweat and sebum. All destructive disease processes of the corium with intact epidermis (i.e. without ulceration) leave behind atrophy. An atrophic patch may or may not be accompanied by scaling, pigmentation and telangiectasia.

Burrow : It is a straight or tortuous, slightly elevated, flesh-coloured or slightly darker line found on the wrist, hand or genitalia in scabies. It represents the path or tunnel of the Acarus scabiei in the stratum corneum of the skin. At the deeper end of the burrow an acarus can be demonstrated.

Cyst : It is a circumscribed collection of fluid or semi-solid substances in the skin surrounded by well-defined walls. Its size, shape, consistency, translucency, depth, and whether or not it is adherent to the skin and underlying structures, should be studied. The common cause of cutaneous cysts are :

Sebaceous cyst	Milia
Implantation cyst	Mucous cyst
Dermoid cyst	Benign cystic epithelioma
Pilonidal cyst	Hydrocystoma

Comedone (blackhead) : It represents a plug at the pilo-sebaceous opening. It consists of dried sebum and epithelial debris. To begin with, it is white. With the passage of time, the sulphur of sebum is converted into sulphide and the colour becomes black. Comedones are usually found on the face, shoulders, sternal region and back in acne vulgaris and acneiform eruptions due to iodides and bromides. Tar, chlorine and oils, by contact, produce comedones on exposed parts like the face, arms and legs.

Circinata : It implies a circular lesion shaped like a coin or disc. If there is central clearing and spreading at the periphery, the lesions are called annular. Common examples are :

Tinea circinata	Psoriasis
Impetigo	Infective eczema
Discoid dermatitis	Erythema multiforme
Lupus erythematosus	Granuloma annulare

Syphilides	Seborrhoea corporis
Leprosy	Drug eruption
Lichen planus annularis	Pityriasis rosea

Further special configurations may occur in different skin diseases, viz., half circle (Arciform), multiple circles joined together (Polycyclic) or circular with central dots (Iris). The latter is typically seen in erythema multiforme.

Erythema : It implies redness of the skin due to dilatation of blood vessels. It is a common early sign of most cutaneous diseases, but may be difficult to make out in dark people.

Erythroderma : It implies generalized redness and infiltrtion of the integument as is evident in pityriasis rubra pilaris, generalized dermatitis due to drugs and reticuloses. When accompanied by marked scaling and exfoliation of the skin, the term exfoliative dermatitis is employed. In reality, both terms mean more or less the same thing.

Erythemato-squamous : It means a combination of erythema and scaling, e.g., psoriasis, tinea, syphilis, lichen planus, parapsoriasis, pityriasis rosea and exfoliative dermatitis.

Elephantiasis : It is a clinical term signifying elephant like swelling due to extreme lymphoedema and fibrous hypertrophy of a part of the body. The common causes are : filariasis, streptococcal lymphangitis, congenital lymphoedema. The parts commonly affected are the feet, legs and the genitalia.

Granuloma : It is a chronic swelling usually in the form of a well defined, deep-seated, dermic nodule. Clinically it is marked by chronic induration and scarring; histologically, histiocyte infiltration in the corium is its special feature. They are very common in the tropics. There are several causes of granulomas :

Infective

Tuberculosis
Syphilis, granuloma inguinale and lymphogranuloma inguinale
Leprosy
Yaws

Leishmaniasis
Septic
Deep fungi like actinomycosis, etc.
Sarcoid.

Drugs

Bromides
Iodides.

Neoplastic

Epitheliomas
Secondary metatases
Reticuloses like mycosis fungoides, Hodgkin's disease etc.

Keratosis : It is a circumscribed hyperplasia of the stratum corneum (horny layer) of the skin, e.g., senile eratosis, arsenical keratosis, seborrhoeic keratosis. Keratoses have predisposition to malignancy. Follicular keratoses are seen in lichen spinulosus, keratosis follicularis, Vit A, C or fatty acid deficiencies, pityriasis rubra pilaris, Darier's disease, lichen planopilaris, lichen scrofulosorum, etc.

Keratoderma : It signifies diffuse plaques of hyperplasia of the stratum corneum of the skin, particularly of the hands and feet, e.g., tylosis, congenital, arsenical, menopausal, chronic eczema, syphilis, psoriasis, avitaminosis, pityriasis rubra pilaris, etc.

Koebner Phenomenon : It means linear lesions produced by scratching a primary lesion, which results in new lesions developing along the line of the scratch, e.g., lichen planus, warts and psoriasis.

Lichenoid : Violaceous or purplish, solid, firm papules, resembling lichen planus but not due to it. This term is loosely used till a proper diagnosis is established. Similarly terms like pemphigoid, leucodermoid and psoriasiform have been coined to describe cutaneous lesions morphologically.

Telangiectasia : It represents groups of fine, dilated capillaries. The common causes are : rosacea, spider naevus, alcoholism, liver disorder and X-ray burn.

Vegetations: They are cauliflower-like growths in moist areas like the ano-genital region, groins and axillae. If the stratum corneum is absent, vegetations look eroded — erosive vegetations. If the stratum corneum is hypertrophic, the vegetations are termed verrucous vegetations. The common causes are condylomata lata, pemphigus vegetans and pyoderma vegetans.

Zosteriform: Grouped lesions along the course of a nerve, usually unilaterally. Common example is herpes zoster. But zosteriform grouping may also be seen in naevi and vitiligo. Further zosteriform grouping should be distinguished from linear, retiform, herpetiform and corymbiform grouping.

PRECIS OF CASE-TAKING IN DERMATOLOGY

History

(a) Name, age, sex, occupation — Exact nature with list of substances handled in occupation dermatoses only.

(b) Complaints.
Duration.

(c) History of present illness; emphasis on :
1. Site of onset
2. Primary lesion
3. Manner of spread
4. Eruption — active or quiescent
5. Subjective symptoms, if any; also whether the symptoms preceded or followed the eruption.
6. Patient's own idea of cause and aggravating factors.
7. History of any illness preceding or accompanying the skin disorder.

(d) Personal history—Hobbies, special habits, etc.
(e) Past history of any skin disorders, duration and response.
(f) Family history of skin and allied disorders.
(g) General health — Any specific disorder and its relationship to the skin ailment.
(h) Treatment tried — In order of use, and the response to it.
(i) Special history, in particular ailments to find out the cause.

1. Use of drugs (habit or temporary), tonics, sleeping tablets, cough medicines, opening medicines, etc.
2. Emotional stress.
3. Contacts in contact eczema, etc.

Examination

(a) Local

1. Inspection — Clinical nature of lesions — Primary, Secondary, special term.

   Distribution — regional, general or local; grouped or polymorphous.

   Particular examination of scalp, mouth, nails, genitalia and feet.

2. Palpation, scraping, diascopy, sensations,etc.

(b) General physical examination — Patient ill, toxic, conscious, cyanotic, febrile, anaemic, debilitated or not. Mental make-up, bearing, clothes, mannerisms.

DIAGNOSIS

Case-taking is an art acquired with experience. A routine case-taking on the lines suggested above, helps to collect all data and removes the likelihood of oversight in any respect.

As the skin is available for close examination, the examiner must have a sharp eye, an acute power of observation and a clear, imaginative mind for the correct analysis of facts. The examination should be done in natural light; where this is not possible, an examination under daylight bulb or fluorescent tube lighting should be insisted upon. It is advisable to wear gloves while examining a skin patient, particularly in cases of suspected infections like syphilis. Regardful of his complaint, ask the patient to take off all his clothes, and then examine him from head to foot paying special attention to the scalp, mouth, nails, genitalia and feet. A magnifying lens is useful in the study of individual lesions.

Scraping with a pointed dissection forceps, helps to study the scaling process in scaling lesions, particularly those of pityriasis versicolor and the silvery scales of psoriasis,etc.

Three important steps in dermatological diagnosis are :

1. **Morphological diagnosis** — Based on morphological study, localization and distribution.

2. **Clinical diagnosis** — Establishment of disease entity based on history and signs.

3. **Etiological diagnosis** — Establishment of cause or causes in the individual patient.

The ultimate aim of the treating homoeopath should be to establish the etiological diagnosis. Having established the diagnosis, information regarding activity, severity and acuity of the disease process (prognostic criteria) should be elicited and collected before treatment is prescribed.

Localization of Common Dermatoses

Acne vulgaris — Face, shoulders, upper back and chest.

Atopic dermatitis — Eyes, face, neck, front of elbows and back of knees.

Chilblains — Fingers and toes.

Contact dermatitis — Site of suspected contact.

Dermatitis herpetiformis — Scapular region, lower back, chest and forearms.

Dermal leishmaniasis — Exposed parts : face, hands and elbows.

Erythema multiforme — Hands, forearms, face and mouth.

Erythema nodosum — Front of legs.

Herpes simplex — Lips and genitalia.

Herpes zoster — Unilateral lesions : Trunk, face, neck and extremities.

Intertrigo — Flexures : groins, axillae, infra-mammary region.

Lupus erythematosus (chronic) — Butterfly distribution : Face.

Lichen planus — Legs, wrists, forearms, genitalia and mouth.

Neurodermatitis — Back of neck, forearms, legs, ankles and ano-genital region.

Psoriasis — Scalp, elbows, knees, back, legs and nails.

Pityriasis versicolor — Chest, back and upper parts of arms.

Pediculoses — Scalp, trunk and pubic region (according to variety).

Rosacea — Central part of face.

Scabies — Hands (Interdigital spaces, palms), front of wrists, elbows, penis, buttocks and abdomen.

Seborrhoeic dermatitis — Scalp, retro-auricular region, eyebrows and eyelids, sternal region, interscapular region and flexures.

Sycosis barbae — Beard region.

Tinea pedis — Interdigital spaces of feet, soles.

Tinea cruris — Inner sides of thighs near the groins, scrotum.

Varicose ulcer — Ankles (inner surface).

Regional Differential Diagnosis of Common Dermatoses

Scalp — Pityriasis capitis, psoriasis, seborrhoeic dermatitis, infective eczema, tinea capitis, pediculoses and diseases of the hair.

Face — Contact dermatitis and eczema, sycosis, impetigo, rosacea, acne vulgaris, atopic dermatitis, seborrhoeic dermatitis, herpes simplex and zoster, lupus vulgaris (L.V.), dermal leishmaniasis, lupus erythematous (L.E.), chloasma, vitiligo.

Nose — Rosacea, dermal leishmaniasis, L.E., L.V., chloasma, rhinoscleroma.

Ear — Leprosy, seborrhoeic dermatitis, infective eczema.

Neck — Back : Sycosis nuchae, contact dermatitis, neurodermatitis.

— Front : contact dermatitis, pityriasis versicolor, actinomycosis, pyoderma, scrofuloderma.

Lips — Cheilitis, cheilitis glandularis, deficiency disease, contact dermatitis, angular stomatitis, syphilis, lupus erythematous, lichen planus.

Mouth — Stomatitis, pemphigus, lichen planus, epithelioma, syphilis, tuberculosis, deficiency diseases.

Chest — Pityriasis versicolor, pityriasis rosea, seborrhoeic dermatitis, pediculosis corporis, acne, herpes zoster, dermatitis herpetiformis, pemphigus.

Back — Pityriasis versicolor, pityriasis rosea (along the ribs), psoriasis, seborrhoeic dermatitis (interscapular region), acne vulgaris (upper part), herpes zoster, dermatitis herpetiformis (scapular region), pemphigus.

Armpits — Contact dermatitis, tinea, seborrhoeic dermatitis, infective eczema, hidradenitis suppurativa, Fox-Fordyce's disease, trichomycosis axillaris, flexural psoriasis.

Abdomen — Pityriasis versicolor, pityriasis rosea, herpes zoster, pemphigus, tinea, lichen planus, pediculosis pubis.

Groins — Intertrigo, infective eczema, flexural psoriasis, tinea cruris, scrofuloderma, lympnogranuloma inguinale, chancroidal pulp, moniliasis.

Anal region — Condylomata lata, condyloma acuminatum, neurodermatitis, contact eczema, pruritus ani, fissure-in-ano.

Genitalia — Chancre, secondary syphilis, contact dermatitis, granuloma inguinale, chancroid, herpes progenitalis, lichen sclerosus et atrophicus, leukoplakia, kraurosis vulvae, epithelioma, phagedaena, scabies, lichen planus, neuro-dermatitis, pediculoses.

Arms — Tinea versicolor, herpes zoster.

Forearms — Discoid dermatitis, lichen planus, erythema multiforme, psoriasis, tinea circinata, dermatitis herpetiformis.

Elbow — Atopic dermatitis (front), psoriasis (back), dermal leishmaniasis, lupus vulgaris.

Hands — Dyshidrosis (palms); trade eruption, contact eczema, infective dermatitis, nummular eczema, pustular bacterides, psoriasis, tinea, drug allergy, keratoderma, syphilis, chilblains, Raynaud's disease, leprosy, warts, tuberculosis verrucosus.

Thighs - Contact dermatitis, tinea, folliculitis.

Knees - Atopic dermatitis (back), psoriasis (front), lupus vulgaris.

Legs - Psoriasis, lichen planus, neurodermatitis, discoid dermatitis, folliculitis, Henoch-Schoenlein purpura, erythema nodosum, Bazin's disease.

Feet - Tinea, contact dermatitis, dyshidrosis, bacterides, discoid dermatitis, leprosy, actinomycosis madurae, post-traumatic infective eczema, warts, varicose ulcer, neurodermatitis, chilblains, Raynaud's disease, Buerger's disease, keratoderma, tuberculosis cutis verrucosus.

NATURAL HISTORY OF DISEASE

A good clinician and an intelligent patient are of enormous help in studying natural history of disease, thereby assisting in making a correct diagnosis, because different diseases follow different and varied courses depending of course, on climate, patient's resistance and virulence of disease process, etc. A few important examples are listed.

Exanthemata like smallpox, chickenpox, herpes zoster have limited course of 12-15 days unless secondarily infected. Pyodermas are of short duration, unless they become chronic as in folliculitis. Anthrax, tropical ulcer and pyoderma gangrenosum develop rapidly.

In comparison, fungus affections in tropical countries are common in summer and more so in warm, humid season of monsoon. In the cold weather, they become dormant to recur again in the hot weather unless properly treated. History extends over years. Scabies is more frequently seen in winter and insect bites in the summer and monsoon on exposed parts.

Warts spread slowly by auto-inoculation except in the beard region (spread fast by shaving) and moist areas (condyloma acuminatum).

History of dermal leishmaniasis is usually in weeks in endemic areas. Syphilitic chancre develops a few weeks after exposure, while herpes progenitalis and gonorrhoea within 1 to 3 days and chancroid in 3-5 days, granuloma venereum in 2-6 days and lympho granuloma in 1-2 weeks. History of epithelioma on glans penis extends to months and warts only a few weeks. Syphilitic gumma has history of months, while natural history of tuberculosis and leprosy extends over years.

Psoriasis has usually winter aggravation; but some cases do show summer flare-ups when prickly heat becomes psoriasiform. Seborrhoeic dermatitis tends to increase in autumn and spring and the history is chronic. Lichen planus has a sudden or insidious onset depending upon the cause. Drug eruptions are usually acute in onset and short-lived unless caused by heavy metals like arsenic or produce erythroderma-like picture.

Amongst the neoplasms, history of basal cell epitheliomas is in years, squamous cell epitheliomas in months, while malignant melanomas develop in weeks to months.

IMMUNITY AND ALLERGY

During the last three decades, concept of immunity has undergone revolutionary changes and has widened its scope immeasurably. WHO report defines immunity as follows : "The immune response comprises all the phenomena that result from the specific interaction of cells of the immune system with antigen."

Immunologic response involves two separate mechanisms, mediated by two types of cells — T. Lymphocyte (Thymus dependent) and B. Lymphocyte (Bursa equivalent of Fabricius). Source of these two types of cells are the precursor stem cells of bone marrow. T. cells migrate to thymus, modified here and released into blood. They are long-lived and comprise 60 to 80% of the lymphocytes in circulation. B. cells are independent of thymus. The B. lymphocytes can proliferate, differentiate and mature into plasma cells which synthesize humoral antibodies (Immunoglobulins).

Cell Mediated (T. Cell) Immunity

Here cells directly approach the antigen wherever it is localized, may destroy it and become sensitized. On a second or continued exposure to the antigen, the sensitized lymphocytes may become attached to it. This form of immunity is responsible for the rejection of foreign cells, resistance to many viral and fungal infections, delayed type of hypersensitivity and rejection of tissue transplants. T. cells have a complex reaction and release soluble factors, lymphokines, which take part in cell mediated immunity and can destroy antigen, attract leucocytes, slow down the work of macrophages, may be killer cells which are cytotoxic for graft target cells and co-operate with B. lymphocytes to antibody production. Failure of T. cell system will lead to defective cell mediated immunity.

Humoral (Antibody Mediated) Immunity

On antigenic stimulation. B. cells (lymphocytes) transform to plasma cells which produce antibodies (immunoglobulins) that are released in the circulation. Immunoglobulins are serum proteins and there are five major types IgG, IgM, IgA, IgD and IgE. Any defect which limits the number of B. lymphocytes will lead to deficiency of immunoglobulin synthesis.

Immunoglobulins IgG can pass through the placental barrier and can reach into foetus to neutralize bacterial toxins. IgA prevents adherence of micro-organisms to cell surface. Finding of raised IgM in a person's blood indicates previous infection. IgE normally binds with mast cells and basophils and releases histamine, bradykinin, acetylcholine, serotonin and other chemical substances.

Human Leucocyte Antigens (HL-A)

The major histo-compatibility system of man is referred to as Human Leucocyte Antigen (HL-A) system and on the basis of leucocyte typing it appears that there are more than 30 transplantation antigens. Transfer of tissue or cell from one member of species to another always induces an immune response. HL-A antigens are present on leucocytes on the cell surface and are richest on lymphoid cells. It is essential to type H antigen of donor and recepient as is done in case of red cell antigens (Blood grouping in ABO and Rh system). In transplantation of skin, kidneys and other organs HL-A antigens have to be matched. Autologous grafting of skin from one site in the body to another site presents no immunologic problem. Rejection of graft principally involves cell mediated immunity and to some extent also humoral antibody. A detailed discussion is beyond the scope of this book and the interested reader is referred to books dealing with modern Immunology and Allergy.

Allergy and Hypersensitivity

According to modern immunologists these two terms are synonymous. The concept of hypersensitivity was first introduced by Portier and Richet in 1902. The term allergy was coined by Von Pirquet in Vienna in 1906. Allergy means altered energy (*Allos* — other, *ergon* — energy). Simple scratching of the skin causes the triple response of Lewis (Sir Thomas Lewis, 1927). This consists of erythema, weal and flare reaction. Flare is due to dilatation of arterioles by a local axon reflex and the liberation of vasodilator substances (Histamine like — H substances, serotonin, bradykinin, acetylcholine, prostaglandin, etc.) from the injured cells like mast cells and basophils, etc.

The manifestation of hypersensitivity may be immediate (anaphylactic) or delayed (late) tuberculin in type. Richet (1902) coined the term anaphylaxis to describe that certain injected substances, diminish instead of increasing the defences of an animal to their harmful effect.

Arthus phenomenon is local anaphylaxis. Arthus demonstrated that each successive inoculation of a foreign protein initially harmless, leaves the tissue more sensitized eventually leading to the necrosis of the surrounding tissue.

Cutaneous Allergy

In the skin, there are two important but different allergic reactions. One as in urticaria, the causative antigen reaches the skin through ingestion, inhalation or injection of protein substances and the reacting antibodies circulate in the serum. Allergic reaction takes place in the dermis — Dermal Reaction. In this type of allergy, Prausnitz-Kustner-passive transfer reaction is positive, and only the intradermal (injection or scratch) tests show reactivity. The response is weal formation which occurs in few minutes.

The second type of allergic cutaneous reaction is Epidermal Reaction, as is seen in allergic dermatitis or eczema. Causative substances reach the skin by contact. Intradermal allergic tests are negative; on the contrary, patch tests show reactivity. Prausnitz-Kustner reaction is also negative. Sensitizers vary from simple substances (chromate and nickel) to complex chemicals (plastics) or even bacterial products (streptococci, fungi).

Allergen + Epidermal protein — Conjugation — Antigen formation — Antibodies production (probably in lymph glands) — Circulation — Fixed in epidermal cells.

Next occasion.

Allergen + Antibodies — eczematous reaction (in the epidermis).

A severe local reaction may result in auto-intoxication and dissemination of eczematous reaction to distant parts.

Delayed hypersensitivity is believed to produce lymphomas, sarcoid. Allergy to immuno-chemically related substances has also been proved. Further it is believed that in cases of severe allergic states, a state may develop when the patient becomes hypersensitive to even unrelated substances, e.g. Status Eczematicus or Status Urticatus. This is comparable to status asthmaticus in the practice of internal medicine.

Further it must be realized that epidermal or dermal sensitization affects the entire integument, and this sensitization once acquired, is lifelong. According to some, a degree of blunting in reactivity may be seen with the passage of time.

To deal with cutaneous reaction of allergy is a challenge to a homoeopath in establishing the offending cause of the allergic reaction. Successful treatment produces dramatic results which are satisfying both to the suffering patient and the treating homoeopath.

Classification of Main Types of Hypersensitivity

Intolerance	:	Exaggeration of normal pharmacological action, without qualitative abnormality, e.g.,quinine.
Anaphylaxis Allergy	:	Lower animals, accelerated serum reaction in human beings.

1. Hereditary — Atopic.
2. Urticaria.
3. Contact eczema.
4. Bacterial — Dermatophytid, Henoch Schoenlein purpura, erythema nodosum, lepromin test, tuberculin test.
5. Serum and drug reaction.

SYSTEMIC DISEASES PRODUCING CUTANEOUS DISORDERS

Cutaneous lesions are occasionally produced by systemic disorders, so they may help in the diagnosis of the latter. On the other hand, a cutaneous disease may affect the internal organs. Hence, it should never be forgotten that skin is an organ of the whole body and should be considered as such, in the practice of dermatology. Important examples of systemic diseases producing cutaneous disorders are :

(a) *Nutritional*
Pellagra, avitaminosis.

(b) *Metabolic*
Diabetes — Pruritus, moniliasis, furunculoses, carbuncle, xanthomatosis, necrobiosis lipoidica, trophic ulcers, gangrene.
Amyloidosis cutis.
Cirrhosis — Spider naevi, sallow complexion, pruritus.
Porphyrinuria — Pigmentation, hydroa aestivale.
Xanthomatosis.
Bronze diabetes or Haemochromatosis.

(c) *Endocrine*

Thyrotoxicosis — Pigmentation.
Myxoedema — Alopecia, myxoedematous skin.
Cushing's diseases — Flame shaped stria.
Pituitary cachexia (Simmond's) — Alopecia.
Addison's disease — Pigmentation.
Menstrual disorders — Pigmentation, chloasma, alopecia, hirsutism.

(d) *Focal Sepsis*

(In teeth, ears, sinuses, tonsils, lungs, gall bladder, kidneys, prostate etc.)

Pyaemic abscesses
Bacterides
Discoid eczema
Urticaria
Dermatitis herpetiformis
Lupus erythematosus
Rosacea
Acne vulgaris
Erythema Multiforme
Dyshidrosis

(e) *Vascular disorders*

Raynaud's disease
Arteriosclerosis
Polyarteritis nodosa
Buerger's disease

(f) *Carcinomatosis*

Secondaries in skin
Pruritus
Pigmentation
Acanthosis nigricans

(g) *Naevi*

Haemangioma of skin — Associated with angioma of brain.
Adenoma sebaceum — Associated with tuberous sclerosis.
Neurofibromatosis — Associated with lesions in bones, nerves and eyes.

(h) *Collagen Diseases*

Lupus erythematosus, scleroderma, dermatomyositis.

(i) *Fever and Rashes.*

CHAPTER 4

Laboratory And Other Aids In Dermatological Practice

The skin is available for close examination and clinical study; reliance on clinical acumen could never be unduly emphasized in dermatological practice. In a certain number of cases there is a definite need and indication for laboratory and other aids, either to confirm the diagnosis or to clear up doubts in case the diagnosis is not certain. But the need also arises to establish the etiology of a disease entity, and so, to establish the ultimate prognosis. In all these instances, laboratory aids take second place to clinical diagnosis. *Firstly*, the homoeopath must be sure of this fundamental principle before ordering any laboratory investigation. *Secondly*, only the absolutely essential laboratory investigations should be ordered. *Thirdly*, the clinician must make sure of the reliability of the laboratory reports before he bases any opinion on them.

BACTERIOLOGICAL STUDIES

They are useful in finding out the exact causative organisms, both in acute and chronic cases of bacterial infections and infective granulomata.

Smears and Stains : Discharge from an infected area is smeared on glass slides and stained with Gram's stain for ordinary organisms, and Ziehl Neelsen stain for acid-fast bacilli.

Dark field examination is done to demonstrate T. Pallidum in the primary and secondary lesions of syphilis.

For examination of L.T. bodies, the edge of the suspected lesion is firmly grasped with the thumb and forefinger of the left hand, and by means of a thin-blade scalpel, a knife point of the tissue from the edge of the lesion is removed and smeared on a slide. The oozing blood is wiped off successively until clear serum begins to exude. A slide of the serum is also made. With some experience, the serum can be sucked into a pipette from the edge of an intact lesion without the use of a knife. The slides are stained with Giemsa's stain. L.T. bodies are seen as blue cytoplasm, pink nucleus and deep red — kinetoplast.

A nasal smear for lepra bacilli is made by firmly scraping the roof and sides of the anterior part of the nose by means of a swab stick, and smearing the material on a slide and staining with Ziehl Neelsen stain.

A slit biopsy in leprosy is performed by firmly holding the edge of a suspected cutaneous lesion or ear lobe (posterior surface to conceal the scar of the slit) between the thumb and index finger of the left hand. This will make the part avascular and numb. Then with the help of a thin blade scalpel, the tissue is slit open superficially. Bleeding should be avoided. The bottom of the slit is scraped along with the oozing serum and smeared on the slide by means of the blunt edge of the scalpel.

Cultures : They are made routinely, on blood agar plates to identify the types of organisms; biochemical examinations also may be required for this purpose. With the help of a flamed platinum loop, a specimen of the pus from the lesion is inoculated at one end of the plate and spread. Plates are incubated at 37° C in an incubator for 24 hours or longer.

Tubercle bacilli are grown on a special medium — glycerine egg medium. L.T. bodies are cultured on N.N.N. medium.

MYCOLOGICAL STUDIES

The most important confirmatory evidence of clinical diagnosis of dermatomycosis can be obtained by scraping the lesion and by the microscopic demonstration of fungus. The procedure is very easy to perform and does not take much time; preferably, it should be done by the physician himself.

Collection of Material

1. Skin : Scrapings are obtained by scraping the growing edge of the suspected lesion, where it merges with the normal skin, with a scalpel, the blade of which should neither be too sharp nor too blunt. It is advisable to wet the scalpel blade with a swab of 70 per cent alcohol when the scraping is being done.

The edge of the scalpel blade is gently agitated in a drop of 10 per cent potassium hydroxide solution taken on a slide to release the scales adherent to it. It is advisable to prepare two coverslip preparations from each lesion, and if there are a number of lesions, it is better if specimens from two or more lesions are obtained. If vesicles are present, the domes should be snipped off with a pair of scissors, and the contents examined in a potassium hydroxide preparation.

2. Hair : Areas showing thinning or scaling of hair with broken-off stumps should be selected. The stumps of the broken-off hair should be epilated and a coverslip preparation of the material placed in a drop of 10 per cent potassium hydroxide should be microscopically examined.

3. Nails : All nails which are discoloured or lustreless or ridged with hyperkeratotic debris should be fully examined. The nails are cut away, and the debris from under the nail is removed, placed in a potassium hydroxide solution and examined microscopically.

4. Pus : From granulomata like actinomycosis and sporotrichosis is collected aseptically and examined directly, or a smear is made and stained with Giemsa's or Gram's stain and then examined under the microscope.

Microscopic Examination

The preparation is gently warmed, or allowed to stand for 20 minutes to half an hour. This helps to soften the keratinous tissue and allows the fungus to stand out more clearly. The preparation is first examined under the low power and then the high power dry objective of the microscope.

In the skin, the fungus appears as a set of parallel septate lines, which show branching in some places. In some areas, the fungus may be seen segmented into a number of separate cells all in the same line. Absence of mycelia does not rule out tinea.

It must be clearly understood that this picture is common to all the dermatophytes infecting the skin, and the identification of their species is impossible from a coverslip preparation. Only by culturing can different species be identified. In the hair, the fungus appears in the form of rounded spores which may be small or large in size. Furthermore the spores may be present around the shaft of the hair. When situated thus, they are known as ectothrix spores; when present inside the hair shaft, they are called endothrix spores.

Culture : Sabouraud's medium is the one very commonly used. For culture work, the aim is to reduce bacterial contamination to the minimum.

After the affected area has been cleansed, with 70 per cent alcohol, scraping is done with the usual technique, the material so obtained is removed from the scalpel with the point of a straight needle and inoculated on the surface of the medium to be used. At least two petri dishes and two slopes of the medium prepared in test tubes or screw-capped bottles are used for each case, and about 4 inoculations of the material on each medium is made. The culture is kept at room temperature or best at 26° C and examined every alternate day. No culture should be discarded as sterile unless kept for at least three weeks.

Another difficulty to overcome is to know whether a growth which is taking place is saprophytic or pathogenic. A working rule in this connection is : any growth which takes place within three days and grows rapidly is likely to be saprophytic. The growth, however, should be investigated before being so labelled. With experience in the identification of saprophytes, however, this difficulty could, in due course be overcome.

Staining : The two reagents commonly employed are : lactophenol blue for the staining of fungus smears routinely and periodic acid Schiff's stain for the staining of fungus in tissues.

WOOD'S LAMP EXAMINATION

A Wood's lamp is a mercury vapour lamp with a special Wood's filter made of nickel oxide. It allows only certain wavelengths of ultraviolet rays (3650_ A) to filter through.

In Wood's lamp light, microsporon infection of the hair is visible as a greenish fluorescence. The scalp must be thoroughly washed of all medicaments before it is examined under the Wood's lamp. It helps to pick up early cases of tinea capitis amongst contacts especially school children, and aids in following up a treated case and declaring it cured.

The colour of the fluorescent light, seen best in a darkened room is characteristic in the following conditions :

Condition	*Fluorescent Colours*
Tinea capitis	Bright yellow green
Erythrasma	Coral red or pink
Vitiligo	Cold bright white
Albinism	Blue white
Leprosy	Blue white
Tuberous sclerosis	Blue white
Pseudomonas infection	Greenish white
Porphyria	Pink/orange
Tinea versicolor	Golden yellow

SEROLOGICAL TESTS FOR SYPHILIS

The commonly used blood tests for syphilis are : The Kahn test, the V.D.R.L. and the Menicke's slide tests. It is advisable to do all the three tests for the sake of accuracy, and to separate the positive from the biologically false positive reactions. It must be remembered that these tests can become positive in leprosy, yaws, chronic malaria, jaundice, etc.

HISTOLOGICAL STUDIES

Dermal histology has played an important role in the study of skin disease.

Biopsy should be done whenever possible. For most tumours and many inflammatory conditions a definite diagnosis may be made with certainty by light microscopy; many diagnosis by the clinical findings alone, will be excluded by the histopathological findings.

Commonly Used Tissue Stains

Tissue	*Stain*	*Result*
Tissue section routine	Haematoxylin and Eosin	Nuclei blue, cytoplasm pink
Collagen and muscle	Van Gieson	Collagen red and muscle fibres yellow
Elastic fibres	Verahoeff	Elastic fibres black
Reticulin	Gomori's	Reticulum fibres black
Amyloid	Congo red	Amyloid stains red
Glycogen fungus and basement membrane	P.A.S.	Glycogen red; fungus purple, red or black; basement membrane pale to deep pink
Acid fast bacilli	Fite — Faraco Stain (Z-N stain)	Bacilli stain red
Leishmania	Giemsa stain	L.D. bodies — red
Iron (haemosiderin)	Perl's ferrocyanide reaction	Pigment stains blue
Melanin	Mason's ammoniacal	Melanin black
Calcium	Von Kossa	Dark brown to black.

Technique of Biopsy

It is important to select the right material for a biopsy; it should either be from a fully developed primary lesion or the edge of such a lesion. Involuting lesions or secondary lesions or secondarily infected lesions should not be selected. It is strongly advisable to do excision biopsies in cases of melanomas. Incision or excision should be arranged along cleavage lines to avoid disfigurement. There are several types of skin biopsy punch biopsy, incisional biopsy, excisional biopsy, shave biopsy,etc. Incisional biopsy is preferable to punch biopsy. Punch sizes vary from 3 mm, 4 mm, 6 mm and 8 mm. Punch biopsy of 4 mm size is suitable for most purposes. In skin sterilization, colourless disinfectants are to be used.

The lesion should not be infiltrated with the anaesthetic but only the surroundings.

Once the specimen has been removed it is placed epidermis upward on a blotting paper. This is then placed in the jar or plastic container with fixative (10% neutral buffered formalin solution) which being a protein coagulant helps the specimen to stick to the blotting paper and comes to the laboratory unwrinkled. Unusually no suture is needed for 4 mm size punch biopsies. After approximately 12 hour's fixation, specimen is ready for processing.

Cytological Examination

It is useful in office practice.

L. E. cell in Acute Lupus Erythematosus. The study is made either with a bone marrow smear, or a smear of the buffy cell layer of centrifuged, heparinized blood. The smear is stained with Leishman's stain. A longer period of staining (10 minutes) is required in this case than in blood smears.

In positive preparations, three features are observed :

1. The L. E. cell which is a large neutrophil leucocyte, distended by a large, homogeneous, globular inclusion body pushing the cytoplasm and the nucleus into a thin rim at the periphery.

2. Rosettes of polymorphonuclear leucocytes surrounding the L. E. cell.

3. Extra-cellular masses which consist of globular masses resembling the inclusion bodies of L. E. cells lying outside the cells. The L. E. phenomenon implies demonstration of L. E. cells in normal blood when the serum from a lupus erythematosus patient has been added to it. L. E. cells are typically demonstrable in acute and subacute lupus erythematosus (systemic variety).

Tzanck test : It is a simple, cytological procedure employed to demonstrate acantholysis in pemphigus.

The procedure consists of snipping off the roof of an early vesicle or a bulla with a sterile knife, wiping off the serum, scraping the base and smearing the scraped material on a clean slide. Smears are fixed in methyl alcohol and stained with Giemsa's stain. The pemphigus cell (Tzanck cell) is a separate detached and rounded cell with a large, pyknotic nucleus and a deeply staining cytoplasm which is pushed to the periphery.

Smears in Skin Cancers : Microscopic examination of smears made from basal and squamous cell epitheliomas is a speedy and inexpensive method of diagnosis in expert hands. Typical cancer cells can be rapidly seen while the biopsy is being undertaken.

Histochemistry

Histochemical methods have been described for detecting many inorganic substances. Formalin fixed and paraffin sections are satisfactory for this purpose.

Stains for mucopolysaccharides, glycogen, lipids, mucins, nucleic acids and various enzymes can be studied by histochemical methods.

Immunofluorescence

Immunofluorescence is a technique for detecting the position and presence of substances in tissue sections.

Unfixed cryostat cut sections are necessary (frozen sections). Certain fluorescent dyes like fluorescein, isothiocyanate, Rhodamin B, Auramine O or Acridine orange,etc.,when exposed to ultraviolet light emit fluorescent radiation. By direct and indirect immunofluorescent techniques, Ig class antibodies other globulins, tissue antigens — bacterial, viral, fungal, protozoal, helminthic,etc.,can be identified. In the field of autoimmunity, demonstration of antinuclear antibody in the sera of patients with various collagen diseases by this technique is now possible.

This technique has been used as a diagnostic tool in certain bullous diseases, bullous pemphigoid can be differentiated from dermatitis herpetiformis and erythema multiforme. Immunofluorescence of the basal lamina can be seen in lupus erythematosus but not in lichen planus.

ALLERGY TESTS

Allergies cover a wide field. Allergy tests can be of great value to a dermatologist in the objective evaluation of an allergic patient.

Patch Tests.: They are done in cases of contact dermatitis to establish the etiological agent or agents. It is simply a reproduction in miniature of a small area of contact dermatitis.

It is artificial and does not necessarily duplicate the clinical exposure in which sweating, maceration and multiple applications play great roles.

Test reading should be taken 20 minutes to 1 hour after removal of patches. This time interval allows pressure effect and erythema from tape removal to subside.

The original dermatitis of the patient must be completely under control before the tests are undertaken. The patient should not be taking any drug, especially antihistaminics and corticosteroids. The back or the forearms are the sites of choice, preferably as close to the original site of the disease as possible. The affected part is cleaned with alcohol and allowed to dry. Patches are placed at distances of 2 to 3 inches in rows; about 20 patches can be applied at one time. The material for testing should be cut to about 5 mm. in diameter and moistened with normal saline or distilled water; liquid contactants can be applied directly. The testing material is covered with a piece of lint one square inch in size and an adhesive tape applied firmly, each patch being labelled or numbered. A control patch of lint dipped in normal saline is also applied.

The patient should be advised to report after 48 hours or earlier if itching starts, and again after 96 hours. Tests will have to be modified according to tested agents. The reading is done when the patient reports after 48 hours or earlier in case of acute sensitivity. In every patient, there is mild redness and folliculitis under the adhesive tape. Unless severe, this is a normal reaction to adhesive tape. A binder bandage may be employed for patients allergic to adhesives and Scotch tapes. The small area in the centre of the patch should be examined and recorded.

+	Mild redness.
++	Marked redness but smooth skin.
+++	Marked redness, swelling and papules.
++++	Redness, oedema and vesicles.

If there is no reaction in 48 hours, the patches should be re-read in 96 hours for delayed positive reaction. Sometimes, the original healed area of contact dermatitis flares up during a test, particularly when there exists a severe degree of hypersensitivity.

Intradermal Tests for Allergies to Foods, Inhalants and Drugs : In the majority of cases, the history of a definite allergy is more important than laboratory tests. Besides, these tests are not very accurate. Hence, they should be undertaken only in a limited number of cases where history and examination do not entirely help. The skin conditions in which these tests are helpful are : urticaria, endogenous eczema, atopic dermatitis and drug sensitivity. The response is a weal reaction.

Foods : An eliminative diet diary is much more useful than allergy tests, since few positive skin reactions can be correlated with clinical symptoms, and negative skin reactions may appear in the definite allergic patient. But in the hands of experts, the tests do give some vital information, like for instance, the presence of a constitutional alergic diathesis, and thus help to determine the lines along which the diet should be ordered. Scratch tests should be ordered first, and in cases of negative reactions, intradermal tests should be done to avoid severe complications and fatal reactions in hyperallergic patients.

Inhalants: They cause nasal and respiratory allergic symptoms; only very rarely do they affect the skin. The results of inhalant tests are more reliable than those of food allergy tests. The important inhalants employed for the tests are :

1. Animal danders — Cat, dog, cow, horse, sheep.
2. House dust.
3. Vegetable gums.
4. Pollens — Grasses, trees, flowers, wood.
5. Moulds.
6. Miscellaneous — Feathers, kapok, oris roots, tobacco, silk, wool.

A properly prepared antigen is scratched into the skin; the reactions are read at the end of 20 minutes, as follows :

+	Erythema less than size of IP[1].
++	Erythema more than size of IP.
+++	Erythema with weal in the centre.
++++	Weal with pseudopodia and surrounding erythema.

BIOLOGICAL TESTS

Basophil Degranulation Test (Shelley): It is based on the principle that basophils exhibit degranulation in the presence of antigen — antibody reaction of allergy. Sensitivity to drugs, foods and contactants has been established by this technique; it is also helpful in cases of atopic dermatitis.

Technique consists of mixing basophil leucocytes, the patient's serum, solution of antigen and the stain on a slide. Test is read microscopically 10 minutes later. In case of positive reaction, rapid movement of granules first inside the cell and later out of the cells is seen.

The Tuberculin (Mantoux) Test :This test is made with solutions of old tuberculin (1 in 100,000; 1 in 10,000 and 1 in 1,000) in descending order. The test is helpful as a prognostic, less so diagnostic, index in skin tuberculosis and sarcoidosis. The test is read after 72 hours.

The Lepromin Test : It is made by the intradermal injection of emulsion of lepra bacilli and tissues. It is a prognostic test and has no value in the diagnosis of leprosy.

The Frei Test :It is an intradermal biological test conducted with Frei's antigen or lygranum in cases of lymphogranuloma inguinale. 0.1 cc is injected, and the test is read 48 hours later.

The Leishmania Vaccine Test :This is made with the solution of leishmania tropica culture on N.N.N. medium. 0.1 cc of solution is injected intradermally. The test is read 48 to 96 hours later. Similarly, biological skin tests can be done for filariasis, syphilis and granuloma venereum.

Kveim Test :There is doubt regarding its specificity in sarcoidosis for which it is employed. The antigen consists of suspension of ground-up sarcoid lymph node. 0.1 cc is injected intradermally; the test is read after 2 weeks. In positive cases, an infiltrated macule or papule or nodule or even an ulcer may be produced. A biopsy of this nodule will show the typical histology of sarcoid.

Ito-Reenstierna Test :Carried out for chancroid, this test is made with a solution of pure culture of Ducrey's bacilli and read after 48 hours.

Haematological studies are important; most of these tests are of a routine nature, viz., haemoglobin, R.B.C. count, total and differential leucocyte count, and erythrocyte sedimentation rate. Others like blood chemistry — proteins, cholesterol and its esters, sugar and vitamin A, calcium and sodium content, cortisol, calcium, sodium, copper and zinc content are done in certain metabolic disorders. Their relative significance is discussed in subsequent chapters.

Cryglobulin Test :It is positive in several dermatoses particularly systemic lupus erythematosus, lymphogranuloma inguinale, cold sensitivity and purpura. Of course, multiple myelomatosis must be excluded. Cold precipitating serum globulins (cryoglobulins) can be demonstrated as gelatinous precipitate by collecting patient's blood in a warm syringe, separating the serum at 37° C and then cooling in a refrigerator.

Urine Analysis.: It is important in cases of chronic pruritus, moniliasis and porphyrinurias. The urine should be tested for sugar and albumin whenever diabetes and nephritis are suspected as causing cutaneous symptoms. In endocrine disorders, urine should be examined for 17 ketosteroids.

Stool Examination.: It is made for ova, amoeba, cysts, cellular reaction and digestive disorders in cases of vitiligo, urticaria, endogenous eczemas, dermatitis, enteropathica, etc.

Radiological.: Since bony and visceral involvement may be associated with several cutaneous diseases, a radiological investigation may be indicated, viz., syphilis, sarcoidosis, neurofibromatosis, tuberculosis, xantomatosis and actinomycosis.

CHAPTER 5

The Principles Of Dermatological Treatment

Remarkable progress has been made in therapeutics; scientific rational measures are replacing specific remedies. Skin surgery has opened up new vistas.

Treatment must be individualized to suit every patient. Skin is a superficial subject, and being an ectodermal structure takes time to heal; besides, nothing is hidden from either the patient himself or society at large. Hence, great care should be exercised in prescribing the right constitutional remedy.

Principles of dermatological treatment are :

1. Correct diagnosis, establishment of the cause and sincere attempt to individualize the case.

2. Reassurance to the patient and relatives so as to allay their anxiety about infectivity, severity, scarring and chances of recovery.

   (a) General measures — Diet, rest, environments.

   (b) Internal — Constitutional remedy.

GENERAL MEASURES

The integument is a part of the body, so when it is affected, the whole body has to be considered and treated accordingly.

Mind

To begin with, a patient's mind should be set at rest. Simply ordering the patient to relax is not enough. Psychogenic stresses and emotional conflicts are responsible for, originally causing and secondarily complicating, quite a few skin diseases. If the cause is simple, bedside psychotherapy is enough. In complicated cases and in psychotic patients, the help of a psychiatrist is very valuable.

Diet

It has an important role to play. Spices, hot condiments, non-vegetarian foods, tea, coffee and alcohol predispose to sense of heat and to several dermotoses. Simple nourishing and wholesome food is recommended in all skin diseases, except in allergic conditions, seborrhoeic conditions, chronic pyoderma, erythroderma and pemphigus.

Diet in Allergic Dermatoses (Urticaria, allergic and atopic eczema): It is needless to enforce diet restriction in every case of allergic dermatosis. Only when an allergy due to foodstuffs is suspected in history, should a special diet be prescribed, both as a diagnostic and therapeutic measure. It gives more valuable information, than even food allergy tests. The single factor eliminative diet and a diet diary are two useful measures. In the former, we start the patient on one foodstuff, like boiled milk. If the disease persists, he is given, to start with, boiled rice and sugar. It is rarely that a patient is sensitive to both rice and milk. If the allergy is due to dietetic factors, the disease should be controlled with this diet alone (mind you, without the help of drugs). After the disease has been controlled on boiled milk or rice, every three days, one more foodstuff is added, starting with essential ones like wheat (chapatis and bread), fats (butter and ghee), mutton, eggs, peas, carrots, bananas, potatoes, lentils, till either an allergic attack develops, meaning that the patient is sensitive to the last added foodstuff or the normal diet is reached. Usually, patients are sensitive to protein diets or vegetables and fruits or to the synthetic chemicals used for preserving food; starches, fats and minerals make poor allergens. In underdeveloped countries adulterated foodstuffs cause a lot of mischief.

Diet Diary: A specimen chart is maintained for a month or two depending upon the case. Every foodstuff taken during the day is marked by a cross (X), and at the bottom of the column, the patient puts down whether he felt better or worse or suffered from an acute flare-up or none at all. The examiner studies the chart every week or fortnight or month depending upon the individual case. By finding a common denominator which explains the worsening of the condition or the acute flare-up, the cause can be discovered. The diet diary is a simple and non-cumbersome procedure through which the cause of diet allergies can be found out.

Diet in Seborrhoeic Conditions (Acne vulgaris, seborrhoeic dermatitis and rosacea): Patients are advised to consume more milk, eggs, fish, mutton, chicken, and also to add green vegetables and fresh fruits. They should cut down and only in severe cases strictly avoid, concentrated, starchy and fat-rich fried stuffs like *puris* white bread, porridge, rice, potatoes, bananas, mangoes, cakes, puddings, pastry, sweets and cheese. Condiments, sauces and pickles should also be avoided. I may add a word of caution; there is no place for a rigid menu since a strict diet never cures a seborrhoeic condition but on the contrary demoralizes the patient restricting his social activities unnecessarily. Restricted diets should not be continued for very long periods.

Diet in Chronic Pyoderma: Recurrent folliculitis and furunculoses do well when there is restriction of sweets, stodgy, concentrated starches and mangoes, etc., on the lines recommended above.

Chronic Erythroderma, Pemphigus and Leprosy: Extra proteins and minerals should be added to the diet to keep up the body's strength and make-up for the loss of these from the skin in the form of scales and serum, particularly in the first two dermatoses.

Disseminated and Acute Eczemas: They heal quicker on restricted salt and light diet. It is customary with the author to give a restricted diet, i.e., milk and rice for 3 days at least, to patients with acute and disseminated eczema and urticarias, bland vegetarian diet with restricted tea, coffee and alcohol is helpful. It should be continued for at least 4 to 12 weeks.

Rest

Complete bed-rest is seldom necessary. Only patients with debilitating diseases like pemphigus, erythroderma, generalized eczema, psoriasis and lepromatous leprosy require rest at home, and may stay in bed if they feel weak. Cases of infectious leprosy should be isolated completely — separate room, separate utensils, separate linen and no visitors. Cases of scabies and impetigo contagiosum should be isolated at home till these diseases are completely controlled.

Localized contact, dermatitis and eczema warrant, local protection with bandages and masks to exclude all irritants and sensitizers till the affected part has healed; these measures also protect the affected part from being scratched. If the eczema is extensive or generalized, it is advisable to isolate the patient in a simple, non-allergic environment, such as a clean room with simple and limited furniture, without carpets, rugs, no flowers, no chemicals,etc. Daily bandages in these patients are cumbersome, expensive and painful to change.

External Environments

A skin patient should be nursed in homely and clean environments; fresh air and mild sunlight help to heal the affected skin. The atmosphere should be free from dust and chemicals. Atopic eczematous patients must be kept, to start with, in pollen free rooms unless declared insensitive to pollens; they are "tricky" patients. External temperature plays an important part in the healing of the skin. In tropical countries, the external atmosphere temperature needs to be regulated with an airconditioner, particularly for chronic illnesses. If airconditioning is not available, the patient should be removed to a more suitable climate. A climatic change may be the only therapeutic measure available for certain cases of chronic and atopic eczemas, severe ichthyosis and prickly heat. Besides a change in climate, a move to a different place provides a change in mental outlook, and helps the mind to relax.

CHAPTER 6

Aids To A Healthy Skin

The prevention of death is a fine ideal, but the prevention of disease is still finer.

A healthy skin is a source of pleasure, not only to its owner but also to the one who looks at it. To possess a nice skin is to have great social and economic advantage. Besides, the positive health of the skin is an insurance against disease the ideal of every individual as well as every medical man.

The normal healthy skin is clear, smooth, supple, elastic, uniformly pigmented without wrinkles, and does not sag; the stratum corneum (horny layer) is thin, translucent and invisibly cast off, the pores are hardly visible, secreting an imperceptible amount of sebum and sweat (except in summer, in hot environments and when exertion takes place), and there is no evidence of active bacterial or fungal growth. This tone and glossiness is noticeably absent in the skin of the sedentary town worker.

The integument being the external covering of the human body is put to great stress and strain by the external environments involving factors like climatic changes, dust, irritants, non-pathogenic and pathogenic micro-organisms, etc. Hair and nails grow constant. Grease (sebum) of the skin is daily washed off. These agents have to be controlled. The following factors are important in keeping the skin healthy.

Diet :It should be balanced and digestible. A fair amount of animal proteins and vitamins are essential. The daily diet should contain liberal helpings of meat, fish, eggs, milk and its products, butter, green vegetables and fruits, concentrated, starchy food should be avoided. Spices, condiments, tea, coffee and alcohol should be consumed as less as possible. They produce a sense of heat hence predisposition to allergic conditions and dermatoses. Occasional fasting is good for health. Keep your digestion healthy.

Gluttons and dyspeptics tend to be greasy, flushed, sallow, pasty and pimply. They later, tend to develop seborrhoeic dermatoses. Besides overeating results in obesity which produces side-effects.

Atmospheric Effects : Fresh cool air, exercise and mild sun are potent natural skin restorers. They stimulate the skin and thereby the thyroid, adrenal and sympathetic system on which are dependent the well being and vitality of the skin and the body. This point can be stressed with an example : A holiday in a hill station or on the coast with a cool climate spent in loose, comfortable clothes, will tone up the skin, stimulate the musculature and improve the well-being of a person so much, that if he happens to suffer from dermatoses like chronic furunculoses, intertrigo and recurrent herpes, they will most probably disappear. This aspect of nature cure and physiotherapy has been developed on scientific lines in many countries for the prevention and cure of many diseases, both cutaneous and systemic. Intertrigo and tinea are rare in individuals who indulge in regular exercises in cool, fresh surroundings.

A moderately cold climate, is the most potent natural stimulus to the integument. Exercise in fresh, cool air is very stimulating. *Yogic* exercises are beneficial because they exercise and relax the musculature in a scientific manner. Extreme cold is injurious, so a person should have the right clothing to protect himself from it. Several tropical conditions can be directly attributed to the scorching heat of the tropical climate causing hyperhidrosis and maceration. Due precautions, therefore, should be taken to keep the body cool. Air conditioning, whenever possible, is the answer.

While mild sun-bathing is beneficial, the strong sun produces degenerative changes and even neoplasms especially in white people. The integument must be protected from the strong sun and direct heat. An umbrella, solar hat and sun protective agents are useful aids.

Clothing : The clothes worn should be the very minimum, and neither the clothing nor footwear should contain sensitizers. Avoid very tight-fitting and nylon clothes, especially in the summer weather; only wear loose cotton clothes and soft sandals/ chappals. Nylon clothes interfere with the absorption and evaporation of sweat. Furthermore, the chemicals dissolved by unevaporated sweat can cause contact dermatitis. The same applies to footwear (especially of rubber and plastic), spectacle frames, furs, artificial jewellery, etc.

Bathing : In tropical countries, daily bathing with clean and cool water is essential in the summer. In cold weather, one should bathe in warm water as often as possible. Clean the various body folds, genitalia and feet properly. The skin should be thoroughly dried after washing.

A hot bath followed by a cold one is stimulating to the skin and the vital organs. To begin with the difference in between the two baths should not be great but in course of time, as a person gets used to the difference he will greatly enjoy such baths with benefit. These baths have been recommended with success in cases of chilblains, thermal urticarias and certain selected cases of atopic dermatitis.

Soap : A simple, least alkaline, soap should be employed. People with greasy skin need more soap than those with dry skins. People with dry skins should use superfatted soaps. Medicated soaps are the least useful as medications, and can be great sensitizers.

Oil : It nourishes the skin and hair; it makes them smooth. Coconut, mustard and olive oil are in common use. Medicated and perfumed oils are great sensitizers. In cold, dry weather, as for example, in the North Indian winter, it is a good habit to massage vaseline or lanoline or milk cream on the exposed parts of the body before retiring to bed. It helps to keep the skin smooth and fresh.

A good substitute for oil is butter, *ghee* or lanoline. In India, the first two are used abundantly to massage the skins of children. They are very useful for chapped lips, hands and feet. Butter is animal fat, rich in vitamins. Many modifications are available.

Shaving: The following points should be kept in mind when shaving:

(a) Do not shave too finely by stretching the skin.

(b) Shave in one direction.

(c) Use clean, sterilized and sharp instruments and avoid repeated shaving on the same part.

(d) The beard should be properly softened with soap or shaving cream before shaving. After shaving rub in a little cream to lubricate the degreased skin.

Strongly alkaline or sensitizing shaving soap and cream should be avoided. The same applies to after-shave lotions.

The electric razor is a useful innovation, particularly for people with disorders on the beard region, since it avoids both trauma and the use of alkaline soap.

Cosmetics: Cosmetics contain chemicals to which individuals may be sensitized or may become sensitized to them; hence, care should be exercised while selecting them. In Europe and America, cosmetics are responsible for a great deal of contact eczema. In Asiatic countries, the incidence is fortunately still low. Chemicals in cosmetics may harm the skin, cause blockage of pores and invisible slow degeneration; hence avoid cosmetics as much as possible.

Whenever one desires to change one brand for another in cosmetics, it is advisable to do a patch test.

CARE OF THE HAIR

It consists of :

Washing with soap or shampoo. Regarding the choice of a shampoo, the same statements apply as have already been made for soaps. Sometimes beaten egg white is employed to give glossiness to the hair. Savlon, Cetavlon and Selsun suspension are useful in controlling dandruff. In India, certain indigenous plant products like *aritha* and *amla* are used for washing the hair. They are cheap and effective. Greasy hair need frequent washing and less oil application. Dry hair require less frequent washing and good oil massage. Frequency of washing depends upon the climate and the length of the hair, daily, alternate days or weekly. Often bland soap and water are sufficient.

Greasing or oil application is essential for effective lubrication and grooming choice depends upon individual taste.

Combing and brushing of the hair is normally done once or twice a day. No force should be used in either combing or brushing. Combs and brushes tend to irritate the scalp; often injure and atrophies the hair.

Singeing of the hair ends is often employed by beauty parlours and hair-dressers to treat splitting. It has no advantages over cutting, and is by no means curative.

Dyeing grey hair with vegetable dyes (henna, chamomile), metallic dyes (bismuth, silver, lead) and chemical dyes (Paratolyendiamine, paraphenyl nediamine, etc). Several dye preparations are available in the market. Vegetable dyes are usually the safest, but there is limited choice of colour in them. Patch test to the dye must be applied before its use.

Hair ornaments — Pins, clips and nets. These are employed to keep the hair in a desired shape and also to enhance looks. Only rarely do such accessories cause dermatitis. Nickel and plastic materials should be used with caution to prevent irritation. Wigs are worn, particularly by women, to conceal alopecia or for improving appearance.

UNDERSTANDING MIASM

It is essential to have a sound understanding of miasm to study various skin diseases and also how to apply the same in a sick individual.

The Miasmatic theory of chronic diseases propounded by Hahnemann has become the most controversial in the history of Homoeopathy.

It has polarised the homoeopathic profession; at one extreme we find a group who holds that the theory is a delusion, at the other end is the group who affirms that all that Hahnemann, Allen, Roberts, Kent wrote on the subject amounts to a priceless pearl given only to intuitive minds and that lesser minds should accept the theory on faith.

I personally feel that if Hahnemann was alive, then he himself would have preferred his theory and clarification of Miasm to be examined dispassionately, objectively under the light of modern science.

Phenomenological Approach

When we study the therapeutics of skin, we include skin and its appendages,viz., hair, nails.

Like any other disease, the signs and symptoms of the patient should be analyzed into :

(1) *Location* — Epidermis, dermis, hair follicle, sweat glands, sebaceous glands.
(2) *Sensations* — Itching, tingling, formication, burning.
(3) *Modalities* — Hot application, cold application, rubbing, scratching.
(4) *Concomittants*.

The next step would be to classify the disease nosologically, e.g.,skin can be affected primarily or it could be a local manifestation of systemic disease, viz., Viral exanthemata, Diabetes mellitus, Hodgkin's disease, SLE, etc. Also many a time one gets the skin symptoms which only come in alternations, e.g., the psora tries to throw eruptions out on the skin and its appendages with its characteristic discharges clinically known as Primary Psora. Whenever these eruptions come out the internal trouble is relieved and the patient feels better. The appearance of boils and the reappearance of eruptions and discharges under treatment is a reliable index of good action of a well selected remedy.

When these peripheral expressions of Primary Psora are blocked through suppressive measures, the road is clear for progressive internalisation of trouble with increasing involvement of more vital organs. That is to say, various other systems, e.g., metabolism, nutrition, CNS, CVS, etc., get affected. The symptomatology is known as Secondary Psoric expression. There is minimal structural alteration of a reversible type with maximum functional disturbance.

Hypersensitivity reactions that follow vaccination are a typical manifestation of psoric miasm. At this juncture I would like to clarify that even though the phenomenon of alternation (or alternating states) is characteristic of psoric miasm, the expression of the state that follows alternation may be of any miasm depending on the pathology of that particular disease. e.g., scabies alternates with asthma. The phenomenon of alternation between the two is characteristic of psoric miasm. But the expression of the two states is as follows : (1) Scabies is classified under tubercular miasm (infective) and (2) Asthma (aggravated in damp weather with greenish offensive expectoration) is classified under sycotic miasm.

Similarly, whenever any skin lesion, irrespective of its nosological classification is suppressed, by any agent — physical, chemical drugs (Homoeopathic, Ayurvedic, Allopathic, Unani, etc.) the manifestation that follows could be classified from psora to sycosis to tubercular to syphilis, e.g., suppression of exanthemata leading to encephalitis is typical of tubercular miasm.

For simplicity, I have classified the diseases according to the Hahnemannian miasmatic evolution of sickness. The most important thing to remember in this classification is that no sickness is ever under a fixed miasm. The miasmatic background changes (Psora to sycosis to tubercular to syphilis) as the disease evolves from functional to structural changes. Taking Acne Vulgaris as an example, one sees that to start with there is only a slight papule with itching, so characteristic of psora; followed by slight induration (sycotic); which is followed by pain and purulent discharge (tubercular); then rupture with necrosis (Syphilis).

THE SKIN

Psora

Vesicles of the itch, voluptuous tickling, itching.

Patient rubs and scratches better for a few moments, after which there is long continued burning of the affected part.

Skin is dry, rough, dirty or unhealthy looking; has an unwashed appearance.

Pruritus

Very little suppuration in psoric skin diseases.

Apt to be dry with scanty suppuration. Seropurulent and occasionally bloody.

Eruptions often papular in form accompanied by intense itching, usually colour of skin unless an inflammatory process is present.

Itching, scales and crusts thin and light, fine and small, and usually quite general over affected part.

Boils

Itching without eruption

< **night, heat bed**

>scratching —> **burning**

> hot application.

Sycosis

All facial skin diseases in barber's shop with exception of Taenia favosa.

Thickening — Lichenification — wine coloured spots.

Subcutaneous nodules. Chafing with peculiar sycotic discharge.

Scales patchy and in circumscribed spots.

Psora	*Sycosis*
Eczema — Papular eruptions : dry. Urticaria. Anhydrosis *Psoriasis* — Have a *SYCO-PSORIC* Variola base. Allergic dermatitis Neurodermatitis (Lichen simplex chromicus). Scabies	*Eczema* — exfoliata-erythematous. Circinatus herpes and herpes zoster. Lichen = SYCOSIS AND PSEUDOPSORA Tinea barbae; Tinea tonsuraus. Tinea vesicular Warts and warty growths. Condylomata — Syphilis and Sycosis also verruca accuminata, pointed papillary growths, coxcomb and warts. Skin lesions in tertiary stage, warty eruptions or growths verruca filiformis
	Verruca vulgaris, verruca plana.
Acne Vulgaris	*Acne Vulgaris*
	Verruca filiformis comes as a tertiary lesion in an acquired form of SYCOSIS.
Suppressions aggravates widespread internal disorders.	Verruca plana is another hereditary form, found more or less upon the backs of hands and faces of children and young people. The filiformis appears in adults with acquired sycosis who have had it suppressed. Usually appear on sexual parts,

Psora

(Nat. Mur., Hep and Sil. good examples)

Acne Vulgaris
Abscess and ulcerations after

Sycosis

trunk — small in diameter; one-eighth of an inch long, often shorter, brownish or greyish pointed with spindle-like attachment.

A form of acne — large red, angry, blunt pointed papules at about menstrual period; they do not suppurate but are sore to touch and sensitive — quite isolated and separate from each other. Lupus — whether of erythematous or of the common form — belong without doubt to the tubercular family of skin diseases with a sycotic element present. The malignancies develop at any age. Malignancies of the skin are more violent and intractable in proportion as the sycotic taint is increased.

All forms of facial skin diseases that are contracted in Barbers' shop except Tinea favosa.

In scalp and beard Tinea circumscripta which causes in form of alopecia.

Acne Vulgaris
Verruca Vulgaris in children

Psora	*Sycosis*
injuries. Bees or bugs affect these patients badly.	with congenital syphilis.
Impetigo The patients often have benign or malignant tumours.	

In TUBERCULAR and SYPHILITIC patients we see much scarring and increase in cicatricial tissue.

Psora	*Sycosis*
Leprosy In the lymphatic temperament we see the malignancies — we find here rich soil for gonorrhoea and syphilis. In tubercular patients we have so much difficulty in eradicating acquired syphilis or gonorrhoea. Gonorrhoea runs to a gleety discharge and strictures, pockets and metastasis forms or we have metastasis to ovaries, broad ligaments, tubes, uterus, rectum and all such complications. It is the tubercular diathesis that complicates all our skin diseases and makes them so difficult to remove. Impetigo. Herpes zoster.	All forms of ringworm. The suppression of ringworm brings rheumatism, chronic headaches, stomach troubles, chronic bronchitis, chronic cough, melancholia, mania, hysteria in women and malignancies. Variola and varicella in all their different forms have very marked characteristics of the sycotic element present or of Syphilis and Sycosis combined.
Vaccination < Sensitivity Reaction	The serum of vaccination has, without doubt both of these elements present. Erythematous eczema: erysipelas, especially in the phlegmonous variety; herpes zoster and impetigo contagiosa. Psoriasis has

Psora	*Sycosis*
	the gouty element so characteristic of sycosis.
	The spider dot (tertiary) occurring on the upper portion of face usually about half an inch below the lower eyelid or over centre of malar bone consists of little sprangle of dilated capillaries resembling somewhat the meshes of a spider's web. In children - pale or bleached or quite red and prominent. Red mole (Naevi) — a tertiary symptom, pinhead to pea— smooth, round, shiny, often red as blood, appearance of polka dot on skin.
	If sycotic element is present, in abdominal operations, the possibility of a stitch abscess is increased. Condylomata.
	Keloids
	Vaccination leads to Keloid.
Tubercular	*Syphilitic*
	Squamous copper coloured eruptions. Crescentic formations Pustular eruptions — dermatoses.
Impetigo Leprosy	Impetigo Eruptions found about the

Tubercular	*Syphilitic*
	joints flexures of the body, or arranged in circular groupings, ring or segments of circles. Copper coloured or raw ham colour, brownish or very red at their base. No itching and very little soreness. No pain. Vitiligo. Scales and crusts thick and heavy, patchy and in circumscribed spots.

Skin eruptions with glandular involvement will necessarily have Syphilitic or tubercular element to conform with the glandular involvement.

In varicose veins, the tubercular taint predominates and it is in these patients that we see the varicose ulcers, the last skin lesion to make its appearance in a case of ancient or hereditary syphilis that has already become and now is largely Psuedo-Psora.	Cracks, fissures, rhagades, ulceration; serpigenous, spreading phagedenic. Varicose ulcers painless
In ecchymoses or any form of purpura, there is a tubercular basis.	
Eczema Pustule — above ears with cracks, gangrene. Herpes Urticaria Hyperhidrosis and Bromidrosis Anidrosis.	Gangerene or gangrenous spots (could be TUBERCULAR). In dry gangrene, Syphilis is always present.
Abscess and ulcers (painful undermined edges). Freckles	Condylomata — Syphilis and Sycosis also verruca accuminata, pointed papillary

Tubercular	*Syphilitic*
Fine, smooth, clear skin Goose flesh	growths, coxcomb and warts.
Suppress any form of ringworm and there often follows tubercular disease. (Sycosis on a TB base)	
Vaccination —> Encephalitis —> Epilepsy —> Suppuration	Vaccination —> ulcer.

N.B. All skin diseases are triple miasmatic.

In Ichthyosis (fish skin) we find all the chronic miasms and where we find them all present, we usually find an incurable skin disease — especially if hereditary.

In Ichthyosis we see the dryness of psora, the squamae of syphilis and often the moles and warty eruptions of sycosis.

All miasms are present in erysipelas-carcinoma-epithelioma-lupus.

In nevus or congenital markings of the skin we have all the miasms as in elephantiasis.

CHAPTER 7

Affections Due To Physical Agents

The physical agents which can affect the integument vary from friction, pressure and maceration to cold, heat, sun etc., They produce a large percentage of dermatoses seen in general practice; the majority of these dermatoses are minor problems, only a very small percentage is serious. Apart from the intensity and quality of the physical agent, the sensitivity and vitality of the individual also plays an important part in bringing about skin disorders.

FRICTION AND PRESSURE

Abrupt and intense friction or pressure produces erythema and sometimes, a blister. A common example is the blister produced on the heel by tight shoes. Continuous light pressure or friction produces pigmentation which is commonly seen around the waist where the sari string or the trouser belt is tied. If the belt or string is tightly tied over a long period, it will roughen the skin, even ulcerate and result in depigmentation. Other examples of such depigmentation are the sites of the truss, corset, brassiere and the hat band.

CORNS AND CALLUSES

Diagnostic Hallmarks

1. Distribution : bony prominences of the feet.
2. Absence of black dots and pinpoint bleeding when lesions are pared.

Clinical Presentation

The ***volar epithelium*** of the palms, soles and digits is embryologically designed to undergo a proliferative hyperkeratotic response as a protective reaction against chronic trauma. Repeated iritation to these tissues results in massive thickening of the stratum corneum. This histologic change is reflected clinically by the presence of corns and calluses.

Corn appear as sharply marginated, square shouldered, firm papules 3 to 10 mm in diameter. They have a slightly roughened surface and are skin coloured to yellow in appearance. They are classically found on the dorsi-lateral aspects of the fifth toe but also occur on the lateral side of the fourth toe. These latter lesions are sometimes called "soft" corns. A translucent core lacking blood vessels will be visible if the top of any corn is pared with a scalpel blade.

Calluses are larger lesions with more diffuse, slope shouldered margins. They too are skin coloured or slightly yellow in appearance and have a slightly roughened surface. Calluses are most commonly found on the medial side of the great toe, around the edges of the heel and over the plantar surfaces of the metatarsal heads. Calluses occurring on the hand generally reflect trauma related to one's job or hobby. Calluses, when pared, may or may not reveal a translucent central core but, in any event, no black dots (thrombosed capillaries) or pinpoint bleeding spots are present. The absence of these changes assures the examiner that the lesion is not a wart. Small corns and calluses may be a symptomatic but larger ones often are quite painful.

Course and Prognosis

Corns and calluses occur when chronic rubbing or pressure squeezes volar epithelium against a firm bony surface. This irritation causes an increased mitotic rate in the epithelium which in turn leads to massive production and retention of stratum corneum cells. It is the widened stratum corneum layer which accounts for the bulkiness of the lesions.

There is no inherent biological difference between corns and calluses. Corns occur when sharply localized pressure develops over the narrow radius of the phalanges. More diffused pressure especially when it occurs over flatter bones better protected by a connective tissue cushion, results in the formation of calluses.

Therapy

The first step in the treatment of corns and calluses requires removal of the source of chronic trauma. For instance, ill-fitting shoes can be discarded, arch supports can be inserted where necessary and metatarsal bars can be added to the sole of the shoes.

On rare occasions orthopaedic procedures are required in order to repair underlying bony abnormalities. Surgical excision of corns and calluses is to be avoided since it does not get at the cause of the disease and the resultant scarring may only complicate it.

Corn and Callus

Intermittent pressure and friction over a long period is likely to produce a callus or a corn. It represents hyperkeratosis formed by nature to protect the sensitive part of the skin and the underlying structures from such pressure and friction. A callus is a raised, uniform, painless plaque of hyperkeratosis appearing on the hands and the dorsum of feet. A corn, on the other hand, represents a conical, painful hyperkeratosis appearing on the soles over the toe joints. Because of the body's weight and shoes, the hyperkeratosis of a corn gets pushed into the skin causing pressure on nerve endings which produces pain. Callosities are indicative of a person's occupation and habits. Unless they are unduly uncomfortable or unsightly, they demand no treatment. On the other hand, a corn is painful, and needs attention. First of all, a corn must be differentiated from a plantar wart by the following facts : A corn is at a pressure site (Over heads of the first and fifth metatarsal bones). It is painful when pressure is applied from above as well as from the sides, and there are no papillary prolongations, nor any verrucous surface. Clinically, a corn is seen as a polished, flesh coloured and circumscribed papule. Ill-fitting shoes and deformed feet are the two important causes.

HOMOEOPATHIC APPROACH FOR CORNS AND CALLUSES

Introduction. Corns arise not only from tight-fitting footwear and deformities of bony arch of foot but also from a certain disposition with some persons, who have tendency to develop recurrent corns.

Here I would like to stress that even though the cause is external, it is only the judicious use of internal remedy which will cure the cause permanently.

Causation. Since the most important cause of the corn is tight-fitting footwear, patients should be advised to wear comfortable footwear preferably a sandal, also wearing of narrow pointed shoes should be strictly prohibited.

Foot deformities must be corrected by exercise advised by orthopaedic surgeon or by expert physiotherapist.

Following points should be noted for case taking :

1. **Causation** : Wearing tight shoes with repeated shoe bites (Arn, All-cepa, Paeonia).

2. **Previous treatment** : It is essential to know whether patient had attempted to cauterize with the help of following :
   (a) Acetic acid
   (b) Caustic potash
   (c) Fluoric acid
   (d) Silver nitrate
   (e) Burning with the help of incense stick (Agarbatti)
   (f) Manual removal of the corns with the help of pedicurist or surgeon (Arn).

3. **Location** : Palms, soles.

4. **Characteristic** : Flat,
soft,
hard.

5. Whether corns are associated :
   (a) With or without Inflammation.
   (b) With or without Itching.
   (c) With or without Bleeding.
   (d) With or without Suppuration.
   (e) With or without Ulceration.
   (f) Tender or Non-tender.

6. Important characteristic sensations should always be inquired, e.g. :
   Burning
   Pulsating
   Stinging
   Stitching

   This is very important when the corn is isolated.

   It is strongly advised not to recommend any local application for the treatment of corns, e.g. :

   (a) Application of lime.
   (b) Application of Homoeopathic mother tinctures.
   (c) Application of ointments.

   Instead relief may be obtained by bathing the feet in warm water and applying Arnica ointment.

7. **Treatment review** : As clearly demonstrated pathologically, corns represent a conical, painful, hyperkeratosis appearing on the soles and over the toe joints. Because of body's weight and shoes, hyperkeratosis of a corn gets pushed into the skin causing a pressure on nerve ending which produces pain. This clearly demonstrates a dominant sycotic miasm with a mechanical exciting cause, i.e., trauma due to tight footwear, hence the drug selected should preferably have a sycotic base and also should act on the nerve ending.

Discussion

Patients usually consult us for :

(a) Painful tender corns, or

(b) Recurrence.

The following cases demonstrate various approaches and use of remedies in the corn :

Case 1

Mrs. S.P. aged 42 years, consulted me for multiple, painful corns on the soles of both the feet. She was in the great agony due to pain. The above condition was present since last four years. In the past, when the corn used to be painful she used to consult a pedicurist who in turn would scrape the skin and remove the corn, as corns used to recur she decided to start Homoeopathic treatment.

On examination I found the corns were very tender to the slightest touch. They were hard and were rough to feel.

Her other symptoms were :

(i) Menorrhagia with dysmenorrhoea — sometimes she fainted due to pain.

(ii) Constipation with frequent ineffectual effort.

(iii) She was a chilly patient.

(iv) Headache by strong odours.

(v) She was depressed due to her condition.

BEFORE **CORN**

I selected *Hep. sulph* 1 M as the corns were very sensitive to touch. After a week she reported that she had only partial relief. I repertorized the case using the above symptoms and selected *Ignatia*. Few doses were given followed by placebo which not only removed the pain but also gave her relief in her menstrual symptoms and headache.

AFTER **ANT-CRUD**

Time and again I have verified that whenever *Hep sulph* fails or partially acts in a tender painful corn drugs like *Ign, Sulph, Rann-s.,* usually cures the condition.

Case 2

A young man consulted me for painful corns on both the palms. He was going to the Gymnasium and used to lift heavy weight, due to constant friction of the palms with the iron rods he developed corns on his palms. There was a burning sensation in the corns. He had no other characteristic symptoms. I prescribed him *Radium bromide* 200 for a prolonged period, gradually his corns started disappearing.

Indication for its use was : Burning sensation in the corn.

Case 3

A lady consulted me for painful corn on her soles. On examination I found that surrounding the corns there were small blisters with ulceration. The corns were very tender.

Patient received *Rann scleratus* 30 on the indication "Painful corns with ulceration and formation of blisters." I have personally verified this on many occasions that *Rann scleratus* dissolves the corn if there is presence of blisters or ulcers.

HOMOEOPATHIC TREATMENT FOR ACUTE PAINFUL CORNS

(1) ***Antim. crud*** : Corns inflamed, large horny placed on soles of feet close to the toes — Thickened skin of soles and feet.
Corns on soles and toes.
Inflamed corn with great sensitiveness of soles on walking.
Aching, stitching pains in corns.

(2) ***Arnica*** : Corns on heels and toes. Very sensitive. Very painful, stinging, stitching, smarting pain.

(3) ***Bryonia*** : Painful corns. Slightest touch pains very severely, stinging, smarting, burning pain. For aching, tearing, stitching pains in the corns. Soles sore with lameness and every spot is painful on pressure.

(4) ***Camphor*** : Corns with skin parchment like sore, painful corns which are very sensitive; soreness especially in toe joints and corns.

(5) ***Carbo. an*** : Sensitive corns with stinging pain. Corns are very painful to touch.

(6) ***Hep-s*** : Inflamed corns, pricking and sticking in affected parts.
Great sensitiveness to slightest touch.

(7) ***Ignatia*** : Painful corns as if sore.
Bruised or stinging sensation in soles of feet.
Burning and soreness in the corns.

(8) ***Ran. b*** : When the corns are sensitive to touch. Hard excrescences. Horny skin. Smarting and burning pain in corns.

(9) ***Ran. scleratus***: Acute painful corns. Acrid exudation which makes surrounding parts sore. Corns on ball of 1st and 2nd left toes, sensitive to touch and pressure, smart and burn; very painful when letting leg hang down, they also throb and especially painful by flexing toes. Better by extending them, wearing thick soled boot at times. Numbness in corns, knocking toes against anything so as to cause boot to grate against corns, causes great pain and burning.

(10) ***Silicea*** : Inflamed corns with stitching, burning pains. Soreness of soles. Stitches in the corns, jerking up the feet.

(11) ***Sulphur*** : Corns and callosities from pressure. If a shoe presses anywhere on the skin, a great corn or bunion develop. Burning, aching, tearing and stitching pain.

For Recurrent Corns

(1) ***Ferr. picrate*** : Corns with yellow discolouration. Multiple corns which are very painful.

(2) ***Graph.*** : Rough, hard, dry and unhealthy skin. Thin sticky, glutinous discharge. Soreness and aching in corns. Horny skin on toes.

(3) ***Lycopodium*** : Corns that are very sensitive with tearing pain. Skin becomes thick and indurated. Painful callosities on soles, toes and fingers contracted. Inflammation with stitching and soreness.

(4) ***Nat. mur*** : Corns, painful scars. Greasy skin. Boring, tearing and stitching pain. Worse walking and standing.

(5) ***Phos.*** : Corns bleed very much; they heal and break out again.
Boring pains with aching.
Corns on toes.

(6) **Sulphur** : Corns and callosities from pressure. Desquamation excoriation of skin, skin application after local medication. Burning, aching, tearing and stitching pain.

REPERTORY OF CORNS AND CALLOSITIES

Acet-ac, Agar, Ambr, Am-c, Anac, Ant-c, Arg, Arn, Bar-c, Bor, Bov, Bry, Calc, Calc-s, Carb-an, Caust, Chin, Cist, Coloc, Cur, Elaps, Ferr-pier, Graph, Hydr, Hep, Ign, Iod, Kali-c, Kali-n, Lyc, Lyss, Mag-s, Nat-c, Nat-m, Nit-ac, Nux-v, Petr, Phos, Ph-ac, Puls, Radm, Ran-b, Ran-s, Rhod, Rhus-t, Ruta, Salc-ac, Sars, Sep, Sil, Spig, Staph, Sulph, Symph, Ter, Thuj, Ver-a.

Aching — *Ant-c, Lyc, Sep, Sil, Sulph.*

Boring — *Bor, Calc, Caust, Hep, Kali-c, Nat-c, Nat-m, Phos, Puls, Ran-s, Rhod, Sep, Sil, Spig, Thuj.*

Burning — *Agar, Alum, Am-c, Ant-c, Arg-m, Bar-c, Bor, Bry, Calc, Calc-s, Carb-v, Caust, Graph, Hep, Ign, Kali-c, Lith, Lyc, Mag-s, Meph, Nat-m, Nat-s, Nux-v, Petr, Ph-ac, Phos, Puls, Ran-b, Ran-s, Rhus-t, Sep, Sil, Spig, Staph, Sulph, Thuj.*

Cracks deep with — *Cist, Graph.*

Formation of tendency to — *Lyc, Sil.*

Hanging down agg	—	*Ran-s*
Horny	—	*Ant-c, Graph, Ran-b, Sulph.*
Inflamed	—	*Ant-c, Bor, Calc, Hep, Lyc, Nit-ac, Phos, Puls, Rhus-t, Sep, Sil, Staph, Sulph.*
Jerks	—	*Anac, Cocl, Dios, Mag-s, Nux-v, Phos, Puls, Rhus-t, Sep, Sulph, Sul-ac.*
Numbness	—	*Ran-s*
Painful	—	*Agar, Alum, Am-c, Ambr, Ant-c, Arn, Aster, Bar-c, Bov, Bry, Bufo, Calc, Calc-s, Calad, Camph, Carb-ac, Carb-v, Caust, Hep, Ign, Iod, Kali-c, Lach, Lith, Lyc, Mag-s, Meph, Nat-c, Nat-m, Nit-ac, Nux-v, Petr, Phos, Puls, Ran-s, Rhus-t, Sep, Sil, Spig, Staph, Sulph, Sul-ac, Thuj, Verat-a.*
Touched when	—	*Bry, Kali-c.*
Ulcerated as if	—	*Am-c, Bor.*
Pinching	—	*Bar-c*
Pressing	—	*Agar, Anac, Ant-c, Arg, Bov, Bry, Calc, Calc-s, Carb-v, Caust, Graph, Ign, Iod, Lyc, Phos, Ph-ac, Ruta, Sep, Sil, Staph, Sulph, Verat-a.*
Pressure slight from	—	*Ant-c*
Pulsating	—	*Calc, Kali-c, Lyc, Sep, Sil, Sulph.*
Sensitive, Sore	—	*Aesc, Agar., Am-c, Ambr, Ant-c, Arn, Bar-c, Bar-c, Bov, Bry, Bufo, Calc, Calc-s, Camph, Carb-an, Fl-ac, Graph, Hep, Ign, Kali-c, Lith, Lyc, Mag-s, Med, Nat-c, Nat-m, Nat-p, Nit-ac, Nux-v, Petr, Phos, Puls, Ran-b,*

		Ran-s, Rhus-t, Sep, Sil, Spig, Staph, Sulph, Sul-ac, Thuj, Verat.
Shooting	—	*Alum, Am-c, Arn, Bry, Bov, Calc, Caust, Cocl, Ign, Kali-c, Lyc, Nat-c, Nat-m, Nux-v, Rhus-t, Sep, Sil, Sulph, Sul-ac.*
Skin hard like callosities	—	*Am-c, Ant-c, Arg-n, Ars, Bar-c, Bor, Bov, Chin, Cic, Clem, Dulc, Graph, Kali-c, Lach, Led, Lyc, Par, Phos, Ran-b, Rhus-t, Sil, Sep, Sulph, Thuj, Verat-a.*
Parchment like	—	*Acon, Aeth, Ars, Camph, Chin, Crot-h, Dig, Dulc, Kali-c, Led, Lith, Lyc, Oop, Phos, Rhus-t, Sars, Sil, Sulph.*
Peeling off	—	*Am-c, Ant-c, Bor, Dulc, Graph, Lach, Ran-b, Rhus-t, Sep, Sil, Sulph.*
Thickening *with*	—	*Am-c, Anac, Ant-c, Ars, Bor, Calc, Cic, Clem, Dulc, Graph, Hydr-ac, Kali-c, Lach, Lyc, Par, Phos, Ran-b, Rhus-t, Sep, Sil, Sulph, Thuj, Verat.*
Soft	—	*Sil*
Sticking, stitching, Stinging	—	*Agar, Alum, Am-c, Ant-c, Arg, Arn, Arum-t, Bar-c, Bov, Bry, Calad, Calc, Calc-s, Carb-an, Carb-ac, Caust, Cocl, Hep, Graph, Ign, Kali-c, Kali-n, Lyc, Mag-m, Mag-s, Nat-c, Nat-m, Nat-p, Nit-ac, Petr, Ph-ac, Phos, Ptel, Puls, Ran-s, Rhod, Rhus-t, Rumx, Sele, Sep, Sil, Spig, Staph, Sulph, Sul-ac, Thuj, Verat.*
Stitches while sitting	—	*Verat*
Stitches during day	—	*Sep*
Smarting soreness	—	*Agar, Amb, Ant-c, Arn, Bry, Calc-c, Camph, Caust, Fl-ac, Graph, Hep, Ign, Kali-c, Lith,*

		Lyc, Mag-s, Nat-m, Nux-v, Phos, Ph-ac, Puls, Rhus-t, Sep, Sil, Staph, Sul-ac, Verat-a.
Tearing	—	*Am-c, Arn, Bry, Calc, Calc-s, Cocc, Kali-c, Lyc, Sep, Sil, Sulph, Sul-ac, Thuj.*
Tender	—	*Med*
Throbbing	—	*Calc, Kali-c, Lyc, Sep, Sil, Sulph.*
Upper limbs	—	*Ant-c, Bor, Calc-f, Graph, Merc-i-r, Nat-m, Sil, Sulph, Thuj.*
Hands	—	*Phos*
Horny on hands	—	*Am-c, Graph, Kali-ar, Rhus-v, Sil, Sulph*
With deep cracks	—	*Cist, Graph.*
Feet	—	*Ant-c, Bar-c,, Caust, Graph, Lyc, Ran-b, Rhus-t, Sep, Sil, Sulph*
Balls of	—	*Ant-c*
Soles on	—	*Ant-c, Ars, Calc, Plb, Sil, Sulph.*
Tenderness	—	*Alum, Lyc, Med, Nat-s.*
Horny	—	*Ant-c, Ars, Calc, Kali-ar, Sil.*
Heels	—	*Arn, Lyc, Phos.*
Toes corns	—	*Acet-ac, Anac, Ant-c, Arn, Cinch, Coloc, Graph, Nat-m, Nux-v, Phos, Ran-s, Tereb.*
Applied locally aching	—	*Sulph*
Joints of	—	*Ign, Mag-s.*

Between second and third of left — *Psor*

Burning alternately right and left — *Apis*

On right violent pains — *Agar*

HOMOEOPATHIC APPROACH OF BUNION

It is a circumscribed swelling consisting of a callus covering a fibromatous growth. A bunion is nature's protection against constant pressure and friction. Bunions commonly appear over the metatarsophalangeal joint — the first and fifth, and in deformed feet that have been confined to ill-fitting shoes. They look ugly, but are generally painless.

Bunions

Patient suffering from bunions comes to a physician only when they are inflamed and painful as bunions are painless. It is always important to remember that the patient's habit of sitting should be changed because it is the pressure and friction which is the important cause. If there is any associated bone deformities it has to be corrected surgically.

It is very essential to enquire about sitting habits of the patient and the type of footwear.

Agaricus

The bunions of Agaricus are extremely sensitive and painful. There is a burning, itching and redness in the bunion which is worse in winter and draft of air. The bunion is prone to develop ulcer. There is a sensation in the bunion as if pierced by needles of ice.

Benz-ac

The characteristic site in Benz-ac is great toe. Bunion of the affected part due to constant friction, burning sense. < open air cold > heat. Bunion in person with uric acid diathesis. Pain in bunion alternates with urinary symptoms.

Graphites

The appearance of bunion is rough, horny and dry. There is foul odour which comes out with burning sensation < heat. Bunion have tendency to bleed and crack with thin, gluey offensive discharge.

Paeonia

Bunions are extremely sensitive < touch, pressure and friction. Formation of bunion especially after ill-fitting footwear. Shooting and splitting type of pain in bunions.

Repertory of Bunions

Agar, Am-c, Benz-ac, Graph, Hyper, Kali-chl, Kali-iod, Kali-m, Paeon, Ph-ac, Phos, Plb, Rhod, Sil, Ver-vir, Zinc.
Excruciatingly painful — *Hyper*
Frost : bite after *Calc.*
Soles : *Calc*
Ulcerated — *Calc*
On big toe — *Agar, Benz-ac, Bor, Hyper, Iod, Kali-iod, Rhod, Sang, Sars, Sil, Ver-v.*
On little toe and ball of foot, with stinging pain on walking — *Zinc.*

CRACKS IN SKIN

It is seen mostly on the hands and feet in dry weather, particularly in the dry cold of the Indian winter which dries up the integument, roughens and cracks it because of its diminished elasticity. If the cracking is severe, fissures may be produced. The hands are further predisposed to cracking by poor general health, avitaminosis and frequent washing with soap and water. Cracking itself is uncomfortable; besides, it predisposes to secondary infection and pyoderma.

The treatment consists of :

1. Lubricating the parts with Nivea cream or pure fat (ghee). These soften the integument and help it to retain moisture.

2. Avoiding frequent washing with soap and water.
3. Improving the general health.
4. Protection from dry climate by proper clothing, gloves, air-conditioning,etc.

CRACKING OF SKIN - HOMOEOPATHIC APPROACH

It is essential on the part of a Homoeopath to inquire in detail about the general health of the patient, as avitaminosis and poor general health predisposes the person to develop cracking. Also since cracks are prone to secondary infection, patient's general condition should always be taken care of.

Homoeopathic approach

(1) Too frequent washing of hands with soap and water should be prevented; however normal hygiene should be maintained.

(2) The affected parts should be kept moist by applying a mixture of half ounce of Calendula extract Q in one and half ounce of olive oil to be applied three to four times a day.

Tendency to develop cracks indicates dominant syphilitic miasm. Hence remedies which are primarily anti-syphilitic should be used.

For repertorial reference rubrics like fissures, rhagades, chaps, cuts, cracks, etc., should be used.

Homoeopathic remedies discussed :

Alumina : Chapped skin, scurf and tetters which itch or become moist chiefly in the evening. Symptoms recur periodically at every new or full moon. Intolerable itching when getting warm in bed, must scratch till it bleeds; then becomes painful; cracks especially in winter. Development of cracks especially after frequent washing of skin.

Anthrakokali : The cracks of *Anthr.* are of a chronic nature. The parts on which cracks are

mainly found are nostrils, hands and feet.
Itching is worse at night. The cracks are prone to ulceration.

Ars. Sulph Flav : Characteristically skin of *Ars., Sulph Flav.* is dry and cracked. There is intense itching in the cracked skin. The itching is better by steam or hot water.

Baryta Carb : The skin of *Baryta carb* is hot and dry. There is itching, pricking and burning in the cracks which is not better by scratching. Infact, more often it is worse due to scratching. The cracks do not heal readily. Associated with cracks is cold foul perspiration and multiple warts on the skin.

Cactus Grandiflorus : Dry, scaly skin with much itching. The itching is quite troublesome and appears in the evening. Itching is reduced when the person retires to rest. The affected part is icy cold to touch.

Cistus-Can : Characteristically, the cracks are deep; most often found on the hands and tips of the fingers. The skin of the hands — hard, thick and dry. There is much itching, so much so, that the person cannot sleep.

Cracks of mercuro syphilitic origin with hardening of the surrounding skin. Tendency to cracks in scrofulous diathesis. Tendency of cracks to ulcerate. It is especially indicated in persons who lift heavy objects with their hands as a result of which there is hardening of the skin with subsequent development of deep oblique cracks.

Condurango : It is specially suited to cracks about the muco-cutaneous junctions. Painful cracks in the corner of the mouth. Tendency to develop cracks in individuals with syphilitic and cancerous diathesis.

Hepar-Sulph : Skin of the hands and feet shows deep cracks which are very sensitive. Also affects the wall of the hand. Cracks suppurate easily and gives off a foul or sour odour.
The axillae are dry and cracked. The itching in the cracks is worse when the body becomes heated.
Cracks of skin after the use of mercury or its compounds.
Stinging, burning pains; generally worse in cold.

Lycopodium : The Lyco. skin has a tendency to become chapped and cracked. Cracks in skin due to frequent washing. The cracks of *Lyco.* patient tend to be distributed on fingers, toes, palms, soles and heels. The palm is dry and hot; soles are moist and cold. There is a sensation of soreness in the cracks from which oozes a watery fluid. The cracks are associated with urinary, gastric and hepatic disorders.

Malandrinum : Dry, rough, unhealthy cracked skin which has occurred after vaccination. Deep rhagades on the palm and soles which are worse in cold weather and worse washing with any kind of soap.

Merc-I.F. : There is troublesome itching associated with cracks. The cracks are painful with some pricking pain; worse in the night and worse on pressure. Also there is intolerable itching at night.

Merc-I.R. : The cracks of *M.I.R.* patient are small and multiple chiefly involving skin of palm. They are sore in touch and are prone to suppuration and also they tend to ulcerate easily. The discharge from the cracks is yellow, sticky and offensive.

Nat-Mur : The sphere of action of *Nat-mur.* cracks is in between toes, around the nails, knuckles and heels. It also affects flexures of skin. There is a violent itching with raw and sore sensation. There is a tendency to develop cracks after excessive consumption of salt.

Nit-Ac : The cracks are characteristically found on hands and also on various mucocutaneous junctions. They are deep, sensitive to touch and bleed easily. The cracks become worse when patient is exposed to slightest cold weather, from wetting the skin, after washing and from use of mercurial compounds. The cracks are prone to suppuration and ulceration. The discharge from the ulcer is bloody purulent and offensive. There is splinter-like pain in the cracks which is worse by cold; better by heat, by covering at night. Tendency to formation of cracks in patients with syphilitic miasm as predisposing cause.

Petroleum : The sphere of action of petroleum patient to develop cracks is as follows : (a) angles of mouth, (b) folds of skin, (c) nipples, (d) finger-tips, (e) heels, (f) palms. The cracks tend to develop in winter or they develop whenever a patient is exposed to cold weather. The cracks may also get worse on washing. There is sensation of burning and itching in the cracks; the patient scratches violently till it bleeds. The area around the cracks is hard rough and thickened.

Pix-Liquida : Typically affects the back of the hands with violent itching at night. When scratched, leads to bleeding.

Sarsaparilla : The site for development of cracks in *Sarsaparilla* are as follows : (a) sides of fingers, (b) sides of toes, (c) thumb, (d) feet. They are deep and bleed easily. Cracks tend to develop especially after washing the part with water. There is a peculiar burning pain which is worse in the night. It is especially indicated in persons with gouty diathesis or persons who had suppressed gonorrhoea. Cracks may also be caused after administration of vaccines.

Silicea : The person tends to develop cracks on : (a) hands, (b) around nails, (c) first finger, (d) between toes, etc. The cracks are painful and very sensitive when exposed to cold weather. Patient feels better when the affected part is covered. The cracks tend to suppurate very easily. There is sensation of itching in the cracks only during day-time and evening. The tips of the fingers are dry. Tendency to develop cracks in a patient with : (a) scrofulous diathesis, (b) after improper vaccination, (c) after injury.

Sulphur : The sites for development of cracks is as follows : (a) between fingers and toes, (b) hands, (c) arms, (d) near and around joints, (e) feet, (f) heels. There is an itching and burning sensation which is worse at night, in warmth of bed, worse washing. Even though a hot patient, a sulphur patient tends to develop cracks in winter. Cracks bleed very easily and easily ulcerate and suppurate. The discharge is offensive, thick, acrid. The cracks are also very sensitive to touch and are very painful. Pain is worse by heat and at night. Formation of cracks on or near joints is very characteristic of this remedy. A person to whom the above remedy is best suited are those with a psoric constitution and who have suppressed eruptions in the past by strong ointments or those who have indulged in excessive vaccination.

Xerophyllum : Skin is rough and cracked. Skin feels like leather. Intense itching, stinging and burning.

X-Ray : Deep cracks and fissures on the hands, feet, knees and extensor surfaces of joints. Skin is dry, scaly, cracked with much itching which is worse in bed, in the evening and at night. Itching is better in the open air. There is much swelling of the part which is sensitive to touch. It antidotes abuse of sulphur.

REPERTORY OF CRACKS, CHAPS, FISSURES AND RHAGADES

Aesc, Aloe, Alum, Am-c, Anthrak, Ant-c, Ant-t, Arn, Ars, Ars-s-fl, Aur, Bad, Bar-c, Bov, Bry, Buf, Calc, Calc-fl, Calc-s, Carb-a, Carb-s, Carb-v, Caus, Cham, Cist, Com, Condur, Cycl, Eug-j, Ferr, Fl-ac, Graph, Hep, Hydr, Ign, Iris, Kali-ar, Kali-c, Kali-s, Kreos, Lach, Led, Lyc, Mag-c, Malandr, Mang, Mar, Merc, Merc-i-r, Merc-pr. rub, Mez, Mur-ac, Nat-m, Nit-ac, Olnd, Osm, Paeon, Petr, Phos, Pix , Psor, Puls, Ran-b, Ratan , Rhus-t, Rut, Sanic, Sars. Sep, Sil, Sulph, Teucr, Viol-t, Xerophy, X-ray, Zinc.

Air-exposed to if — *Alum*
Burning — *Petr, Sars. Zinc.*

Deep bloody — *Alum, Graph, Merc, Nit-ac, Petr, Puls, Sars, Sulph.*
Delicate skin on — parts covered with — *Sil.*
Discharges serous fluid — *Como*
Fetid — *Merc.*
Humid — *Aloe*
Ichorous fluid, irritating surrounding parts — *Cond.*
Itching — *Merc, Petr.*
Joints in bends of, brownish fluid oozes and gets ulcerous — *Hippoz.*
Mercurial — *Hep, Nit-ac, Sulph.*
New skin cracks and burns — *Sars.*
Orifices at — *Sulph*
Painful and bleeding — *Merc*
Painful — *Graph, Mang, Zinc.*
Sequela of itch — *Calc*
Small — *Merc-i-r*
Sleeplessness — *Pix*
Ulcerated — *Bry, Merc.*
Washing after — *Alum, Ant-c, Bry, Calc-c, Calc-s, Cham, Kali-c, Lyc, Nit-ac, Puls, Rhus-t, Sars, Sep, Sulph, Zinc.*
Winter in — *Alum, Calc, Calc-s, Carb-s, Graph, Petr, Psor, Sep, Sulph.*
Wounds : Cuts — *Arn, Led, Merc, Nat-c, Ph-ac, Sil, Staph, Sulph, Sul-ac.*
Yellow — *Merc*

Eruptions

Herpetic : chapping — *Alum, Aur, Bry, Cadm, Calc, Cycl, Graph, Hep, Kali-c, Kreos, Lach, Lyc, Mag-c, Mang, Merc, Nat-c, Nat-m, Nit- ac, Petr, Puls, Rhus-t, Ruta, Sar, Sep, Sil, Sulph, Viol-t, Zinc.*
Pustules : cracked — *Rhus-t*
Vesicular : cracked, breaking — *Bry, Crot-h, Lach, Phos, Vip.*
Head : Eruptions : cracks — *Graph, Petr.*
: fissures on — *Mag-c, Rut.*
Eyes — *Alu, Arn, Bar-c, Bry, Calc-c, Carb-v, Caust, Colo, Croc, Euphr, Iod, Kali-c, Lyc, Nat-m, Nit-ac, Nux-v, Phos, Sep. Sil, Stap, Sul.*
Eye : cracks canthi in — *Alum, Graph, Iod, Lyc, Merc, Nat-m, Nit-ac, Petr, Plat, Sep, Sil, Sulph, Zinc.*
Outer — *Nat-m, Sulph, Zinc.*
Tarsi — *Graph*

Ear : eruptions : cracked and desquamating a substance like powdered starch — *Corn.*

Ears — *Calc, Chel, Mag-c, Mar, Sep.*

Nose : chapped — *Ant-c, Arum-t, Bell, Carb-an, Graph, Merc, Nit-ac, Petr.*

: nostril — *Aur.*

: angles of nostrils — *Ant-c*

: cracks in nostrils — *Ant-c, Anthro, Aur, Aur-m, Graph, Nit-ac, Petr.*

: corners — *Graph, Merc.*

: septum — *Merc*

: tip — *Alum, Carb-an.*

: wings — *Aur-m, Caust, Hep, Merc, Sil, Thuj.*

Face : chapped — *Arum-t, Graph, Lach, Petr, Sil.*

Lips dry and cracked — *Nat-m*

Lips : chapped — *Agar, Ail, Aloe, Alum, Ambr, Am-c, Am-m, Ant-c, Ant-t.*

Lips : cracked — *Apis, Arn, Ars, Arum-t, Aur, Bapt, Bar-c, Bell, Bism, Bov, Bry, Calc, Calc-s, Caps, Carb-ac, Carb-an, Carb-s, Carb-v, Cham, Caust, Chel, Chin, Chin-a, Cimic, Clem, Condur, Cop, Colch, Con, Cor-r, Croc, Cupr, Dros, Echin, Fl-ac, Graph, Glycerin, Guare, Ham, Hell, Hep, Ign, Iris, Jatr, Kali-ar, Kali-bi, Kali-c, Kali-i, Kali-p, Kali-s, Kalm, Kreos, Lach, **Mag-m**, Merc, Merc-c, Mez, Nat-a, Nat-c, Nat-m, Nicc, Nit-ac, Nux-v, Ol-an, Par, Ph-ac, Phos, Plat, Plb, Puls, Rhust, Sabad, Selen, Sil, Spig, Squil, Staph, Stram, Sulph, Tab, Tarax, Ter, Verat, Zinc.*

Lower lip — *Apis, Cham, Cimic, Nat-c, Nit-ac, Phos,* **Sep.**

Middle of — *Agar, Am-c, Aur-m, Cham, Dros, Graph, Hep, Nat-m, Puls, Sep.*

Upper Lip — *Bar-c, Hell, Kali-c, Nat-c, Nat-m, Tarax.*

Upper Lip Middle — *Hep,* **Nat-m**, *Sel.*

Corner of mouth — *Ambr, Am-c, Ant-c, Apis, Arum-t, Calc, Caust, Cinnb,* **Cond**, *Eup-per, Graph, Hell, Hydr, Ind, Merc, Mez, Nat-a, Nat-m, Nit-ac, Sep, Sil, Zinc.*

Face : eruptions : fissures — *Calc, Graph, Merc, Nicc, Nit-ac, Petr, Psor, Sil, Sulph.*

Mouth cracked, fissured — *Ph-ac, Phos, Ambr, Bism, Bufo, Cocc, Lach, Merc-c.*

Gums — *Plat.*

Tongue : fissured — *Ail, Anan, Apis, Ars,* **Ars-i**, *Arum-t, Aur, Atro, Bar-c, Bar-m, Bapt, Bell, Benz-ac, Bor, Bry, Bufo, Calc, Calc-p,*

Calc-s, Camph, Carb-ac, Carb-s, Carb-v, Cham, Chel, Chin, Chin-a, Cic, Clem, Cob, Crot-h, Cupr, Cur, Fl-ac, Hell, Hyos, Iod, Kali-b, Lach, Lyc, Mag-m, Merc, Mez, Mur-ac, Nat-a, Nit-ac, Nux-v, Ph-ac, Phos, Plat, Plb, Podo, Puls, Pyrog, Ran-s, Raph, Rhus-t, Rhus-v, Sacc, Sinap, Spig, Stram, Sulph, Tub, Verat, Zinc.

In all directions — *Fl-ac, Nit-ac.*

Centre — *Bapt, Bufo, Cob, Cub, Lept, Mez, Nit-ac, Raph, Rhus-v, Sin-n.*

Across — *Cob*

Edges — *Anan, Clem, Ferr-p, Lach, Nux-v, Thuj.*

Left — *Bar-c*

Painful with hard **margins — *Clem*, tip — *Lach*.**

Cracks : on surface of abdomen — *Sil*

Rectum : fissure — *Aesc, Agn, All-c, Alum, Ant-c, Arg-m, Ars, Arum-t, Berb, Calc, Calc-f, Calc-p, Carb-an, Caust, Cham, Cond, Cur, Fl-ac, Graph, Grat, Hydr, Ign, Kali-c, Lach, Med, Merc, Merc-i-r, Mez, Mur-ac, Nat-m, Nit-ac, Nux-v, Pacon, Petr, Phos, Phyt, Plat, Plb, Rat, Rhus-t, Sep, Sil, Sulph, Syph, Thuj.*

Perineum : fissure — *Graph*

Urethra : cracks in meatus — *Nat-c, Nit-ac, Phos, Ph-ac, Thuj.*

Genitalia : cracks gland — *Ars, Kali-c, Mosch, Rhus-t.*

: prepuce — *Merc, Sep, Sulph.*

Eruptions : scrotum : rhagades — *Petr*

Cracks : female genitalia — *Carb-v, Graph, Nit-ac, Urt-u.*

Chest — *Arn, Calc, Caust, Cham, Graph, Ham, Ign, Lil-t, Lyc, Merc, Nux-v, Psor, Puls, Sang, Sep, Sil, Sulph.*

Cracks of nipples — *Arn, Cast-eq, Caust, Cur, Fl-ac, Graph, Hydr, Lyc, Mer-c, Mill, Phyt, Rat, Sep, Sil, Sulph.*

Painful — *Graph, Phyt.*

Eruptions : axilla : **cracks** — *Hep*

Cracks : skin joints bends of — *Hippoz, Graph.*

Upper limbs — ***Cond**, Graph, Kali-ar, Kali-c, Kreos, Phos, Sil.*

Shoulder — *Petr*

Wrist — *Kali-ar*

Hands : chapped — *Alum, Aesc, Apis, Am-c, Anan, Ant-c.*

: cracks — *Arn, Aur, Aur-m, Bar-c, Calc, Calend, Carb-ac, Carb-s, Castor, Caust, Cench, Cist, Cud, Graph, Ham, Hep, Hydr, Kali-c, Kali-s, Kreos, Lach, Lyc, Mag-c, Mang, Maland, Merc, Nat-a, Nat-c, Nat-m, Nit-ac, Petr, Phos, Psor, Puls, Rhus-t, Rut, Sars, Sec, Sep, Sil, Sulph, Sulph-ac, Zinc.*

Burning — *Petr, Sars, Zinc.*
Cold from — *Sanic, Zinc.*
Deep and bleeding — *Alum, Merc, Nit-ac, Petr, Sanic, Sars.*
Itching — *Merc, Petr.*
Wetting from — *Alum, Ant-c, Calc, Cist, Kali-c, Nit-ac, Puls, Rhus-t, Rhus-v, Sars, Sep, Sulph, Zinc.*
Winter in — *Alum, Calc, Cist, Merc, Petr, Psor, Sanic, Sep, Sulph.*
Working in water — *Alum,Ant-c, Calc, Cham, Hep, Merc, Rhus-t, Sars, Sep, Sulph.*
Back of — *Cist, Kreos, Merc, Nat-c, Petr, Rhus-t, Sanic, Sep.*
Ball of — *Hep*
Palms of — *Alu, Cist, Graph, Kreos, Merc-i-r, Petr, Sulph.*
Fingers — *Am-m, Bar-c, Calc, Cist, Hep, Kali-c, Mag-c, Merc, Nat-m, Petr, Phos, Sars, Sil, Zinc.*
Between — *Aur-m, Ars, Graph, Sulph, Zinc.*
Joints of — *Graph, Mang, Merc, Phos, Sanc, Sulph.*
That ulcerate — *Merc*
Nails on — *Ant-c, Ars, Nat-m, Sil.*
Nails about — *Nat-m*
Tips — *Aur-m, Bar-c, Graph, Petr.*
First — *Sil*
Thumb — *Sars*
Lower limbs — *Alum, Aur, Aur-m, Bar-c, Calc, Chin, Coff, Croc, Cycl, Hep, Lach, Merc, Nat-c, Nat-m, Petr, Plat, Puls, Rut, Sars, Sulph, Val, Verat-a, Zinc.*
Feet — *Aur-m, Com, Hep, Sars, Sulph.*
Heel — *Graph, Lyc.*
Soles — *Ars*
Toes on — *Lach*
Toes between — *Aur-m, Carb-an, Graph, Lach, Nat-m, Sars, Sil.*
Deep — *Hydr*
Violent itching — *Nat-m*
: under — *Sabad*
Extremities : eruptions cracked — *Phos*
Eruption - elbow bend of : fissures — *Kali-ar*
: wrist : fissures — *Kali-ar*
Eruption : hand : cracked — *Alum, Lyc, Merc, Petr.*
Eruption : hand back of : cracks — *Merc*
Ulcers : hand : cracked — *Merc*

CASES

Homoeopathy Journal
Vol. III- No. 5
Page No. 148 - Case No. 3

Lady over 60 years consulted me on February 10th 1934, about her hands. These were cracked, oozing with serum and bleeding. There were also pustules. There was a history of this having lasted for four years, accompanied by boils and carbuncles on body.

Petroleum 30 given. Ten days later hands had greatly improved. A further ten days, more improvement; then next visit showed no further improvement and the hands had become hot and burning, and *Sulph.* 200 given.

She signed off April 10th 1934, with hands in a normal condition.

Homoeopathy and Comparative Medicine
Vol. 2—No. 9 (1950)
Page No. 657 - Case No. ii(a)

Cracked Skin of the Palms

In one of the villages approximately 9 miles from Kanpur, a woman of 35 showed her hands to me, the palms of which were very badly cracked all over. There was intense itching and a burning sensation in the palms and feet which hindered her sleep and compelled her to put her hands and feet out from the blanket. She said the cracked palms appeared three years ago after she had given birth to a child. I gave her *Sulphur* 200 with instructions to take early in the morning. This was on 5-12-1949. I went again the next Sunday and was told that there was much relief in the heat of the hands and feet as also in the itching. I gave a few doses of placebo and promised to see her again next Sunday. On 19-12-1949, I saw her hands and noticed that the skin had almost regained its natural tone and colour but for the appearance of an eczematous eruption on the left hand thumb. I gave her *Psorinum* 200 which was my last prescription, and the eczema cleared off within another week's time.

MACERATION

Prolonged moisture produces two effects : (1) Maceration, (2) Paronychia. The former is seen in the flexures, like the inter-digital spaces, the groins and the axillae during the monsoon where it results in intertrigo.

Interdigital maceration is common in people who wear shoes for long hours. Paronychia, due to maceration, is frequently seen in domestic servants, washermen, housewives, cooks and barmen. Macerated skin predisposes to monilia, tinea and streptococcal infection. In the case of patients confined to bed continuous pressure and maceration results in necrosis of the tissues as is seen in bed sores.

The treatment of all these conditions consists in correcting the basic causes and keeping the affected parts dry.

Homoeopathic Approach to Macerated Skin

Maceration of the skin usually takes place in the folds of the skin e.g. axilla, groin, in between toes and fingers. Hence one should refer the rubrics skin folds, flexor where the following drugs have got marked affinity.

Ars, Calc-c, Carbo-veg, Graphites, Hepar-sulph, Lyc, Merc-sol, Nat-m, Oleum-an, Petro, Psor, Puls, Sele, Sep, Sil, Sulph.

The macerated skin is highly prone to develop secondary infection, hence every care should be taken to clean the affected part either with *Calendula* Q or *Ecchinacea* Q diluted with water in 1:10 ratio. Also since moisture aggravates the condition hence the affected part should be kept dry.

Simple maceration is an example of psoric miasm but when gets secondary infection with formation of pus, it represents tubercular miasm.

If the macerated skin leads to ulceration and necrosis it indicates syphilitic miasm. The importance lies in prescribing appropriate anti-miasmatic remedy.

The following remedies are useful :

Carbo-Veg : The macerated skin has got burning sensation which is worse at night and in bed. The skin is raw, ulcerated with an offensive odour with tendency to suppuration and ulcer formation. It is specially indicated in old broken down constitution with chronic illnesses who are bed-ridden. The burning is much relieved by heat.

Graphites : It affects folds on the skin throughout the body characterised by great itching, worse at night. There is a burning sensation. There is a characteristic thin sticky acrid offensive gluey discharge which oozes from the skin. The affected part burns after scratching and there is tendency to form cracks and fissures. When skin is cleaned with warm water it aggravates. Better in open air.

Merc-Sol : The macerated skin of *Merc* is full of itching. Itching becomes pleasant on scratching more at night in bed on getting warm. After scratching there is burning and skin becomes rough and secretes a thin acrid fluid with small vesicle formation. Surrounding lymph nodes are enlarged and tender. Affected part may bleed when scratched. Part is dirty and odour is offensive. Part affected is prone to suppuration and ulceration. Burning is worse from scratching and warmth.

Nat-Mur : The appearance of *Nat-mur* skin is oily greasy, dirty looking, withered. There is a sensation of rawness and soreness. The site affinity of *Nat-mur* is near the edges of hair, on genitals and groin. Excessive itching in affected part leads to secretion of acrid, thin discharge with formation of cracks. There may also be formation of crust on the scratched area. Patient feels worse in warm room, on exposure to sun and better in open air. Eating salt also aggravates itching.

Petroleum : The appearance of *Petroleum* skin is dirty, hard, rough thickened. This is especially true with the folds of the skin. There is a tendency for the patient to develop deep painful cracks in the affected part. There is violent sensation of itching and one must scratch until it bleeds. Parts become cold after scratching. The skin symptoms of *Petroleum* tend to be worse in winter and patient feels better in warm air and dry weather.

Psorinum : Characteristically, the skin of *Psorinum* is inactive with want of perspiration. Skin has a dirty dingy look as if patient never washed. There is sensation of itching in macerated skin which is worse in bed and from warmth. The patient scratches until it bleeds. There is a peculiar offensive odour emitted by the lesion. Also, due to scratching, one gets typical offensive sticky discharge which is aggravated before midnight and in open air. The maceration of skin may be as a consequence of skin disease suppressed by sulphur ointment.

CHILBLAINS

Synonym : *Erythema pernio.*

People with poor peripheral circulation, and sometimes with poor general health, are the victims. It is more common among females than males. It occurs on the fingers and toes only during the cold weather. It usually subsides completely in summer. When there is exposure to cold, itching, tenderness and burning sensations develop. The fingers and toes become dusky red and cold. Itchy swellings also develop; occasionally, these ulcerate. On healing, there is no scarring except where there has been ulceration.

Chilblains may be associated with acrocyanosis, erythrocyanosis, crurum and acrosclerosis.

Differential diagnosis : It is distinguished from lupus erythematosus, which may even complicate chilblains. In lupus erythematosus of the hands, bluish-red, slightly infiltrated and scaly lesions develop on the backs of fingers, accompanied by typical lesions on face. When one comes across chronic whitlows and erosions on fingers the possibility of chilblains must be considered.

AFFECTIONS DUE TO COLD

Acrocyanosis

It implies cold and clammy extremities of the body — hands and feet, less commonly the tip of the nose and the ears — in people with poor peripheral circulation. The parts are cold and dusky red; often accompanied by oversweating. Acrocyanotic individuals are usually young, emotionally sensitive, with rather unstable vasomotor systems. The condition becomes accentuated in the cold weather, improving as it becomes warmer.

When this circulatory disturbance affects the legs it is called erythrocyanosis crurum. It is seen as a cold, dusky or bluish-red swelling over the outer side of the lower parts of the legs. The only subjective complaint is an ache. The condition is common in people who wear skirts and no stockings; hence, it is rather uncommon in Asiatic countries where people wear garments down to the ankles.

The treatment consists of exercising the affected parts, keeping them warm with proper clothing — gloves, thick stockings and footwear and a good, nourishing diet.

Frost-bite

It implies the destruction of tissues of the hands and the feet, less frequently, the ears and the tip of the nose, by exposure to extreme cold (usually below freezing point). Any part of the body being wet, strong winds and poor general health predispose to frost-bite. Cold temperatures lead to contraction of the arterioles, later, to dilatation of capillaries and last of all, to the freezing of parts. On thawing, necrosis of the frozen tissue and blood vessels occurs; the latter results in thrombosis and gangrene. Frost-bite is uncommon in south Asiatic countries except in the mountains.

Almost similar to frost-bite are the effects of **Immersion Foot**, a condition brought on by immersion of the feet in **cold water** for long hours as in sea accidents.

Clinical Features. The affected part first appears cold, and bluish-red. Then as freezing sets in, it becomes white and numb. On thawing, it becomes swollen, bluish-red and painful, and may develop bullae or ulceration due to the sloughing of the superficial tissue or frank gangrene of the digits.

FROST-BITE AND IMMERSION FOOT

The above condition should be treated on the lines of gangrene. This is purely freezing of the body tissue thereby producing necrosis which leads to gangrene. The appearance of the affected part should be carefully observed especially the colour, the sensation in the local part should be inquired and the peripheral pulsations should be thoroughly examined to rule out ischaemia.

When it is the question of threatened gangrene in the affected part, one should decide whether the individual requires surgical treatment.

Indication for Amputation

(1) Absence of total pulsation in the affected part.
(2) General condition poor.
(3) Severe secondary infections.

Treatment

(1) Gradual warming of the part, that is warm room but not direct heat. Wrapping the affected part in sterile gauze. No massage.
(2) On recovery — gradual exercise to restore the function.
(3) Every care should be taken by a homoeopath to prevent secondary infection and vascular thrombosis in the affected part. Hence, after the initial relief obtained by the short-acting remedy, a deep-acting constitutional remedy be prescribed, preferably a snake venom which acts as an anticoagulant. Kindly refer the therapeutics of chilblains.

CHILBLAINS

There is enough scope of homoeopathic drugs in the treatment of the chilblains. Here once again questions pertaining to general health are quite essential. Because poor general health sometimes predisposes the individual to develop chilblains. Also, poor peripheral circulation can lead to formation of chilblains, hence homoeopathic drugs acting on vasomotor system, skin with tendency to form ulceration should be included in the therapeutics of chilblains.

The above pathology indicates dominant syphilitic miasm. The following are the most common symptoms encountered :

(1) Itching.
(2) Burning.
(3) Ulceration.

The following points should be noted during history taking :

(1) Site — Most commonly fingers and toes.
(2) Thermal modalities
(3) Causative factor and other associated symptoms.
(4) The description of ulcers with its discharge.

The hands and feet must be kept warm with gloves and woollen stockings. Sudden changes of temperature, like exposing parts of the body to cold and then warming them near a fire, act badly on the malady. Locally *Rhus-Ven* Q mother tincture should be applied to give immediate relief.

Treatment

Abrotanum

The characteristic indications allow us to prescribe *Abrot.* is sensation of itching in the lesion (*Agar, Petr*).

The other characteristic symptoms of the skin are : (1) loose and flabby skin, (2) skin becomes purplish after suppression of eruptions, (3) this is specially indicated in persons with tendency towards marasmus, (4) patient in general is worse by cold air, worse wet weather.

Agaricus

(1) Burning, itching, redness and swelling as if frozen.
(2) Itching changes places on scratching.
(3) Pricking as from needles.
(4) Chilblains more painful during cold weather, freezing air.
(5) Worse after consumption of alcohol.

Borax

(1) Extreme dryness of the skin.
(2) Withered, witted, wrinkled skin.
(3) Tendency to develop whitish pimples with red areolar.
(4) Slightest injury suppurates.

Calendula

(1) Tendency to develop chilblains after an injury with formation of ulcers with excessive secretion of pus.
(2) The surrounding part is red.
(3) The pain in the chilblains tend to become worse at night.

Cantharis

(1) Burning pain in the chilblains better by cold application.
(2) Tendency for the chilblain to develop ulceration leading to gangrene.
(3) The chilblains burn when touched.

Carbo-An

(1) Itching in the chilblains especially in the evening in bed.
(2) Burning pain in the chilblains worse at night.
(3) Chilblains associated with glandular enlargement.
(4) Chilblain with tendency to form ulcers which bleed very easily.

Fragaria Vesca

(1) Chilblains associated with urticaria.
(2) Especially tendency to develop chilblains in hot weather.

Hep-S

(1) The skin of *Hep-s* person is extremely sensitive to cold air.
(2) Tendency to develop deep cracks with chilblain.
(3) Better by warm application, warm wraps and heat.
(4) Worse in cold air, winter, cold application.
(5) Easy suppuration developing in chilblains.

Lachesis

(1) Chilblain with bluish-red or bluish-black discoloration round it.
(2) Chilblains tends to develop ulceration leading to gangrene.
(3) Severe burning sensation worse at night and during sleep.
(4) Chilblains are very sensitive to touch.

(5) Chilblains bleed easily and copiously.
(6) Severe excoriation of the affected part.

Ledum
(1) Dryness of skin with want of perspiration.
(2) Itching in chilblains worse after scratching.
(3) Sensation of burning after scratching.
(4) Burning worse in open air.

Mur-Ac
(1) Chilblains burn at the margins.
(2) Chilblains covered with scurf.
(3) Voluptuous itching sensation in chilblains.

Nit-Ac
(1) Dryness of the skin.
(2) Severe pricking, shooting, burning pain.
(3) Worse open air, cold application, nights cold weather.
(4) Tendency to form multiple cracks surrounding the chilblains which are very sensitive and painful to touch.

Petroleum
(1) Itching chilblains with chapped hands and feet.
(2) Slightest injury on the chilblains tends to suppurate.
(3) Severe excoriation of the affected part.
(4) Itching sensation and from it moist discharge comes out which is very acrid.
(5) In general there is aggravation of symptoms warmth of bed.

Psorinum
(1) Burning, itching, smarting pain.
(2) Burning after scratching.
(3) The skin is rough easily becomes thick and scaly.
(4) Cracks break out easily on various parts of the skin.
(5) Offensive odour comes from affected part.

Pulsatilla
(1) Itching with burning worse in the evening at night, warmth of bed, scratching.
(2) Especially indicated when the chilblains turn blue.
(3) Tendency to develop ulcers from chilblains.

Rhus-ven

(1) Chilblains with severe burning sensation.

(2) The affected part looks red, indurated and swollen.

(3) Formation of deep corroding, phagedenic ulcers with offensive discharge.

(4) Itching is worse by warmth and better by cold (locally apply Q for instant relief).

Sulphur

(1) Voluptuous itching sensation.

(2) Burning sensation sensitive to air and wind and washing.

(3) Chilblains alternate with various other bodily complaints.

(4) Skin is dry rough chapped.

(5) Offensive odour of skin, worse at night in bed, scratching and washing.

Tamus

(1) Chilblains and chapped hands.

(2) It takes away black and blue marks that come after bruises and dryness.

(3) It dissolves coagulated blood.

(4) It removes pain when it is applied locally on painful parts.

Terebinthinum

Skin is warm and moist with presence of erythema around chilblain.

Thyroidinum

(1) Tendency to develop crust with chilblains.

(2) Suppuration within the lesion.

(3) Early peeling of skin.

(4) Bluish blackish discoloration of skin.

(5) Skin gets desquamated quite freely.

CASES

Homoeoepathy
Vol. IV - No. 4
Page No. 129 - Case No. 6

Lady aged 21. Chilblains for many years. Started having return of chilblains in September 1934. *Petroleum* has kept her free all the winter.

(With *Petr.* "hands chap, crack, burn and itch intolerably, particularly in winter, itching chilblains: chapped hands." — Ed.)

Vol. IV—No. 4
Page No. 129 - Case No. 7

Lady aged 48. Chilblains cleared up with *Nitric acid.* (Probably a chilly patient with desire for fats and salts. 'Chilblains inflame from slight degree of cold.' — Ed.)

Vol IV—No.4
Page No. 129 - Case No. 8

Lady aged 21. Chilblains on hands and feet. *Nux vom* cured this case. (Bright-red swelling, superficial with burning itching—crack and bleed easily. Patient chilly, choleric and hypersensitive. — Ed.)

CHILBLAINS AND FROST-BITE

Abrot, Acon, Agar, All-c, Alum, Alumn, Aloe, Ant-c, Apis, Arn, Ars, Asar, Aur, Bad, Bell, Bor, Bufo, Bry, Cadm, Calc, Calend, Canth, *Camph, Carn-an, Carb-v, Cham,* Chin, Cinch, Cocl, Colch, *Cop.* Croc, Crot-t, Cycl, Ferr-p, Fragan, *Hep,* Ham, Hyo, Ign, Kali-ar, Kali-c, Kali-chl, Kalm, Lach, Led, Lyc, Mag-c, Merc, Mur-ac, Nit-ac, Nux-m, *Nux-v,* Op, Petr, Plant, Phos, Ph-ac, Puls, Rheum, Rhus-t, Rut, Sep, Sil, Starn, Staph, Sulph, Sut-ac, Tamus, Tereb, Thyr, Thuj, Ver-v, *Zinc.*

Alcohol was used externally — *Mur-ac*
Always bluish — *Ham*
Blue — *Arn, Bad, Bell, Kali-c, Kalm, Puls.*
Bleeding : rhagades — *Nux-v.*
Burning — *Carb-an*
From not severe cold — *Nit-ac*
Crawling in — *Arn, Colch, Nux-v, Rhus-t, Sep.*
Inflamed — *Ars, Bell, Cham, Hep, Lyc, Nit-ac, Nux-v, Phos, Puls, Rhus-t, Staph, Sulph.*
With bluish red swelling and rhagades — *Puls*
Itch and swell — *Zinc*
Itching — *Abrot, Agar, Petr, Zinc.*
Itching inflamed from slight degree of cold — *Nit-ac*

Painful — *Arn, Ars, Aur, Bell, Chin, Hep, Lyc, Mag-c, Nit-ac, Nux-v, Petr, Phos, Ph-ac, Puls, Sep.*
Pulsating — *Nux-v*
Suppurating — *Calc-s, Hep, Sil.*
Throbbing in summer — *Nux-v*
In incipient tuberculosis — *Tub*
Vesicles or bullae with — *Ant-c, Bell, Carb-an, Chin, Cycl, Mag-c, Nit-ac, Phos, Rhus-t, Sep, Sulph.*
Ear itching-burning — *Agar, Alum, Arn, Ars, Arund, Bad, Bry, Calc, Calc-p, Carb-an, Carb-v, Caust, Corn, Lach, Lyc, Mur-ac, Nat-p, Nit-ac, Nux-v, Petr, Phos, Puls, Stry, Sulph, Thuj, Zinc.*
After scratching — *Fl-ac*
Warm room — *Calc-p.*
Discolouration redness : chilblains — *Agar*
Nose — *Agar*
Easily — *Zinc*
Face : itching : frost bitten as if — *Agar, Arg-m.*
Face : burning : frost bitten as "if" — *Agar.*
Foot : bunions after frost bite — *Calc.*
Hands — *Agar, Aloe, Arg-m, Cic-v, Croc, Kali-chl, Nit-ac, Op, Petr, Puls, Stann, Sulph, Sul-ac, Zinc.*
Itching — *Puls, Zinc.*
Mild weather — *Stann*
Swelling — *Zinc*
Fingers — *Agar, Berb, Carb-an, Lyc, Nit-ac, Nux-v, Petr, Puls, Sulph, Sul-ac.*
Itching — *Sulph*
Painful — *Sul-ac*
Feet — *Abrot, Agar, Alumn, Am-c, Anac, Ant-c, Aur, Bad, Bell, Berb, Bor, Bry, Bufo, Cadm, Carb-an, Carb-v, Caust, Cham, Chin, Colch, Croc, Crot-h, Cycl, Hep, Hyos, Ign, Kali-chl, Kali-n, Lyc, Merc, Mur-ac, Naja, Nit-ac, Nux-m, Nux-v, Op, Petr, Ph-ac, Phos, Puls, Ran-b, Rhus-t, Sep, Stann, Staph, Sulph, Sul-ac, Thuj, Zinc.*
Cracked — *Merc, Nux-v, Petr.*
Inflammation — *Lach, Merc, Nit-ac, Petr.*
Purple — *Lach, Merc, Puls, Sulph.*
Suppurating — *Lach, Sil, Sulph.*
Swollen — *Merc*
Heel swollen and red — *Petr.*
Toes — *Agar, Alum, Aur, Bor, Carb—an, Croc, Kali-c, Nit-ac, Nux-v, Petr, Phos, Puls, Rhod.*
Pain toe fifth : as from chilblains — *Aloe*

AFFECTION DUE TO SUNLIGHT

Sunlight when mild, stimulates the integument, but if fair skin is repeatedly exposed to it, over long period, it will produce diffuse pigmentation or freckles (small, spotted pigmentation). Strong sunlight burns the integument: in hypersensitive individuals, certain light or photosensitization dermatoses are produced.

Solar Dermatitis

Exposure to strong sunlight produces dermatitis which may be of an acute or chronic nature. The actual degree of the burn depends upon the intensity of the sunlight and the environments under which the integument is exposed. Snow and water reflect sunlight strongly, especially the ultraviolet beam; hence, sunburns occur easily on the mountains and near the sea. Dark people sunburn less frequently than the white; people used to exposing themselves to the sun, can stand sunlight better than those who do not. Blondes and red heads are sensitive to sunlight.

The signs of sunburn vary from redness to swelling and blistering. The eyelids may swell, if the face is affected. The eruption is usually bilateral and symmetrical. Subjectively, the patient complains of burning and itching. The signs develop several hours after exposure. A mild attack clears up within a couple of days; the inflamed epidermis peels off, leaving behind hyperpigmentation, freckles, and sometimes though rarely, depigmentation. A severe attack may be accompanied by prostration and shock, and will take weeks to subside; it may leave behind some degree of atrophy or scarring.

Chronic sunburn is produced in fair people by exposure to strong sunlight over a period of years. The integument looks like that of a sailor, there being patchy and diffuse pigmentation, wrinkling, atrophy, telangiectasis and keratoses. There is a tendency to develop epitheliomata. Exposed parts like the face, neck, the dorsum of the hands and feet, are the sites chiefly affected.

AFFECTIONS DUE TO HEAT

Mild heat produces erythema due to the dilatation of blood vessels. Excessive dry heat produces various degree of burns, and

BURNS TREATED WITH CANTHARIS

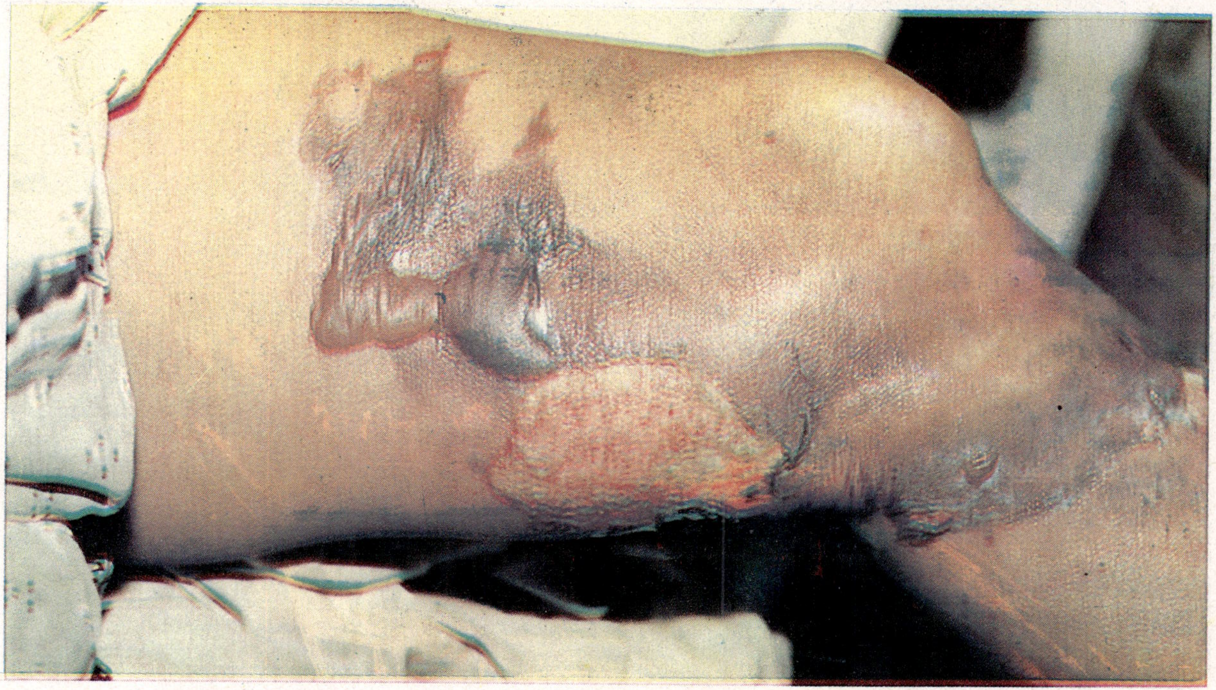

BEFORE

BURNS TREATED WITH CANTHARIS

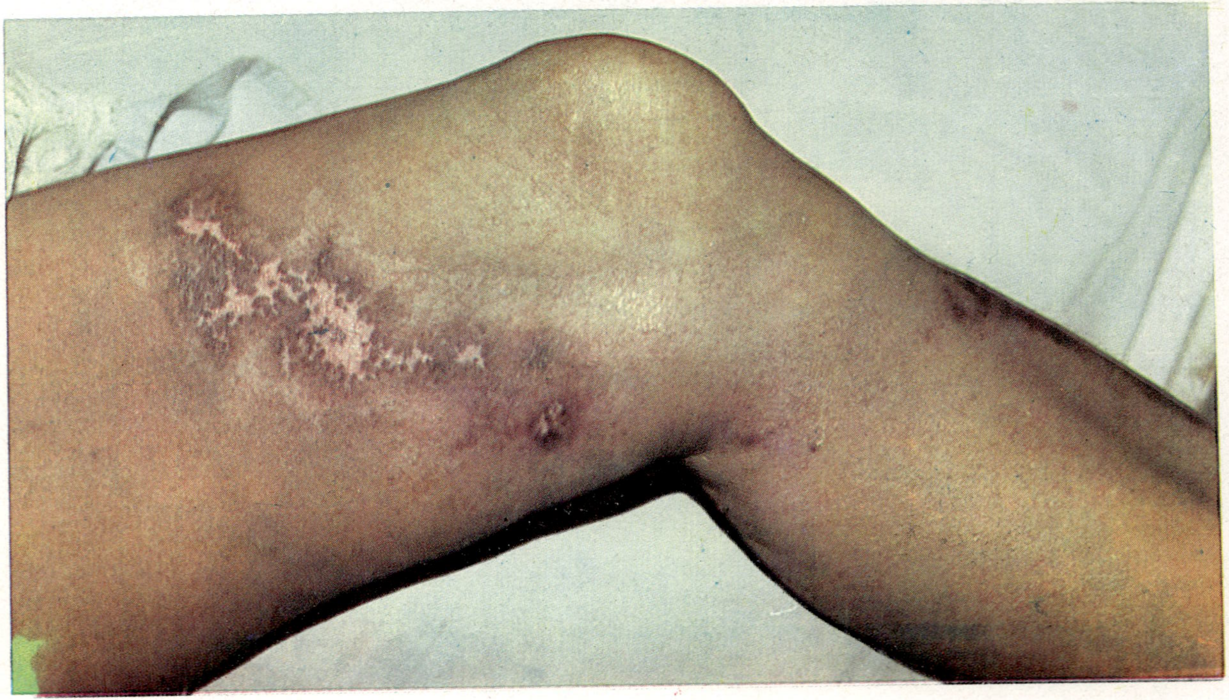

AFTER

moist heat, scalds. They are mainly surgical conditions. Electric burns are deeper than they appear, and are generally slow in healing. Mild degree of electrical burns are occasionally seen following the use of medical diathermy in people wearing metal embroidered saris.

Frequent application of mild heat to any part of body results in pigmentation. It is found for instance, on the legs of cooks, and on the abdomens of people using the kangri (Kashmiris). This pigmentation is dark-brown in colour, and occurs in a network fashion dependent upon the arterial and venous circulation of the blood. This condition is called ephelis abigne.

Exposure to heat produces profuse sweating which may give rise to different types of miliaria or prickly heat.

SOLAR DERMATITIS

As there are two phases of above condition acute and chronic, patient should be treated accordingly. During acute sunburn patient complains of burning and itching. In severe cases attack may be accompanied by prostration and shock. This is the pure psoric manifestation which produces itching followed by redness and finally disappears. In chronic cases one gets diffuse pigmentation with keratosis, hence there are very few local symptoms available for prescription. Therefore general, symptoms in mind has to be considered to prescribe a deep constitutional remedy.

Treatment

Prophylactic — People with light skin blondes, red heads and also with photosensitivity should avoid direct exposure to strong sun. In sunbathing, exposure to the sun should be increased gradually, in stages. Such people should use sun shades, umbrellas and apply evenly on exposed parts, a mixture of urtica urens mother tincture with olive oil in 1 : 4 proportion.

Homoeopathic drugs having aggravation from exposure to sun are considered here.

Treatment

For pigmentary disorder after exposure to sun, *Tuberculinum Bovinum* should be considered.

For acute sunstroke :

Aconite : The characteristic skin of *Aconite* patient is dry with absence of sweat. The skin may be very hot or very cold to touch. There is a sensation of itching which is better by taking stimulants. The three characteristic symptoms which justify the *Aconite* :

(1) Great anxiety.
(2) Agonising fever.
(3) Restlessness.

The other symptoms are head hot, cheeks red and hot. Intense thirst and burning. Palms are hot. Patient feels better in open air and fanning.

Amyl Nitrite : It presents a typical picture of sunstroke. Two symptoms should always be given prime importance while prescribing *Amyl Nitrite*. They are :

(1) Flushing heat.
(2) Drenching sweat.

The other symptoms are throbbing sensation in the head, surging of blood to the head with fiery red face < in heat, closed room > open air by drinking cold water.

Ant Crud : The overall look of *Ant-crud* skin is unhealthy. It is full of various types of eruptions. Whenever a person is exposed to sun, he develops small acne like eruptions which are red in colour and give an appearance of insect-bites. There is a sensation of itching and the skin feels sore when scratched. Also, the solar dermatitis of *Ant-crud* may come up due to suppression of eruptions or ulcers in the past. The solar dermatitis is commonly associated with gastric derangement and there is a tendency for the patient to develop (a) pimples, (b) vesicles, (c) corns, (d) urticaria, etc.

Arnica : The appearance of the Arnica skin is dry, red, oedematous. On exposure to sun, one gets red spots especially on the extremities. There is intense pricking or itching which moves from place to place after scratching. There is a tendency for the patient to develop very sore acne or crops of small boils.

Belladonna : Hot, dry and scarlet red skin points to . The skin is smooth and shiny. It may be accompanied by fever and headache. On exposure to sun, patient may develop the following complaints :

Throbbing, hammering headache worse temples, worse motion.
Redness of the conjunctiva with photophobia.
Dry hot mouth, great thirst for cold water.

Cactus Grandiflorus : On exposure to sun, there is troublesome itching as of a flea-bite. The other concomitant symptoms being compressive dull pain in the head, face red and bloated.

Camphor : The skin on exposure to sun, becomes dry as parchment, hot to touch. Solar dermatitis can occur after suppression of eruptions. Typical head symptoms develop as a concomitant to the solar dermatitis. They are — throbbing pain in occipital region, head feels knotted up. The ear lobes are hot to touch and red. There is sensation of coldness with burning thirst.

Carbo Veg : Exposure to sun-rays causes burning sensation in various areas of skin, there is a sensation of itching. The skin becomes raw and sore when scratched. The other concomitant symptoms would be (a) cold sweat on the forehead, (b) head hot with cold extremities, (c) compressive heavy headache worse occiput, (d) face cold with cold sweat, (e) rancid loud eructations with excessive flatulence, (f) burning sensation in various places.

Gelsemium : On exposure to sun, there is extreme reddish discolouration of face and neck. The skin is hot and dry. There is a sensation of itching all over the body. The other concomitant symptoms are :

Dull heavy pain around occiput to cover the eyes.
Blood rushes to the head.
Heavy drooping eyelids with diplopia, face dusky red, tongue heavy and numb.
Thirstlessness.
Cold hands and feet.
Solar dermatitis associated with gastric and nervous complaints.

Glonoine : Amongst all the remedies having aggravation by sun *Glonoine* hold the position of honour. On exposure to sun, patient develops itching all over, especially on the extremities. The other concomitants are as follows: violent pulsations, ebullitions, blood rushes upwards. Eyes protrude, look wild, flushed, hot face; violent palpitations with profuse perspiration especially on face and chest.

Nat. Carb : The appearance of *Nat. Carb* skin is dry, rough and cracked in places. The skin has a tendency to sweat easily. On exposure to sun, there is a sensation of itching over the whole body as from fleas. Solar dermatitis is associated with gastric as well as nervous symptoms. Other concomitants are : Vertigo and headache from slightest exposure to sun, weak digestion, aggravated by slightest error in diet; weak ankles.

Opium : There is absolute dryness of the skin. On exposure to sun, it turns red. There is a sensation of itching with formation of red blotches after scratching. There is a sensation of heat all over the body with hot sweat. The other concomitant symptoms are drowsy, stuporous condition, internal dryness. Rush of blood to head with throbbing arteries. Ill effects of suppressed discharges. Ailments from exposure to sun.

Veratrum Alb : On exposure to sun, patient develops bluish eruption and rash over the body, especially on face and hands. The skin is cold to touch. Concomitant—ill effects of suppressed exanthemata. Sensation of lump of ice under vertex, craves ice-water, violent retching with cutting colic. Cramps in limbs with rapid prostration.

Veratrum Viride : On exposure to sun itching of different parts of the body. There is a burning sensation which follows scratching. Skin may be cold and moist or hot and burning to the touch. Other concomitants — Vertigo with nausea and sudden prostration. Eyes blood-shot, face is flushed, livid and turgid. Very thirsty but drinks little. Slow heavy breathing.

FOR CHRONIC EFFECTS OF SUNSTROKE

Nat. Carb : Refer therapeutics of solar dermatitis.

Lachesis : The appearance of skin in chronic effects of sunstroke in *Lachesis* is intense itching almost driving to distraction mostly at night but also paroxysms in daytime; often changing to a severe, burning, stinging sensation. The skin is dry and burning. There may be a tendency for the patient to develop multiple swellings with a purplish hue. There may be presence of purpuric spots. The other characteristic symptoms are as follows :

> Mentally the patient is loquacious, suspicious and jealous. There is a sensation of heat in the vertex with flushes. There is a tendency to haemorrhages in various parts of the body. The symptoms develop in sleep and patient wakes up from symptoms; at any time at day or night. Sensation of choking in the throat.

Bad Effects of Sunburn

Bufo : Blisters on palms and soles. Bullae bursts, leaves raw surface with ichorous discharge. Itching and burning. Patches of skin loose sensation.

Cantharis : Burning, scalding with rawness and smarting, better by cold applications, followed by inflammation, Bleb formation. Eruption with mealy scales.

PHOTOSENSITIZATION DERMATOSES

It implies a group of skin disorders produced by susceptibility or hypersensitivity to light — sun's rays and U.V. rays. These disorders can be classified under two headings :

Primary (sensitivity to sunlight is primarily responsible) :
- **(a) Hydroa aestivale or vacciniform.**
- **(b) Xeroderma pigmentosum.**
- **(c) Solar eczema and polymorphic light eruption.**
- **(d) Solar urticaria.**

Secondary (sunlight only secondarily aggravates the condition) :
- **(a) Lupus erythematosus.**
- **(b) Seborrhoeic dermatitis.**
- **(c) Pellagra.**
- **(d) External applications :**
  Dyes — Hexachlorophene, salicylanilide, bithionol etc.

Plants — Phyto-photo dermatitis-Bapchi, bergamot, ragweed,etc. Tar, pitch, flurochromes.

(e) Drugs — Sulphonamides, barbiturates, griseofulvin, ledermycin (P), tetracycline, chlorthazide, hypotensives, anti-diabetics, phenergan (P), chloroquine, psoralens, I.N.H., etc.

(f) Foods — Figs, buckwheat, celery.

(g) Metabolic disorders — Porphyrinuria.

Photo sensitization dermatoses like solar dermatitis occur on exposed parts of the body — the face, V of the neck and chest, back of the neck and the dorsum of hands. If the other parts are also exposed, they can, as well, be affected; for instance, the feet, the legs and arms of poor people who wear only the loin cloth and shirt, the shoulders and waist of women who wear sleeveless dresses and *sari* respectively. The seasonal incidence of photodermatoses is typical, and varies from country to country depending upon the seasonal variation of sunshine. In North India, Photo dermatoses are common in the spring and the winter, because people expose themselves to the sun mostly at these times of the year.

Xeroderma Pigmentosum

It is a rare congenital and heredo familial disorder showing undue sensitivity to light. The disorder starts in infancy, but may begin later in childhood or adult life. The characteristic lesions are : hyperpigmentation, freckles and blotches, atrophic spots and telangiectasis. Later warty growths, keratoses and epitheliomas may complicate the disorder. The exposed parts of the body are the sites of choice. Exposure to sunlight aggravates the condition, which may be accompanied by photophobia and keratitis. The prognosis is bad in severe cases; patients die early, but some live to adulthood.

The treatment administered is unsatisfactory. Patients should learn to live with their skins, respecting its undue sensitivity; they should avoid sunlight and use anti-actinic creams.

Solar Eczema

It implies abnormal sensitivity to sunlight amounting to an allergy which results in a polymorphic type of eruption consisting of erythema, papules, vesicles, oozing, crusting, which may later on turn into pigmented freckles and blotches and even depressed scars on the parts of the body exposed to sunlight. Lesions vary from oedematous papules to frank eczema in different individuals. In others, it consists of only infiltrated, blotchy erythema of the face. The eruption is accompanied by considerable pruritus, which may result in secondary infection and even lichenification in chronic solar eczema. The etiology is unknown. The disorder usually starts in childhood, and lasts for several years. In children, it is usually seasonal and then it is named Juvenile Spring Eruption or Summer Eruption. In adults it is more persistent with only minor seasonal flare ups.

The condition must be differentiated from eczema produced by chemical contact, lupus erythematosus and phyto-photodermatitis.

Solar Urticaria

It is a variety of physical urticaria, caused by sensitivity to sunlight, affecting the exposed parts of the skin. Urticarial lesions begin to develop soon after an exposure has been made to the sun. In the temperate climate, the condition is seasonal, while in the tropics, it may occur throughout the year. The condition is chronic and recurrent. The treatment consists of protecting the skin from sunlight, and in the use of antihistaminics. One could try desensitizing the skin by exposing it by degrees, to the sun.

CHAPTER 8

Virus Infection

Introduction

Viruses are the smallest infectious agents 300-18 nm in diameter (one nm = one millionth part of a millimetre) whose genome is an element of either deoxyribonucleic acid (DNA) or ribonucleic acid (RNA) but never both, enclosed within an outer shell of protein, capsid. Viruses can reproduce only inside living cells and utilise the synthetic machinery of the host cell for synthesis of specialized particles, the 'virions', which contain the viral genome and serve as a vehicle to carry the genome to other cells. When a virion enters its host cell the capsid is stripped off and its nucleic acid is liberated within the host cells entering into an eclipse phase in their reproductive cycle, a characteristic of all true viruses. The surface proteins of the virion have special affinity for specific receptor sites on the host cell. Proteins also contain the viral antigens that stimulate the host's immune responses during infection. Viruses possess the property of haemagglutination.

Interferon, a protein produced by the cell after infection with a virus interferes with the replication of the other viruses. Inactivated virus and also a few other substances (foreign nucleic acids and other synthetic polynucleotides) also induce synthesis of interferon.

Any of the following events may occur following the presence of virus within a cell :

(1) Destruction, e.g., primary herpes hominis virus infection.

(2) Stimulation and multiplication first forming a papule which then undergoes destruction associated with inflammatory exudate forming vesicle, which subsequently evolves into a pustule and finally drying up to form scab, e.g. variola, varicella.

(3) Stimulation of the cells to proliferate indefinitely forming papillomata, e.g., warts.

Skin is one of the principal target organs for viral attack. Rashes (exanthemata) are characteristic of many acute systemic viral infections, where virions in the blood invade the endothelium of the capillaries and venules of the dermis. Viral rash may also be related to antigen — antibody reaction and the circulation of immune complexes. The rash may be an outward sign of the neutralization of circulating virus by antibody. Haemorrhagic rashes may be due to disseminated intravascular coagulation precipitated by the circulating virus antibodies and immune complexes.

Skin probably offers a peculiarly sensitive situation for some viral growth because of its lower temperature.

In dermatologic practice the following group of viruses appear important :

DNA Viruses (Deoxyriboviruses)	*RNA Viruses (Riboviruses)*
1. Herpes viruses: Herpes simplex, varicella, Zoster, Epstein-Barr Vieua.	1. Picorna viruses : Coxsackie: Herpengina, Rubella.
2. Pox viruses: Variola, Vaccinia, Molluaxum xonragiosum Orf, Milker's nodes.	2. Echo viruses: Hand-foot mouth disease (HFMD).

3. Papova viruses :
   Warts.

Virus Inhibitors.: Viruses are resistant to all known antibiotics. Many substances have been synthesized which inhibit their growth in vitro. They have at present, limited clinical use. They are :

(i) Those found clinically useful — Thiosemicarbazones (for small-pox contacts), halogenated deoxyuridines, i.e. IDUR, BDUR, etc. (for herpes simplex) : acrylic doxyguanosine (Acyclovir).

(ii) Those not used clinically — Interferon, Guanidine and HBB, Adamantamine.

WARTS (VERRUCA VULGARIS, PARONYCHIAL WARTS AND PLANTAR WARTS)

Clinical Presentation

Warts can occur at any age but are most commonly seen in children and young adults. They begin as pinhead sized papules which grow quickly to a stable, final size of 6 to 10 mm in diameter. Shedding and subsequent implantation of wart virus into surrounding skin results in the development of new warts in a cluster around the original "mother" wart. Tightly clustered warts may merge as they enlarge, forming mosaic warts 1 to 3 cm in diameter.

Verruca vulgaris is the name used for warts which develop on "non-pressure" dry surfaces of the skin. They are most commonly found on the dorsal surface of the fingers, hands, arms and toes. These warts extend 2 to 8 mm above the surrounding skin surface and are approximately as wide as they are tall. Their margination is extremely sharp; in cross-section they are square shouldered. The surface is verrucous; that is, rough on palpation and somewhat jagged in appearance. Verruca vulgaris are usually skin coloured but sometimes they are somewhat hyperpigmented compared to surrounding normal skin.

Paronychial warts are verruca vulgaris that grow in the paronychial tissue which surrounds the nails. There is a marked tendency for confluent growth such that these warts are regularly wider than they are tall. Otherwise, their appearance is similar to conventional verruca vulgaris.

Plantar warts are those warts which occur on the plantar surface of the feet. Constant pressure from walking affects the appearance of these warts in two ways : *First*, the mass of the wart is pushed into the underlying soft tissue; these warts do not seem greatly raised above the surface of the surrounding normal skin. *Second*, the surface of the wart becomes heavily callused and thus has a smoother than expected feel on palpation. Paring of the callused surface reveals an underlying translucent core peppered with black dots. These black dots represent thromboses in the vertically oriented capillaries which provide nutrition for the warts. Calluses and corns unassociated with warts lack these black dots. Single plantar warts may be only 2 or 3 mm in diameter but there is marked tendency for confluent growth such that mosaic pattern 2 or more cm in diameter are frequently found. Most warts are asymptomatic but plantar warts may be painful on walking because of compression against the underlying tissue.

The diagnosis of keratotic warts is made on the basis of clinical history and examination. Recognition of thrombosed or bleeding capillaries following paring is especially helpful. Biopsy is occasionally indicated to separate warts from other tumours. Electron microscopy will show, if enough fields are examined, the distinctive viral particles.

Course and Prognosis

In children untreated warts almost always disappear spontaneously. Twenty per cent of warts disappear in as little as 1 month and in the majority of children all warts will be gone within 2 to 3 years. Spontaneous resolution also occurs in adults but the average time of disappearance is longer.

Left untreated, warts tend to spread through a process of autoinoculation. Viral particles which are continually shed from the surface of the skin are implanted into small cuts and scratches elsewhere on the body. Warts are also spread from person to person as a result of direct contact.

Pathogenesis

Warts are caused by the human papilloma virus. Several sub-types of this spherical DNA virus have been identified and each appears to be responsible for a different morphologic type of wart. These wart virus sub-types are morphologically identical but differ immunogenetically and in amino acid sequence.

Wart viruses have specific affinity for epidermal cells and they cannot replicate in dermal connective tissue cells. After implantation into the epidermis, the viruses enter the nuclei of lower and mid-epidermal cells. There they take over the machinery of cell reproduction and while replicating themselves, they induce a rapid and greater than normal proliferation of epithelial cells. On electron microscopy viral particles are most numerous between 6 and 12 months of wart growth. Thereafter the number of visible particles decreases to the point where, after 2 to 3 years of growth, they become difficult if not impossible to find.

Like other viral infections the presence of the wart virus in human skin incites an immunological response. In the early months of wart growth IgM is elaborated; later IgG is produced. Antibody measurements suggest that infection with the wart virus is almost universal. By late adult life, 90% of the population have developed antibodies suggesting one or more episodes of earlier infection. Resolution of warts, however, depends on cell mediated immune responsiveness, not on antibody production. The importance of the cell mediated response is reflected by the frequency and severity of wart infections in renal transplant patients and individuals with Hodgkin's disease. In all individuals the immune response which leads to spontaneous resolution of the infection is not long lasting. Reinfection easily occurs within months.

WARTS
(CONDYLOMA ACUMINATA AND FLAT WARTS)

Clinical Presentation

Condyloma acuminata and flat warts lack visible or palpable surface keratin and both demonstrate a marked tendency for clustering. They are otherwise quite different in appearance.

Condyloma acuminata (venereal warts) usually appear as thin, flexible, stalk-like papules. They are taller than they are wide. The distal tip of these warts sometimes has a fine filiform appearance. Multiple adjacent lesions may develop a confluent growth pattern forming a large cauliflower-like nodule. On rare occasions dense mats of the warts can grow over large surface areas so as to almost occlude the vaginal or rectal orifices. Condyloma acuminata can grow on any moist surface but they are most commonly found on the glans penis, at the vaginal introitis and at the anal orifice. Since they transferred venereally, they are found most often in young and middle aged sexually active adults. Condyloma acuminata are asymptomatic. The diagnosis is made on a clinical basis.

Flat warts (verruca plana) appear as square shouldered, flat topped papules 1 to 3 mm in diameter. They are barely raised above the surface of the surrounding normal skin. New warts appear rapidly and by the time patients are first examined dense clusters of the lesions are usually present. Linear clusters are sometimes seen because of implantation of viral particles into scratch marks. Flat warts are generally skin coloured but some may be slightly hyperpigmented compared to adjacent skin. In children flat warts are most commonly found on the face or on traumatized surfaces of the arms and legs. In adults the distribution assumed is often related to shaving. Thus men frequently develop flat warts on the face whereas they are found on the lower legs in women. Flat warts are asymptomatic. The diagnosis is made on a clinical basis.

Course and Prognosis

Condyloma acuminata appear to be more contagious than other types of warts. They not only spread easily on the patient's own skin through autoinoculation but they also can be passed on to sexual partners. Left untreated there is the same tendency for eventual, spontaneous disappearance as is found in varruca vulgaris.

Flat warts, when they occur in c 'ldren, go through a short phase of very rapid growth and spread. This is followed by a plateau period involving little change in growth. The plateau period is, in turn, succeeded by a phase of steady, rapid, spontaneous resolution. Flat warts when they occur in adults are much more stubborn and when left untreated they tend to persist for years. Flat warts are considered as totally benign lesions but here, too, evidence is accumulating to suggest that at least one sub-type of flat wart virus has some oncegenic potential.

Pathogenesis

Condyloma acuminata and flat warts are each caused by separate and distinct sub-types of the human papilloma virus. Implantation and growth of these viruses seems to require some degree of preceding minor skin trauma.

Warts — Homoeopathic Approach

Warts are something very peculiar. Some, specially, if they are numerous, sometime heal very rapidly, whereas others isolated warts, sometimes bid defiance to all treatment. This is one of the important manifestation of sycotic miasm.

The following points should be noted very carefully during case taking :

(A) **Causation**: e.g.,
- (a) After Gonorrhoea — *Thuja.*
- (b) After having consumed too much Salt — *Nitri Spiritus Dulcis*
- (c) After abuse of mercury — *Sarsaparilla*
- (d) After syphilitic infection — *Aurum met*
- (e) After injury — *Bellis Perennis*

(B) **Previous treatment**: It is essential to know whether patient has attempted to cauterize with the help of the following:
- (a) Acetic Acid
- (b) Caustic Potash
- (c) Fluoric acid
- (d) Silver Nitrate
- (e) Burning with the help of Agarbatti (a perfume stick used in India)

If it is so then it should be antidoted as follows:
- (i) Ailments after cauterisation — Causticum, Nitric Acid, Thuja.
- (ii) Use of Acetic acid, caustic potash and Fluoric acid preferably in high potencies.

(iii) For bad effects of Silver nitrate — Use *Nat-mur* in high potencies.

(iv) When Agarbatti is used, then to neutralize its ill-effects, use carbolic acid or causticum.

(v) When electric cautery is used for cauterization, it should be antidoted with drugs like carbolic acid, causticum, radium bromide and X-ray.

(C) **Location**:e.g.,

Face
Fingers
Palms, etc.

(D) **Characteristic**:

Flat
Fleshy
Hard
Horny
Pedunculated
Smooth, etc.

(E) **Whether warts are associated**:

(a) With or without Inflammation
(b) With or without Itching
(c) With or without Bleeding
(d) With or without Suppuration
(e) With or without ulceration
(f) Tender or Non-tender.

(F) **Important characteristic sensations** should always be inquired,e.g.,

Burning
Pulsating
Stinging
Stitching

This is very important when the wart is isolated.

(G) Sometimes the **colour of the warts** also helps us to select remedy indirectly.

Red — *Calc Carb, Thuja.*
Brown — *Sepia, Thuja.*
Greyish Brown — *Conium.*

It is strongly advised not to recommend to the patient any local application for the treatment of warts, e.g.

(a) Application of lime.
(b) Application of Homoeopathic mother tinctures.
(c) Application of ointments — *Salicylic acid, Fluoric acid.*

For the following reasons :

(i) It is against the basic principle of Homoeopathy.
(ii) Recurrence rate is very high.
(iii) Since the cause lie within, it is futile to cure disease externally.

(H) **Treatment Review** :

I have observed that majority of cases get cured, where only, constitutional remedies were prescribed and occasionally those remedies which do not produce warts in its provings have frequently cured the cases at the beginning should be on a constitutional background.

Failing to respond to the above method a drug should be selected taking into account the local signs and symptoms. If this also fails then only one should take help of empirical or specific medicine.

It is always wise to restudy the case at least three times before seeking these specific medicines.

The cases described below should give you the evidence of the treatment review.

(1) A young Gujarati boy Mr. N.B. aged 20 years old, consulted me in 1985 for multiple warts on palms, fingers and foot. He was a student studying in commerce college and he used to cut his warts whenever it became painful or whenever he found the site was ugly. The above symptoms were present since last 5 years.

The following were the characteristic symptoms :

(i) Warts flat, hard, tender.
(ii) Profuse perspiration from slightest exertion.
(iii) Tendency to catch cold very fast.
(iv) Psychologically — he was very talkative and happy-go-lucky type, was not much interested in studies as he

wanted to learn and practise carpentry bu ; because his father didn't like the idea, he was forcibly advised to join a commerce college. He also had difficulty in concentration and comprehension. He had an inability to perform any intellectual task.

(v) Appetite voracious weak, stomach gets easily disordered, especially after consuming milk products.

For just few weeks he was given placebo till the case was repertorised which was followed by *Natrum carb* 1M, 3 doses for 21 days within a fortnight all the warts disappeared. He was advised not to repeat the last dose, till today he is under my observation and he has not developed new warts.

(2) Mr. N.M. aged 43 years consulted us in March 1987 with two chief complaints :

(i) Left-sided renal calculus since April 1985.
(ii) Multiple warts around nose, mouth, thumb and extremities.

Other complaints were :

Craving for lime. Difficulty in digesting milk.
Nausea after eating. Occasional bitter and sour vomiting.
Burning Micturition with strong odour.
Psychologically — He had fear of death due to his illness. He was easily frightened. Got vexed at trifles. Occasionally developed fits of rage with despair.

He had strong family history of asthma, DM and IHD and past history of cataract and typhoid.

His IVP taken on June and November 1985 showed large opaque calculus in left upper ureter.

He was prescribed *Nitric acid* 30 bid followed by *Nitric acid* 200 for more 15 days. For 2 months patient did not report to us. It was only in June 1987 when he had an attack of bilious headache we inquired about his warts and to our surprise not a single wart was present; also there was no recurrence of renal colic. A repeated IVP showed a calculus of same size but it had descended the course of ureter.

(3) Master S.B. 9 years old approached me in May 1988 for a wart on the left index finger — middle phalanyx. He had noticed this only 4 months back. Being a student of 4th standard, he was very conscious of this wart and would pick on it continuously. The following symptoms were taken into consideration :

(i) Extreme restlessness.
(ii) Stubborn — Always retaliates to authority.
(iii) Short-tempered, becomes more angry when contraindicated.
(iv) Disorderly and very haphazard in his work.
(v) Desire for cold milk, chocolates, ice-cream, potatoes.
(vi) Aversion to meat, spicy food.
(vii) Profuse perspiration.
(viii) Dreams of ghosts—fearful.
(ix) Nocturnal eneuresis.

After detailed study of this case *Tub. bov.* 10M one dose every alternate day was prescribed for a period of 7 days. On his second visit there was a slight improvement — the wart had decreased in size. So he was put on *Tub. bov.* 10M one dose every fourth day for one month. Since they were to emigrate to Australia his mother was most adamant to get rid of the wart as fast as possible. To speed up the healing a specific prescription was given and the drug was *Lac-c* 200, 4 pills T.D.S. This was chosen since *Lac-c* was the only remedy with 3 marks in the Kent's Repertory under warts fingers.

WARTS

Acetic Acid : The warts of acetic acid are flat and moist, i.e., on touching the wart one feels a moist sensation. Warts are present especially in persons who are pale, lean, thin, anaemic, debilitated, with lax, flabby muscles. The skin is dry and hot to touch. There is excessive perspiration in skin.

Alumina : The warts of *Alumina* are associated with chapped and dry skin. There is intolerable itching when getting warm in bed. The skin is dry, rough and cracked; the skin symptoms usually become worse in winter, full and new moon.

Anacardium : Warts are present on hands, especially dorsum and eyebrows. There is sensation of intense itching in the warts which is worse on scratching.

Antim-crud : It is the leading remedy for warts, and has great practical use in homoeopathy. The warts are situated especially on hand; they are hard, horny, soft or smooth, with characteristic stinging pain. Warts are surrounded by circle of ulcers. Warts tend to develop which are prone to pressure and friction, especially suited to individuals who have tendency to grow fat. Warts develop in individuals who have suppression of eruption or ulcers.

Arg. Nit. : It tends to develop warts on palate, near anus, the appearance is brownish and hard to touch. The wart tends to ulcerate easily. Tendency to develop warts in patient with mental and digestive symptoms.

Baryta Carb : It develops small warts, especially on hands and fingers, with stinging pain; gradually due to friction. Warts get excoriated and start oozing, it typically affects patients who are dwarfish, mentally and physically with tendency to enlargement of glands with induration; there is strong tendency to take cold.

Belladona : It plays a very useful role whenever warts are inflamed with burning pain. They are hot and tender to touch with characteristic throbbing pain.

Bovista : Warts are present on the upper limb. They are very painful due to inflammation surrounding it; they also tend to suppurate easily.

Calc. Carb : Warts are present on face, neck and upper extremities, male genitalia, canthi, fingers. They are black and fleshy, hard and horny, sometimes inflamed and painful; the warts tend to suppurate. Giving an odour of stale cheese. The skin is icy cold to touch with cold and profuse perspiration. Development of warts in patient having history of suppression of eruption and perspiration. Development of warts in individual with scrofoulous diathesis with faulty development of bones. It has a typical physically constitution, i.e., fat, flabby, fair, perspiring, cold and damp.

Causticum : Warts are present on nose, eyebrows, face, lips, near the nail, tips of fingers, upper limbs. They are large, horny, broad, fat and hard, moist and pedenculated. They tend to bleed easily. They are also prone to easy suppuration. Warts are present in individual after suppressed eruptions.

Dulcamara : Warts are present on face, hands, fingers, close to nail; the warts are smooth, hard; they usually come in crops; they always tend to aggravate when skin is washed with cold water.

Euphorbinum : The warts are covered by erythema with fine bran like desquamation, there is smarting and burning sensation in warts.

Ferrum Pic : Multiple warts, especially on hands; they are usually pedenculated. There is a sensation, as if warts were growing on thumb.

Flu. Acid : The warts are situated on hands and fingers. They are flat and hard; there is presence of elevated red blotches, which resemble fleshy warts. The appearance of skin is dry, harsh, itching with multiple cracks.

Graph : Warts are present around the female genitalia. They have cauliflower shape. They discharge sticky exduation which smells like old cheese or herring brine. The appearance of skin is dry, rough, irritable that breaks easily and exude a gluey moisture which is worse in folds. Warts are present in persons who have tendency to develop erysipelas. The patient is extremely sensitive to cold. Digestive symptoms are important concomitant symptoms to warts.

Hepar Sulph : It is typically indicated in syphilitic warts with burning, sore, stitching and stinging pain in the warts. They tend to suppurate easily. They discharge smell like old cheese. The warts bleed easily.

Lachesis : The warts of *Lachesis* are hard, smooth and small. They have a bluish, purple surrounding. The wart may appear small but it has strong tendency to bleed.

Lycopodium : *Lycopodium* has two types of warts (1) isolated warts, (2) warts in crops. Warts are situated especially on face, tongue, male genitalia, upper limbs and fingers. Warts are associated with terrible itching. They are large, jagged furrowed, splitted and pedenculated; they exude moisture, surrounded by a herpetic areola, with desquamation. The warts have tendency to bleed easily.

Millefolium : It has tendency to develop sycotic warts which bleed very easily.

Medorrhinum : The warts are small, pedenculated resembling small button mushrooms, especially on thighs and other parts of the body. They emit offensive odour. The skin is cold to touch. It affects individuals who have poor resistance due to sycotic tent.

Nat-Mur. : The warts are especially situated on palms, hands and knuckles. There is a cutting pain in the wart, the look of the skin is oily, dry, harsh, unhealthy or yellow. Tendency to develop warts in individual after cautery with silver nitrate.

Nit-Ac. : The warts appear on female genitals, anus, cervical region inside nose, external throat, sternum, eyelids, canthi. They usually develop after abuse of mercury. The following are the characteristics :

(a) Moist
(b) Cauliflower like
(c) Hard
(d) Rhagadic
(e) Large
(f) Indented
(g) Inflamed
(h) Pricking pain < night
(i) They emit foetid discharge
(j) They bleed on touch.

Nitri-spirit Dulcis : Warts after abuse of excessive salt.

Phos-Ac. : Warts are present in mouth, male genitalia. They are hot to touch. They are large, jagged, indented in appearance.

Psorinum : Warts are situated on canthi, around mouth, near male genitalia. There is a sensation of itching < heat of bed. The appearance of skin is dirty rough, scabby, greasy. It breaks out in folds.

Rananculus Bulb : It produces cauliflower-like warts; especially situated on outer side of terminal phalynx of right thumb.

Rhus-Tox : Warts are situated on fingers, hands and upper limb. They are horny, rough and knotty. Thickened epidermis forms hard crust which peels off.

Sepia : Warts are situated on male genitalia, upper lip, fingers, face. They are small, flat, hard, dark colour and sometimes brownish in colour with a horny excrescences in centre. There is a sensation of itching. Appearance of skin blotched, raw, rough, hard or cracked. Tendency to form induration and warts from constant pressure.

Silicea : The warts are situated on throat, upper limb, back and forearm. They are large, fleshy and suppurating. They are painful to touch. Development of warts in individual with scrofulous diathesis. The patient is keenly sensitive to noise, pain and cold.

Staphysagria : Warts are situated on iris, on tongue, on male genitalia. They are moist, pedunculated and are extremely sensitive to touch. Warts appear after abuse of mercury and suppressed eruption. Warts in syphilitic individual.

Sulphur : Warts are situated on face, near eyelids, on upper lip. Warts covered with thin epidermis. The appearance of skin is dry, rough, wringled and scaly. Warts alternate with other complaints. Suppression of warts leads to asthma.

Thuja : Warts are situated on back, cervical region, upper limb, face, nose, eyebrows, eyes and eyelids, external throat. They are

WARTS TREATED WITH NITRIC ACID

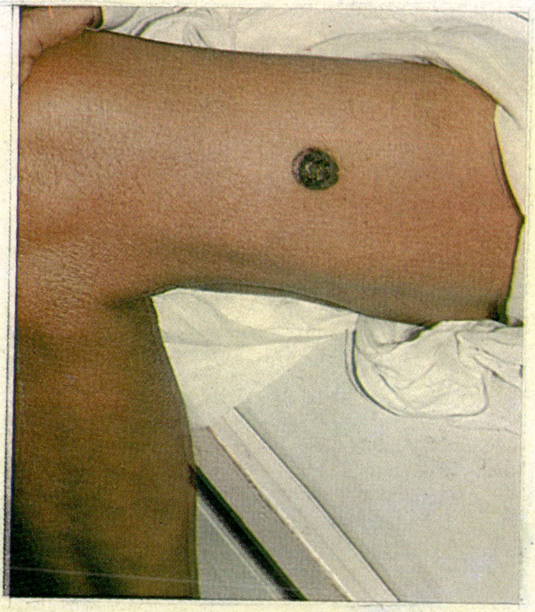

BEFORE

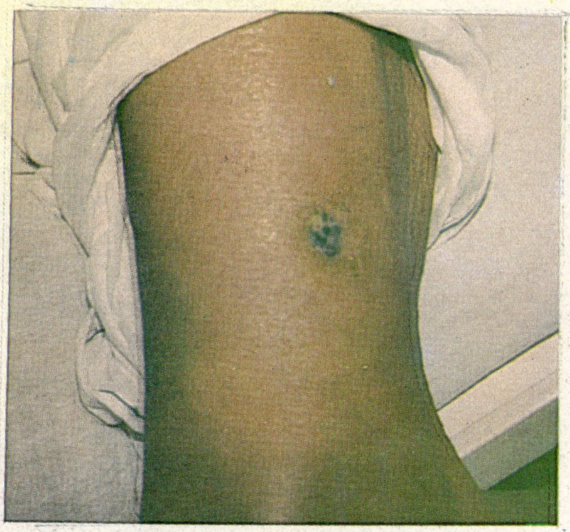

AFTER

WARTS TREATED WITH NITRIC ACID

BEFORE

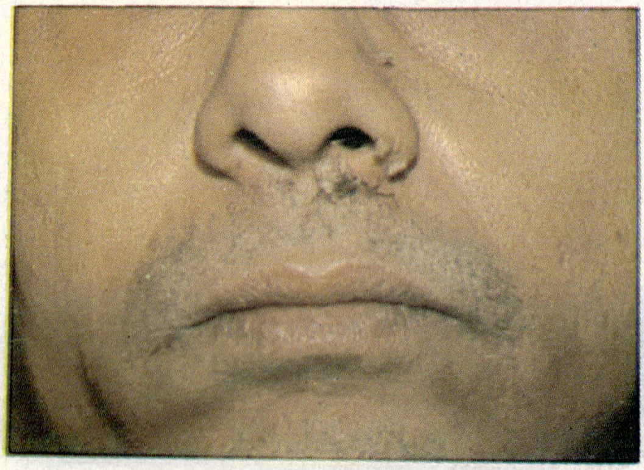

AFTER

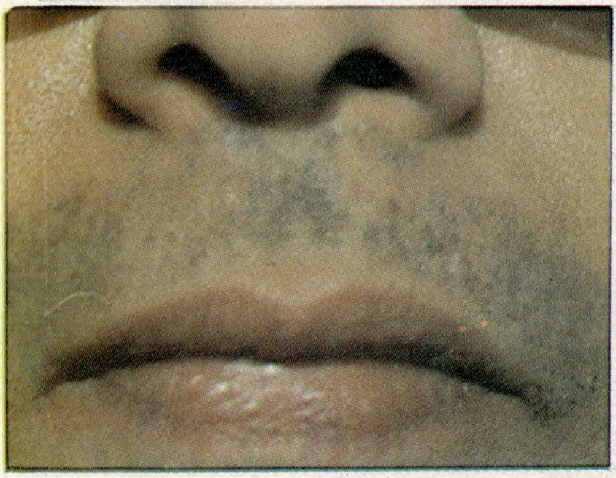

WARTS TREATED WITH NITRIC ACID

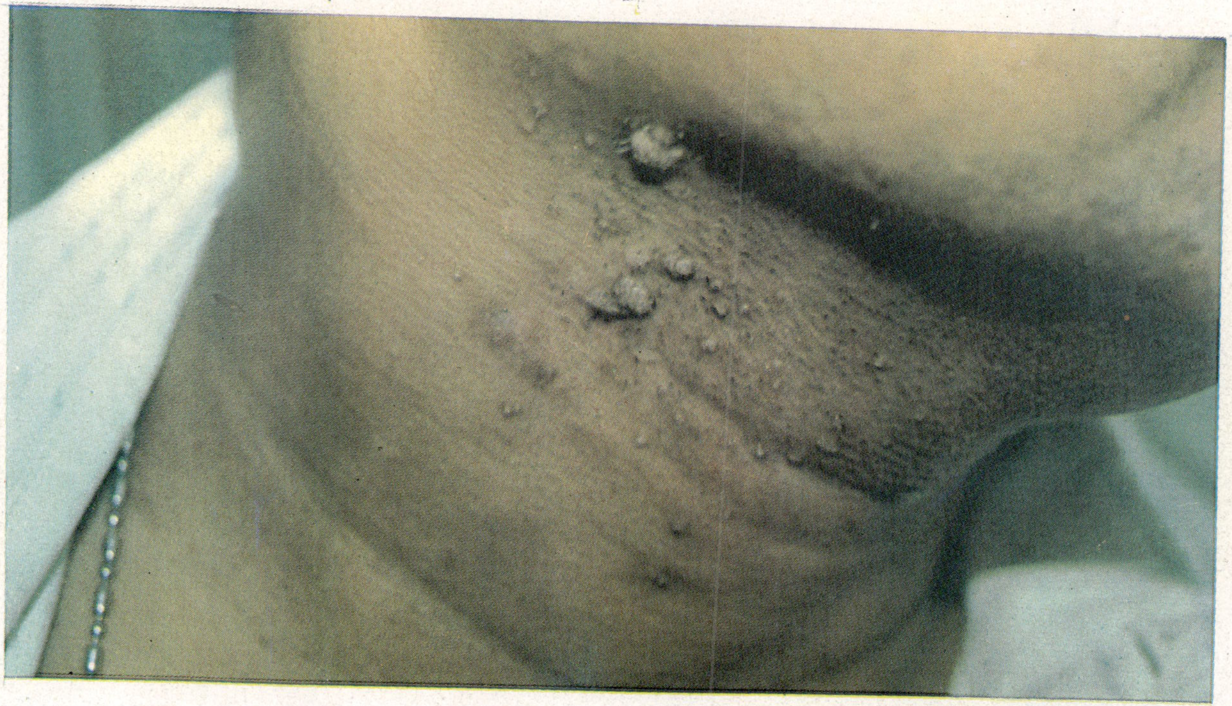

BEFORE

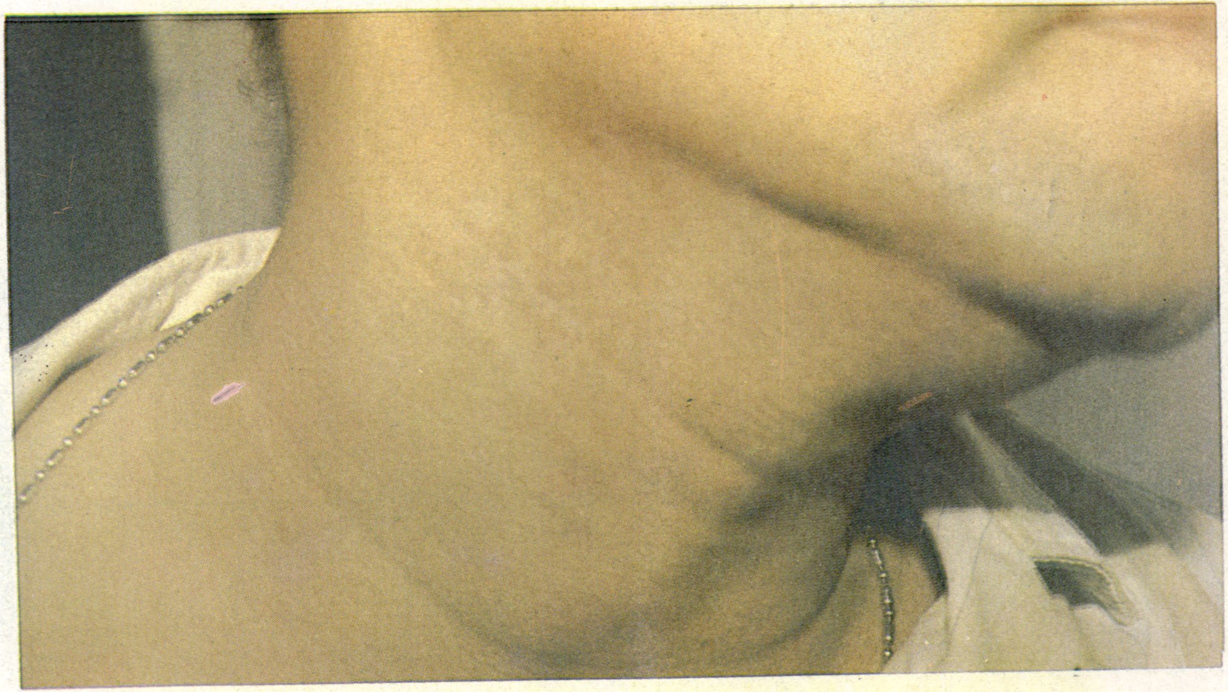

AFTER

WARTS TREATED WITH NITRIC ACID

broad, conical, flat pedunculated, indented, fan shaped in appearance. They are reddish in colour, bleed easily. The warts have a tendency to split from their edge or from the surface.

THE HOMOEOPATHIC HERITAGE
VOL. XII - 1987
Case of the Month - Page 292

The drug was *Thuja.* The condition *Venereal Warts.*

> Treated for gonorrhoea 18 months ago with sulphonamides with apparently a very quick and very successful result. No discharge at all since, but recently, crop of warts on the vulva increasing and spreading. These when examined were typical condylomata acuminata.
>
> *Thuja* 30 T.D.S. was prescribed but without effect. Then one dose of *Thuja* C.M. was given and all vanished. Three months later none at all, and no recurrence.
>
> The cause and origins of these warts is still debatable. They are held to be due to a quite separate infection (a virus infection) and not to the original venereal disease. But here one has a clear-cut case of gonorrhoeal infection followed by a crop of such warts. It is difficult not to associate the two conditions, as was, of course, done in the past. What is the interaction presumed between this virus infection and gonorrhoea is not very clear, but it is interesting to note that *Thuja* the drug here given is stated to be effective in all sorts of warts due, as is stated, to the same virus infection. One would interpolate, however, that it is in the combined state, viz., virus and gonorrhoea that one has seen the most brilliant results, and usually with very highest potencies.
>
> *Thuja (arbor vitae)* : The main action of this drug is on the skin and genito-urinary organs producing conditions which correspond to Hahnemann's sycosis whose chief manifestation is the formation of wart-like excrescences of mucous and cutaneous surfaces. It has been extolled for its effects in suppressed gonorrhoea and vaccination, and is the drug of choice in vaccinosis when constitutional

effects following vaccination are extreme. There is no doubt that here it acts specifically and quickly. One had always felt that a simple experiment to prove the efficacy of potencies would be to administer potencies of *Thuja* for some weeks before vaccination and observe how many cases would show complete resistance to vaccination with cow-pox.

Thuja like *Nat-sulph* has a hydrogenoid constitution, i.e., is susceptible to damp humid atmosphere. Pains (like *Rhus*) are worse in damp and better in dry weather.

The mentals of *Thuja* are strange, rare and peculiar. 'That there is a strange person at his side.' 'That something is alive in the abdomen' cf. *Crocus*

The skin is greasy like *Nat-mur* and *Psorinum*, chronic catarrhal states of eyes, nose, ears are covered by *Thuja* : in the eyes-styes and tarsal tumours; ears — polypi and chronic discharge; nose — ulceration and conditions resembling ozoena. The teeth decay next to the gums as in pyorrhoea. *Thuja* is recommended for tea drinkers' dyspepsia and has an aggravation from eating onions.

The stool recedes like *Silicea* and there are, of course, the anal warts.

In the male *Thuja* is quoted for enlargement of the prostate and for chronic epididymitis and indeed both may be a result of gonorrhoeal infection. In the female *Thuja* covers many manifestations of chronic pelvic infection (not necessarily gonorrhoeal) and again, the warts of vulva and vagina already mentioned. Papillomata of the larynx are of course again covered in the *Thuja* constitution. Papillomata in any situation.

In the limbs the peculiar symptom of 'legs feel like glass or wood' should be remembered and was the guide to the use of *Thuja* in Dr. Fergie Wood's famous 'brittle man'.

Thuja sweats only on the uncovered parts unlike *China* and *Pulsatilla* which sweat only on covered parts.

The skin manifestations have already been described but all sorts of blotches, brown spots, even naevi are noted in the picture besides the warty growth so typical of the drug.

Thuja like *Leuticum* is worse at night; like *Sulph* from the heat of the bed and like *Kali carb* at 3 a.m. (but also at 3 p.m.)

INDIAN JOURNAL OF HOMOEOPATHIC MEDICINE
Page No. 60 - Case No. 3
Plantar Wart - Conium 1M

Mrs. E.B.G. aged 46 years had Plantar Wart of left foot for twenty years. She was cutting the wart off and on but it became much worse during the last six months. Wart was very painful, unable to walk because of tenderness of the affected part. Sensation of pinpricks and stabbing pain. Pain worse on lying down. Worse on keeping leg up and extended, better on letting leg hand down.

The concomitant symptoms were chronic sinusitis. *Conium* was prescribed on the basis of the peculiar modality. The result was a beautiful cure within two weeks. *Conium* is not listed under warts or corns in any repertory.

INDIAN JOURNAL OF HOMOEOPATHIC MEDICINE
Page No, 64 - Case No. 12
Warts Tongue - Kali Sulph 6

Miss P., a five year old girl, had warts on tongue and left tonsils for three months. Tendency to catch colds since birth. Warts were soft, non-bleeding and not painful. They were growing and were more marked on left side.

She was a hot patient throwing off covers even in winter months and was averse to any tight clothing around the neck. She had been given *Thuja* earlier with no change. *Lachesis* 1M was prescribed with no change in the warts.

Then the girl developed a cold with thick yellow, stringy nasal discharge. Obstruction of nose better in open or cold air. She was given *Kali sulph* 6. It was noticed that within 4-5 days a slight reduction had taken place in the size of the warts. Of course the coryza was cured with *Kali sulph* 6 within this period. She was kept on *Kali sulph.* 6, four times a day and gradually the warts were cured in about two months.

THE HOMOEOPATHIC HERITAGE
No. 9 - September 1983
Page No. 420 - Case No. 1065

Mr. B.F. age 35; light complexion, blue eyes and of a mild disposition, follows farming and fruit-growing as a business. Family history : consumption, two sisters and an uncle died of that disease; one of his own children, aged two years, died last summer of marasmus. Father and mother both living and well now, but both are subject to attacks of erysipelas about once a year. Previous to his present trouble his health has generally been good. As long as he remembers has had a wart on the left cheek, near the angle of the mouth, about the size of a small pea. It never gave him any trouble until last September, when, for some unknown reason, it began to grow rapidly. At the end of two months it had grown about one inch in length, and as thick as the little finger, and had already begun to ulcerate and discharge thin, acrid and badly smelling pus; occasionally it would bleed so profusely, as to be somewhat alarming. It was during one of these attacks that he called the attention of a physician to it, who diagnosed it as a cancerous wart, and advised immediate excision. Not satisfied with his decision he consulted two others, who gave him similar advice, when he was advised to consult me about it. On examination of it carefully I came to the conclusion that it was cancer; the ulceration had already reached the cheek, which was very much swollen, infiltrated and angry, with a tendency of the tissues to contract around the growth.

Treatment

From the character of the discharge, which was thin, watery and excoriating, the intense burning, the constantly increasingl thirst, and the nightly restlessness and aggravation after midnight. I prescribed *Arsenicum*, two powders in the cm potency, with no medicine for one week; at the end of one week he returned improved, the discharge had nearly ceased, the inflammation lessened, thirst gone, and the nightly restlessness much better; the growth had now begun to contact at the base. At the end of the second week it had so dried up that it looked as if it was burnt; the contraction had still gone on at the base, so that with a slight touch it broke off close to cheek and was followed by a slight haemorrhage. Continued no medicine and at the end of the third week I discharged the case cured.

HEALTH AND HOMOEOPATHY
Vol No. 1 - No. 2 (1940)
Page No. 92

Warts: (Dr. Diwan Jai Chand).

In the year 1970, when I was in the initial stages of the study of homoeopathy (but not practising it) I encountered in my younger brother — a medical student — a case of warts. He had three warts on the outer ridge and back of the right ear. To test the efficacy of various caustics, I applied glacial acetic acid to one, pure nitric acid to the second and solid silver nitrate to the third. All these applications were made to the warts themselves and to the skin surrounding the roots of the warts. In a few days the warts dried up, leaving pigmented scars in their place. Imagine my horror when within the next few weeks I saw not only the right ear but also the right side of the face and neck (hairy part) studded with many warts. Shaving would result in bleeding points corresponding to the sites of cut warts on the face. The number of warts increased rapidly, making shaving impossible. In addition, he had obstinate constipation which would yield to liquid paraffin (in rather large doses) taken every night at bedtime. No other laxative could be depended upon with certainty of movement of the bowels. Having failed to cure him either of warts or of constipation, I sent him to a homoeopath who cured him of the latter (the bowels began moving daily and regularly, even when the homoeopathic medicine was withdrawn). But the warts remained unaffected. For this, I sent him to another homoeopath who gave him *Graphites* 200 and *Thuja occidentalis* 200, one dose alternately once a week. In four weeks' time, I had the pleasure of seeing every wart disappear, leaving the surface of the skin smooth and clean.

This case made a tremendous impression upon me, of the superior efficacy of homoeopathic treatment, particularly when not only I, but his professors in the King Edward Medical College as well, had failed to cure him of either constipation or warts. Besides, it made a convert of my brother to homoeopathy as after qualifying himself an M.B.B.S., he never practised allopathy for a single day but studied homoeopathy with me for over a year before he started practice of his own as homoeopath in Lyallpur (Punjab) where he earned name and fame as such.

INDIAN JOURNAL OF HOMOEOPATHIC MEDICINE
Vol. II - No. 1 (1977)
Page No. 26 - Case No. 4

Miss H.B. 21 years old.

The outside of the right hand covered with warts since her childhood. No treatment helped.

Very dry around the nails.

Intermittent pain in the right ear.

Shivering from time to time, in the middle of the day.

Palpitations.

She wanted some ointment for warts. After explaining to her that we absolutely don't treat warts with ointment, or unguents, I ordered to replace it, a drop of alcohol each evening on every wart, which she was to allow to evaporate.

In June 1925 she took *Nat-mur* XM.

In October the warts were flattened.

She became touchy, quickly irritable and lived in a dreadful disorder. She didn't like washing.

On October 9, I prescribed *Sulphur* XM. Two weeks after no trace of warts. General state considerably improved and she even started tidying up at home.

INDIAN JOURNAL OF HOMOEOPATHIC MEDICINE
Page No. 62 - Case No. 8

Warts - Calcarea Phos. 10 M

Miss S.S. aged 11 years had big warts on the fingers of both the hands for one year. There were five warts on right index finger and one on right middle finger. On the left hand there was a small wart on the index finger. She often complained of pain in legs and headache on returning from school for which she was given *Crocin* frequently. She was constipated. There was a history of worms since childhood, and eczema on left foot 6 months back. *Calc. phos.* 10M was given.

On 19-9-1975 two warts of right index finger had cleared up and the remaining warts had considerably reduced in size. Headache was less frequent. She was required to take another dose of *Calc. phos.* 10M.

On 19-10-1975 all the warts had disappeared. Her other complaints also improved.

HOMOEOPATHY AND COMPARATIVE MEDICINE
Page No. 59 - Case No. III (2)

A Case of Warts

Mr. Gopalkrishnan aged 48 years, had a number of warts on chin and neck. It was extremely difficult for him to shave for fear of cutting them and consequent pain and bleeding. The warts were soft and pulpy and very sensitive. He also complained of sleeplessness at night. He had been re-vaccinated twice last 2 years back. *Thuja* 200, one dose in three divided parts at intervals of 10 minutes was given. This was repeated after a month. After about six weeks the warts disappeared completely. No wart appeared after that and sound sleep returned.

INDIAN JOURNAL OF HOMOEOPATHIC MEDICINE
Vol. 9 - No. 2 (1975)
Page No. 59 - Case No. 1

Dr. 'A', male aged 30 with multiple pedunculated warts about 50 to 60 on neck and face, of over 2 years' duration; two previous electrocauterizations had failed, more warts coming after each cauterization. As there seemed to be no other symptoms, *Thuja* 1M, 3 doses in 24 hours were given. No response at all even after two weeks. So more information was sought. The patient gave the history that originally there was a small wart on left side of the face which was repeatedly nicked during shaving. Since then not only the original wart has grown but numerous others had arisen. On this basis *Staph.* 200 was given, 3 doses in one day. Apparently for four days there was no change, on the fifth morning the warts looked shrunken and black and many just dropped off on rubbing the face with a towel. 48 hours later all the warts had dropped off. One more dose of *Staph.* was given three weeks later.

For four years there has been no recurrence.

A NEW REMEDY FOR WARTS
Dr. S.R. Wadia, M.B.B.S. (Bombay),
F.F. HOM.(London), D.H.T.(USA).

Name : J.C.P.
Age : 40 years.

(1) This patient was shown to me by a Homoeopathic doctor who had given him all the possible remedies. He was having about 30-35 warts, black in colour, some large and small,

soft in consistency, on the left side of his face and neck. Also stray warts here and there all over the body. This is for the last six months.

(2) There is a past history of scabies, boils, blisters, feet, fungus infection toes, occasional vaccinations and innoculations. Being a high executive, he was treated in the United States but to no avail.

(3) Family history — Father died early, cause not known; mother normal.

(4) Stool, urine, appetite, thirst — normal.

(5) Hot patient — perspiration profuse and foul smell.

(6) Obese patient — Weight 82 kilograms.

No other symptoms were available but he told me that he has used a lot of *Cortisone* preparations orally as well as for external use for his skin condition. As such, on :

26-6-1977 — *Cortisone* 200, 3 doses.

17-7-1977 — When I saw him next, there was no change. Constitutionally, he looked like a *Calc carb* patient. As such I thought of trying a new remedy which was not given so far and that was *Cal calcinata* 30 in repeated doses. The Homoeopathic physician who was looking after him told me that 50 per cent of the warts disappeared or became smaller in about fifteen days. When I saw him again, only three doses of the same remedy in 200 potency were given.

17-9-1977 — All warts all over the body have completely disappeared. All those who were working with him, were really surprised with this magic cure. I have tried this remedy in some other cases also with a good deal of success.

HOMOEOPATHY AND COMPARATIVE MEDICINE
September 1957
Page No. 153 - Case No. 1 (i)

A Case of Multiple Warts
(Dr. S.R. Wadia)

Patient's Name : Master Keotj
Age : 12 years.

This boy was brought to me by his mother somewhere on November 1, 1950. The boy had about 20 or 25 warts mainly on his hands, sides of the fingers and legs. Most of the warts were fairly large, hard and jagged and two or three were soft. The duration was about six months. Being Anglo-Indian and believer in the Modern Science, the mother consulted the Government Doctor. He naturally being ignorant of any other better treatment applied *Silver Nitrate* over all the warts. The result was that the poor fellow's skin was burnt, but the warts remained as they were. I asked the mother to wash them nicely with soap and warm water. Apply nothing externally and watch the wonderful effects of homoeopathic treatment. On taking a careful history I could not elicit any definite symptoms except that the boy while in a boarding school at Deolali was innoculated every year against small-pox, also sometimes against Typhoid, Cholera and lastly he had taken B.C.G. innoculation. I had seen several such cases in my practice suffering from the ill-effects of vaccination, and I presumed that these warts were due to the same.

A dose of *Thuja* 1000 was given in the dispensary and the boy was kept under observation. There was no improvement for about one fortnight. One evening he came alone and told me that while playing and whenever he injured his legs the warts began to bleed and asked me to stop bleeding. I dressed him. This gave me a clue. This boy was put on *Causticum* 30, twice a day. Within eight days he told me that he found the warts had disappeared like magic effect of the minimum dose and told the Government Doctor about the result. But alas, he refused to believe that so many warts could disappear so soon with oral medicine and without any external application. This is the modern trend of thought.

THE HOMOEOPATHIC HERITAGE, MAY 1983
Page No. 229 - Case No. 982

One day in the children's clinic, a child came with warts large and flat — on the tongue, besides warts inside the cheeks and elsewhere. The child had been given *Thuja* 30 without effect. Then whooping cough and other treatment had intervened; but always the warts persisted. They had been previously operated on in an adjacent hospital — cauterized and cut away but had recurred.

Dr. Nash got out his pocket case and put a few tiniest globules of *Thuja* CM on the child's tongue. A month later, all the warts had disappeared except a very small excrescence, which a dose of *Thuja* 10M (the highest potency then procurable) finally caused to disappear.

HOMOEOPATHY
Vol. XI - No. 3
Page No. 37

Warts : Nothing very terrible, one may think : nor are they, as a rule; but when a patient comes with a big wart on lower lid, interfering with vision; or a big wart on cheek just below the eye, or crops of unsightly warts, perhaps painful; perhaps bleeding easily — well the victim is very thankful to find them vanish or drop off after 'The Remedy' : and one is glad to have been able to discover it, and so help.

Burnett gives a case of middle-aged man, who complained of long-standing indigestion, epigastric pain and distress. He also complained of a most uncomfortable state of his anal region which was found to have a number of small warts arranged almost in a ring around the orifice. An old gonorrhoea of many years ago, also several vaccinations led to the prescription of *Thuja* 30, in infrequent doses, which quite cured the dyspepsia and also the anus; for when again examined, the warts had quite disappeared. 'I feel all right there now.'

N.B. Without the knowledge, and the appreciation of the significance of the lurking latent disease, behind the evident symptoms, this case might have gone uncured. *Very interesting.*

Medicine is not dull : but is a matter of recurrent intense interest, where the treatment is not by disease name; but of individual investigation of cause.

Thuja : Warts on any part of the body, with little necks called fig warts; tubular warts; i.e., long warts of the same size all the way out.
Wart-like excrescences on back of hand, on chin and other places.
Warts and condylomata, large, seedy and pedunculated; sometimes oozing and bleeding readily. Effects of vaccination.
Dreams of the dead : of falling.

Nitric acid : Warts : sticking and pricking : on upper lip. Smart and bleed on washing; painful to touch. Soft with thin epidermis and moist: large, jagged, often pedunculated, exuding moisture and bleeding readily : condylomata, etc.
Splinter-sensations anywhere.
Worse : touch, jar, cold at night.

Dulcamara : In black type we find : warts, fleshy or large, smooth on dorsum of hands and on face. *Dulc.* is one of our very great skin medicines. Typical *Dulc.* is worse from exposure to damp cold weather or air — a cellar or dairy. A few years ago, *Dulc.* cured for a patient a big wart on right lower lid, not easy to see over. Big warts on face can be very trying, yet, with 'the remedy', they just drop off. *Dulcamara* in one's mind, stands especially for warts and for umbilical pain or eruptions.

Causticum : Large, jagged, often pedunculated warts exuding moisture and bleeding easily.

Small, non-pedunculated warts all over the body internal and external, and on eyelids.
In *Caust.*, injuries which had healed become sore again.
Years ago there was an epidemic of warts on calves at a little farm — cured by *Causticum.*
Caust. is worse cold, dry weather : rev. *Dulc.*, *Thu.*, in clear, fine weather. Better damp and wet weather.

Castor Equi : We are told by the owner of a herd of some sixty cows that *Castor equi* promptly cures warts on the udders of cows; a troublesome condition leading to painful cracks, which make milking difficult.

Calcarea : Warts : round, soft at base, almost the colour of skin; upper surface hard, rough, whitish, horny.
Wart appears, itches, bleeds and disappears.
Warts : inflamed; stinging; suppurating; form ulcers.
Warts thickly studding mouths of sheep.
Calc. suits phlegmatic people; large head and features; pale skin and chalky look.
Better dry weather, from being touched (*Phos.*)
Worse milk : from suppressed perspiration.

Sepia : Warts on hands, neck, face with horny excrescences in centre : small, itching, flat.
Large, hard seed warts; dark colour; painless.
Sepia is indifferent : with emptiness, with nothing satisfied. Bursting pains or cramping and drawing. Internal pulsations.
A left-sided medicine, generally.
Worse from music : milk; fat pork; perspiration, snow; washing; getting wet.
Better : motion; walking quickly; when alone.

Sulphur : Callous warts; especially around the fingers.
Itching eruptions, or itching skin; 'feels so good to scratch.'

Fantastic illusions : everything seems beautiful : as an old rag or stick.
Redness about anus — red eyelids.
Perspiration of single parts : of back part of body. Flushes of heat. Heaviness, abdomen; as if it needs to be bandaged or supported.
Sulph. sometimes feels small, sometimes large.

Rhus Tox : Warts : especially on hands and fingers; large jagged, often pedunculated, exuding moisture and bleeding readily.
Rhus has irresistible desire to move, or change position, with great relief for a short time.
External coldness of skin : but doesn't mind cold air. Chilly; coldness of single parts; of one side only.
Worse getting wet while perspiring.
Worse from getting wet - even years ago.
Better hot things: in clear, dry weather.

Antimonium Crud : Horny excrescences. Smooth warts, often soft.
Ulcers breaking out around a wart.
Tendency to grow fat.
Worse warm weather — heat of sun.
Children can't bear to be touched or looked at.
Feels as if he had eaten too much.
Heartburn with good appetite.
Characteristic — while coated tongue.

WARTS

Acet-ac, Alum, Ambr, Am-c, Anac, Anag, Anan, Ant-c, Ant-t, Arg-nit, Ars, Aur, Aur-m, Aur-m-n, Bar-c, Bell, Benz-ac, Berb, Bor, Bov, Bufo, Calc, Calc-s, Carb-an, Carb-v, Cast-eq, Caust, Chel, Chrom-ac, Cinn-b, Colch, Cub, Cund, Cupr, Dulc, Euphor, Euphr, Ferr, Ferr-p, Ferr-pic, Fl-ac, Graph, Hep, Kali-ar, Kali-br, Kali-c, Kali-chl, Kali-m, Lac-c, Lach, Lyc, Mag-s, Med, Merc-c, Merc-iod-fl, Merc-iod-rub, Mill, Nat-c, Nat-m, Nat-p, Nat-s, Nit-ac, Ox-ac, Petr, Ph-ac, Phos, Pic-ac, Phyt, Psor, Ran-b, Rhus-t, Ruta, Sabin, Sars, Sang, Semperv-t, Sep, Sil, Spig, Staph, Sulph, Sul-ac, Thuj, X-ray.

Black — *Calc-c, Hecla.*

Bleeding — *Abmr, Caust, Cinnb, Hep, Lyc, Nat-c, Nit-ac, Ph-ac, Phos, Rhus, Staph, Thuj.*

Bleed easily : jagged large — *Cast, Nit-ac.*

Broad — *Caust, Dulc.*

Broad, dry, moist — *Acet-ac*

Brown — *Sep, Thuj.*

Burning — *Am-c, Ars, Hep, Lyc, Peptr, Phos, Rhus-t, Sabin, Sep, Sulph.*

On Canthi — *Calc, Nit-ac.*

Cauliflower-like on outer side of terminal phalynx of right thumb — *Ran-b*

Cold washing agg — *Dulc*

Conical — *Ant-t, Nat-m.*

Discharge pus then heals — *Calc*

Drawing in — *Con*

Fan-shaped on genitals — *Thuj*

Fissured — *Thuj*

Flat — *Acet-ac, Berb, Calc-c, Caust, Dulc, Fl-ac, Lach, Merc-i-r, Nat-m, Ruta, Sep, Thuj.*

Fleshy — *Calc, Caust, Dulc, Sil, Staph, Thuj.*

Granular — *Arg-n, Calc, Nit-ac, Staph, Thuj.*

Hard — *Ant-c, Calc, Caust, Dulc, Fl-ac, Lach, Ran-b, Sep, Sil, Sulph, Thuj.*

Horny : broad — *Rhus-t*

Indented — *Calc, Euphr, Lyc, Nit-ac, Phos-ac, Rhus-t, Sabin, Sep, Staph, Thuj.*

Inflamed — *Am-c, Bell, Bov, Calc, Caust, Hep, Lyc, Nat-c, Nit-ac, Rhus-t, Sars, Sep, Sil, Staph, Sulph, Thuj.*

Internal — *Caust*

Isolated — *Lyc, Thuj.*

Itching — *Carb-an, Euphr, Kali-c, Nit-ac, Phos, Psor, Sabin, Sep, Thuj.*

Jagged — *Caust, Lyc, Nit-ac, Ph-ac, Rhus-t, Sep, Staph, Thuj.*

Large — *Caust, Dulc, Kali-c, Nat-c, Nit-ac, Ph-ac, Rhus-t, Sep, Sil, Thuj.*

Large : Soft — *Mag-s, Dulc.*

Large, fleshy, suppurating — *Sil*

Large, hard, dark colour — *Sep*

Large, jagged — *Caust*

Large, jagged, often pedunculated, exuding moisture and bleeds easily — *Lyc*

Large seedy — *Thuj*

Ludpiod — *Ferr, Pixr.*

Mercury after abuse of — *Aur, Nit-ac, Staph.*

Moist — *Caust, Lyc, Nit-ac, Ph-ac, Psor, Rhus-t, Staph, Thuj.*

Old — *Calc, Caust, Kali-c, Nit-ac, Rhod, Rhus-t, Sulph, Thuj.*

Painful — *Am-c, Bov, Calc, Caust, Hep, Kali-c, Kali-s, Lach, Lyc, Nat-c, Nat-m, Nit-ac, Petr, Phos, Rhus-t, Ruta, Sabin, Sep, Sil, Sulph, Thuj.*

Sore pains — *Ruta*

Pedunculated — *Caust, Dulc, Lyc, Med, Nat-s, Nit-ac, Ph-ac, Rhus-t, Sabin, Sil, Staph, Thuj.*

Pricking — *Nit-ac*

Pulsating — *Calc, Kali-c, Lyc, Petr, Sep, Sil, Sulph.*

Ragged — *Nat-c, Ph-ac, Rhus-t, Thuj.*

Red — *Calc, Nat-s, Thuj.*

Round — *Calc*

Rough : seed warts — *Caust*

Salt : having used too much — *Nitr. Sp-d.*

Scrofulous — *Aur-met*

Seedy — *Thuj*

Sensitive to touch — *Caust, Cupr, Hep, Nat-c, Nat-m, Staph, Thuj.*

Shooting — *Bov*

Small — *Bar-c, Berb, Calc, Caust, Dulc, Ferr, Ferr-p, Hep, Lach, Nit-ac, Rhus-t, Sars, Sep, Sulph, Thuj.*

Small all over body — *Caust*

Small : many — *Calc, Sars.*

Small : pedunculated all over body — *Caust*

Smelling like old cheese or herring brine — *Calc, Graph, Hep, Thuj.*

Smooth — *Ant-c, Calc, Dulc, Lach, Nat-m, Nat-s, Nit-ac, Psor, Ruta, Thuj.*

Soft — *Am-c, Ant-c, Calc, Calen, Nat-s, Nit-ac, Sil, Thuj.*

Sore — *Nit-ac*

Spongy — *Calc, Lyc, Nit-ac, Staph, Thuj.*

Stinging — *Am-c, Ant-c, Bar-c, Calc, Caust, Hep, Lyc, Nit-ac, Rhus-t, Sep, Sil, Staph, Sulph, Thuj.*

Stitching in — *Bov, Hep, Nit-ac.*

Suppurating — *Ars, Bov, Calc, Caust, Hep, Nat-c, Sil, Thuj.*

Suppressed — *Meny, Nit-ac, Staph, Thuj.*

Sycotic — *Alum, Mill, Nat-s.*

Syphilitic — *Aur, Aur-m, Aur-m-n, Hep, Merc, Nit-ac, Staph, Thuj.*

Tearing — *Am-c*

Thick — *Dulc*

Thin epidermis with — *Nit-ac*

Throbbing — *Calc-c, Kali-c, Lyc, Petr, Sep, Sil, Sulph.*

Ulcers surrounded by a circle of — *Ant-c, Ars, Calc, Caust, Hell, Nat-c, Phos.*

Every four weeks — *Calc*

Withered — *Ars, Calc, Camph, Cap, Cham, Chin, Clem, Cocc, Croc, Ferr, Ferr-ar, Ferr-p, Hyos, Iod, Kali-c, Lyc, Merc, Ph-ac, Phos, Rheum, Rhod, Sars, Sec, Seneg, Sil, Spong, Sulph, Verat.*

Location : On forehead — *Castorea*

On general body — *Nat-s, Sep.*

On eyebrows — *Anan, Caust, Nit-ac, Thuj.*

On eyelids — *Caust, Cinnb, Nit-ac, Sulph, Thuj.*

Right lower — *Nit-ac*

Iris — *Cinnb, Merc, Staph, Thuj.*

Eyes around — *Arund, Calc, Cinnb, Merc, Nit-ac, Phos, Staph, Thuj.*

Wart-like growth behind ear, inflamed and ulcerated — *Calc.*

On the ears — *Bufo*

On nose — *Caust, Nit-ac, Thuj.*

Inside nose — *Nit-ac*

On face — *Calc, Caust, Dulc, Kali-c, Lyc, Nit-ac, Sep, Sulph, Thuj.*

Chin — *Lyc, Thuj*

Lips — *Caust, Kali-s, Nit-ac, Thuj.*

Mouth around — *Cund, Psor.*

Mouth — *Ph-ac*

Palate — *Arg-n*

Tongue — *Aur, Aur-m, Aur-m-n, Lyc, Mang, Staph.*

Neck — *Nit-ac*

Throat — *Arg-n, Merc-c, Nit-ac, Thuj.*

Ext-throat — *Nit-ac, Sil, Thuj.*

Rectum — *Arg-n, Aur, Aur-m, Benz-ac, Caust, Cinn-b, Euphr, Jac-c, Lyc, Merc, Merc-d, Mill, Nat-s, Nit-ac, Petr, Phos, Sabin, Sep, Staph, Sulph, Thuj.*

Copious bleeding — *Mill*

Sensitive — *Staph*

Flat — *Euphr, Sulph, Thuj.*

Sore — *Benz-ac, Thuj*

Prepuce — *Cinn-ab, Ph-ac, Sab.*

Female : genitalia — *Crot-h, Cub, Graph, Kreos, Lac-c, Merc, Nit-ac, Sec, Tarent, Thuj.*

Uterus — *Cub, Kreos, Merc, Nit-ac, Sec, Tarent, Thuj.*

Bleeding — *Merc, Thuj.*

Cauliflower — *Crot-h, Graph, Kali-ac, Kreos, Lac-c, Phos, Thuj.*

Wart : Shaped — *Thuj*

On breast — *Castor-eq*

On sternum — *Nit-ac*

Back — *Nit-ac, Sil, Thuj.*

Cervical region — *Nit-ac, Thuj.*

Back of hand — *Thuj*

Fingers — *Thuj*

Upper limb — *Ars, Bov, Calc, Carb-an, Caust, Dulc, Kali-c, Lyc, Merc, Nat-c, Nat-m, Nat-s, Nit-ac, Petr, Phos, Rhus-t, Sep, Sil, Sulph, Thuj.*

Elbow bend on — *Calc-f*

Arm — *Calc-c, Nit-ac.*

Forearm — *Sil*

Black — *Calc-c, Hecla.*

Wrist — *Ferr-ma.*

Hand — *Anac, Ant-c, Bar-c, Berb, Bov, Bufo, Calc, Caust, Dulc, Ferr, Ferr-ma, Ferr-pic, Fl-ac, Kali-c, Kali-chl, Kali-m, Lach, Lyc, Nat-c, Nat-m, Nit-ac, Ph-ac, Phos, Psor, Ruta, Rhus-t, Sep, Sil, Sulph, Thuj.*

- **Flat** — *Berb, Dulc, Lach, Ruta, Sep.*
- **Horny** — *Ant-c, Caust, Sep, Thuj.*

Hand itching — *Sep*

- **Large** — *Dulc*
- **Sensitive** — *Nat-c*

- **Sore** — *Ambr, Fl-ac, Ruta.*

Knuckles — *Pall*

Palm — *Anac, Berb, Dulc, Nat-c, Nat-m, Ruta.*

Flat — *Dulc, Nat-m, Ruta.*

Painful on pressure — *Nat-m*

Fingers — *Ambr, Bar, Berb, Calc, Carb-an, Caust, Dulc, Ferr, Fl-ac, Lac-c, Lach, Lyc, Nat-m, Nit-ac, Petr, Psor, Ran-b, Rhus-t, Sang, Sars, Sep, Sulph, Thuj.*

Joints — *Sars*

Tips — *Caust, Dulc, Thuj.*

First — *Caust, Thuj.*

Horny — *Caust*

Second — *Berb, Lachy.*

Third — *Nat-s*

Nails close to — *Caust, Dulc, Fl-ac.*

Thumb — *Berb, Lach, Ran-b, Thuj.*

Nates — *Con*

Thigh — *Med*

Toes — *Spig*

On face, hands — *Calc, Caust, Carb-an, Dulc, Kali-c.*

On neck, arms, hands, soft, smooth — *Ant-c*

On nose, fingers tips eyebrows — *Caust*

Condylomata, Fig warts — *Calc, Cinnb, Euphr, Kali-iod, Lyc, Med, Merc-c, Merc-s, Nat-s, Nit-ac, Phos-ac, Sab, Sep, Sil, Staph, Thuja.*

URTICARIAL ERUPTIONS

1. Urticaria.
2. Papular urticaria.
3. Urticaria pigmentosa.
4. Angioneurotic oedema.

Urticaria

Synonyms : Hindustani: Chhapaki, Dhapar.

Layman's popular name : "Nettle rash".

It is a common, annoying reaction pattern affecting almost 15% of the population at one time or the other during their lifetime.

No age is exempt, but its incidence is highest at puberty and middle age.

Clinical features : There are two varieties of urticaria, Localized and Generalized, depending upon the distribution of the eruption. The nature of the lesions is identical in both varieties. Localized urticaria is confined to a small part of the body usually a limb and is caused by bites or stings of nettles, caterpillars, weaver fish, jelly fish, whip lash, on site injection or contact with stinging plants known as 'nettles' — Urticaceae family (Bichhu buti). In comparison generalized urticaria is widespread all over the body trunk and extremities asymmetrically. Eyes, lips or hands may be swollen.

The onset is usually sudden and abrupt. The lesions resemble those produced by the sting of nettles. They start as rosy-red, erythematous macules, on which flesh or lighter colour oedematous weals soon develop. The erythema is ill-defined, and fades on pressure. The lesions are usually irregular and asymmetrical. The rash is accompanied by severe, annoying itching, burning and sense of heat. The individual lesions subside within a few hours; at the latest in a day or two. An attack of urticaria can be brought on by exposure to cold winds, baths, or by exposure to heat; also by hot, spicy food and psychogenic stress. The dermographism is usually positive, e.g., scratching the skin produces triple response.

Dermographism can occur as such without being accompanied by the spontaneous weals and irritation of true urticaria (Fictitious Urticaria).

Pathology : Main features are capillary dilatation and accumulation to produce pallor, but at the edge of lesion, capillary dilatation can always be detected. Activation of mast cells and basophils by immunoglobulins Ig E and Ig C and complements and other stimulants results in release of mediators like histamine, serotonin and bradykinin which act on H_1 and H_2 receptors in the skin and its blood vessels.

Etiology : In the author's experience, besides genetic predisposition, there is increased sense of heat, which is increased considerably at the time of attack. This is more often seen in physical urticarias and allergies to food and drugs.

Drugs	:	*Penicillin* (also penicillin in dairy products). *Aspirin* and other salicylates. There is cross sensitization with tartrazine and benzoic acid in aerated drinks and preserved foods. And to Indomethecin.
Food	:	Nuts, shell fish, oysters, prawns, eggs, milk and its products. Strawberries, Zaminkand, Mushrooms. Food additives — preservatives, dyes, flavouring agents — Tartrazine, benzoic acid, azodyes, salicylates, yeast, saccharin.
Plants	:	The 'nettles' — Urticaeceae family — Bicchu buti.
Insect bites	:	Nettles, wasps, jelly fish, weaver fish, caterpillars, trombicula irritants.
Internal disorders	:	Rheumatic fever, SLE reticuloses, hypogammaglobulinemia.
Genetic	:	Hereditary angiodema, familial cold urticaria.
Focal sepsis	:	Teeth, nose, throat, ears, sinuses, lungs, liver, intestines, kidney, bladder, vagina, etc.
Parasites	:	Round worms, tape worms, hookworms, thread worms, hydatid cyst, filariasis.
Psychogenic	:	Resentful frustration, emotional stresses, overwork, etc.
Physical factors	:	Pressure, vibration, heat, cold, sun, exertion.

Acute urticarias are usually due to drugs and foods. They last from a few days to a few weeks and then disappear.

Urticaria which is prolonged over 6 weeks is termed chronic urticaria. These pose a problem and cause considerable strain on the expertise of physician for detection of the cause. With patience, one can detect causative factors like focal sepsis, parasites, psychogenic stresses and physical factors. People consuming large quantities of hot spicy food, tea, coffee, alcohol and non-vegetarian food are more prone to urticarias. Food additives and aspirin are the two common culprits.

Cold urticaria may be familial or acquired; the former may be accompanied by fever, joint pains, and presence of cryoglobulins. Swimming or a cold bath may bring on a severe attack, hypotension and collapse. Ice cube test may be positive.

Heat, exertion and emotional stress cause cholinergic urticaria. These are more common in the Indian winter. Cycling or walking fast or standing in the sun starts a pricking sensation in the skin and an uncomfortable feeling in the body followed by urticaria. These patients complain of a sense of heat with warm clothes and bed covers. They are very uncomfortable and restless in the sun. Weals are small. Mecholyl and nicotine injection produce an attack.

Solar urticaria is confined to exposed parts and is seen on exposure to sun.

Diagnosis : In the handling of urticarias, great emphasis should be laid on history taking and physical examination. Patient's personality, food and drug habits should be thoroughly studied and a search for foci of infection made. Examination of stool for ova and cysts would help in discovering parasitic infestation, urine for kidney infection, ESR for infection, and internal diseases, diet diary and single factor elimination diet for food allergies. In intractable cases standard battery intradermal testing may provide a lead to the cause. This can be supplemented by provocative administration of aspirin, tartrazine, benzoic acid and sun set yellow added one by one with 2-3 days interval in between.

Immunology can be studied by investigative tools like cryoglobulins, ANA, skin tests, etc.

Differential diagnosis is from granuloma (there is infiltration, absence of itching and lesions persist while the urticarial lesions are non-infiltrated and transient typical weals accompanied by marked itching and dermographism).

Prognosis : Acute urticarias have a good outlook; those due to food clear up quickly within a few days, and those due to drugs like penicillin, clear up within a few weeks. This prognosis is good when the specific cause has been established and eliminated. Chronic urticarias, without a traceable cause have a bad prognosis, because in such cases treatment can only be symptomatic. In severe acute urticarias, without a traceable cause have a bad prognosis, because in such cases treatment can only be symptomatic. In severe acute urticarias with swelling of the face, there is always danger of laryngeal obstruction.

Papular Urticaria

It affects infants and children between the age of three months and six years. It is usually seen during the summer months. It is a common condition in tropical countries.

Clinically, the lesions are erythematous macules or whitish weals, surmounted by a central papule or sometimes papulo-vesicle. The weal usually disappears in an hour or two, but the papulo-vesicle may last a few days. Lesions are accompanied by itching and scratch marks. The trunk is the site of choice. The course is chronic with seasonal variations.

According to some authorities, papular urticaria is due to infestation with animal parasite, Trombicula irritans. Lesions are arranged in lines, and may show puncture in the early stages. If an animal parasite is the cause, *crotorax (P)* will cure the condition.

Papular urticaria may also be caused by : sensitivity to food or its digestive products, certain metabolites or focal sepsis. The treatment is on the same lines as for urticaria.

Synonym : Quncke's disease.

It is an acute giant variety of urticaria, characterized by the sudden development of circumscribed swellings of the skin and subcutaneous tissue, the mucous membrane and sub-mucous tissue. The swellings are reddish or skin-coloured; the local temperature is not raised. The consistency is firm. The swellings are single or multiple, usually arranged asymmetrically. The common sites involved are : the eyelids, the tongue, the lips, the glottis, the hands, the trunk, the feet and the genitalia. Angioneurotic oedema of the glottis is a serious condition because it interferes with the respiration and if not controlled in time can prove fatal.

Swelling appears suddenly, and lasts from a few hours to a few days, leaving neither atrophy, scars or stains when they subside. The swellings recur from time to time or in quick succession.

Angioneurotic oedema may be accompanied by urticarial lesions. There are no constitutional symptoms except for local tension, heat, pain, moderate itching and tenderness. If the gastro-intestinal tract is involved, there may be a concomitant attack of colic. Involvement of the glottis, however, produces difficulty in breathing, hoarseness and even death.

Etiology : Young adults are most frequently affected, females more often than males. Heredity is an important predisposing factor. The exciting causes are : psychogenic stresses and allergic offenders, similar to urticaria.

Diagnosis : It is based upon the acute, transient and recurrent nature of these tense, circumscribed swellings. The other local causes of oedema, like insect bites, cellulitis, erysipelas, venous thrombosis, also gravitational oedema, and the kind produced by lymphatic obstruction as in filariasis, should first be excluded.

Prognosis : It is favourable in the acute, cutaneous varieties. Death can occur when the glottis is involved. Recurrent cases are rather resistant to treatment.

Treatment : It is almost on the same lines as in urticaria. The patient must be reassured. The cause must be established, and an attempt made to remove it. Psychogenic cases with chronic emotional problems should be referred to a psychiatrist and/or social worker for help.

Acute cases : Treat with antihistaminics, adrenaline or corticosteroids. If the glottis is involved, and there is difficulty in breathing, a tracheostomy should be done as an emergency measure.

Chronic cases.: Treat with antihistaminics, a simple diet, non-specific stimulants, sedatives and a holiday.

URTICARIA

Urticaria is one of the most common annoying reaction pattern affecting patients of every population sometime during their life-time.

Homoeopathy has maximum scope in the above condition, as modern medicine has nothing more to offer other than anti-histaminics.

Homoeopathic Approach

The following pattern should be observed most meticulously whilst treating the patient :

(i) Confirm whether the lesion fits into urticarial rash. The typical lesion should include a rosy, red erythematous macule with oedematous weals. The erythema fades on pressure.

(ii) The time of aggravation should be carefully enquired. I have found night aggravation more common than during daytime.

(iii) Does urticaria alternate with any other complaint especially asthma or rheumatism?

(iv) Always ask whether urticaria is preceded by any other symptoms, e.g., nausea, chill, menses.

(v) Enquire in which season the patient develops urticaria and at what temperature, e.g., in a hot room, cold room, open air, near the sea shore, etc.

(vi) The most important factor which helps us to eliminate majority of the drugs is the patient's feeling of well being after an application of heat or cold.

(vii) Try and find out which particular foodstuff aggravates the condition, especially shellfish, meat, sweets, chocolates, etc.

(viii) Has the patient got any emotional stress? I have seen many patients of urticaria who have any history of worm infestation. Therefore one should enquire for any history of worms. Also history of insect bites, or contact with any plants or ingestion of any drugs, especially penicillin or salicylates.

(ix) Sometimes physical factors, especially exposure to sun excessive physical exertion and exercise leads to urticaria.

All the above points should be thoroughly scrutinised to get the maximum data from the patient.

I may caution my colleagues here that in very rare cases during an attack of urticaria, patient may develop swelling of the face with laryngeal obstruction. At that time the patient should be shifted to a homoeopathic hospital and his airway should be kept clear with endotracheal intubation and oral drugs like chlorum,etc., should be administered.

The treatment consists of not only giving the indicated homoeopathic drugs, but to eliminate the offending agent, e.g., eliminative diet, withdrawal of causative drug, treatment of the parasitic infestation, correction of the existing physical stress.

During an acute attack, the patient should be kept on a bland diet. Alcohol, tea and coffee are preferably avoided.

Finally, reassurance should be given to the patient who have chronic urticaria.

Drugs — Acute urticaria :

Anthrakokali : The urticaria of *Anthrakokali* increases with general sweat. There is intense itching which is worse at night. The site or urticaria is hands, tibia, shoulders and dorsum of feet. Eruptions always decrease with the full moon.

Concomitant symptoms with urticaria are dropsy and intense thirst.

Antim Crud : The skin of *Antim crud* is dirty, and unhealthy. Urticaria, white lump with red areola which itch. The itching is not continuous, but seems to come and go. There is a marked aggravation after the ingestion of meat and when in bed. The itching makes the patient irritable, hot and thirsty.

Urticaria associated with gastric disorders which is characterised by a thick white coated tongue.

Antipyrine : *Antipyrine* causes an urticaria found chiefly between the fingers. There is troublesome itching. The urticaria appears and disappears quite suddenly and is often accompanied by internal coldness.

Apis Mellifica : The characteristic of urticaria is the stinging and itching as if from bee stings. The itching is always worse at night. The urticaria may consist of isolated elevations which are quite painful and tender to touch; these later become purple or livid. There is slight fever and heat of skin, accompanying urticaria. There is burning pain.

Generalized anasarca as a strong concomitant to the urticaria. Change of weather, warmth, and exercise cause troublesome itching and burning urticaria. The urticaria is worse during both chill as well as fever. The urticaria sometimes accompanies asthmatic troubles.

Arsenicum Album : *Arsenic* causes urticaria with burning and restlessness. It is also useful for persistence of complaints during recession of the urticaria.

The urticaria may occur after eating shellfish. Urticaria gets worse at the sea-shore and due to sea bathing.

Astacus Fluviatilis : It is a short acting remedy having a special affinity for skin, producing urticaria all over the body with violent pruritus. The important concomitant which is the characteristic symptom is liver affection with urticaria. The urticarial rash is so violent that patient may go into a mild miliaria.

Bombyx : The characteristic urticaria of *Bombyx* shows hard, large tubercles with a red areola. The tubercles are most marked near the joints. There is a sensation of a foreign body under the skin, with itching of the whole body. The itching gets worse in the evening but is not relieved in any way. There is a burning heat everywhere.

Bovista : The urticaria of *Bovista* covers nearly the whole body.

There is burning, itching of a type which is not relieved by scratching, and comes on more at night.

Urticaria which is caused by tar: The itching is worse on getting warm.

Urticaria with a disposition to diarrhoea. Each stool is followed by tenesmus. The other concomitant symptoms of urticaria are scorbutic gums, inflammation of the eyes, metrorrhagia and various mental symptoms.

Chloral Hydrate : The urticaria of *Chloral hydrate* is characterised by its periodicity. It disappears by day, and comes on by night, with such intense itching as to prevent sleep.

Urticaria from drinking wine and hot drinks :

There are red blotches on the skin. There is violent stinging itching all over the body.

Copaiva : Urticaria over the whole body with a red face. The skin is dry and hot. There is violent itching. Chronic urticaria in children.

Urticaria from gastric irritation with fever and intolerable itching. The itching is worse at night and during the fever.

Dulcamara : Hives come on at night, especially when the nights are cool, with heavy dew, after a hot day or when weather changes from warm to cool and damp; urticaria with violent cough and oedema of glands; feverish urticaria, obliging one to scratch and burning after scratching, every eruption being preceded by sensation of pricking over whole body; eruption of white, irregular blotches raised upon the skin, surrounded with red areola, appearing in warmth, and disappearing in cold and extremities, face, chest and back, violently itching and burning after scratching, headache, want of appetite; nausea, bitter taste, vomiting, intense aching in pit of stomach and praecordial region, restlessness and sleeplessness, night-sweats turbid, dark urine, diarrhoea, pains in limbs. Urticaria from gastric disorders.

Ichthyolum : Urticaria associated with severe itching sensation. Urticaria which is chronic in a patient who is of uric acid or tuberculous diathesis. Urticaria in alcoholics. Urticaria especially in old people. Most important concomitant is intense appetite.

Medusa : There is burning, pricking, itching sensation associated with urticaria. Urticaria especially on face, arms, shoulders and breaths. Concomitant is oedema of eyes, nose, ears and lips.

Pulsatilla Nitricans : Hives of gastric or uterine origin. Urticaria from pastries or pork or delayed menses. Urticaria with diarrhoea, itching is worse at night. Patient is chilly all the time, even in a warm room.

Rhus-tox : Vesicular urticaria from getting wet, during rheumatism, with chills and fever, worse in cold air. Patient has itching all over; worse on hairy parts with burning after scratching.

Strophanthus : It is usually indicated in chronic urticaria, especially when associated with cardiopulmonary disorders. Urticaria of chronic tobacco smokers.

Triosteum Perfoliatum : It has urticaria with gastric derangement, especially biliousness.

Urtica Urens : Itching and burning of the skin as if scorched; raised red blotches; fine stinging points; Pale rash requiring constant rubbing; consequences of suppressed urticaria; Eruption and itching disappear as soon as she lies down and reappear immediately after rising. There is oedema of the face, chest and limbs without inflammation. Urticaria affects patient every year in the same season. Site of urticaria is face, arms, shoulders, scalp. Vomitting and diarrhoea from suppression of urticaria.

Ustilago Maydis : Urticaria with terrible itching at night. The site of affection is body, arms and legs. The skin is dry and hot. Large pale eruptions. A strong concomitant is menstrual irregularity from ovarian irritation.

Vespa Crabro : Urticaria with intense burning stinging and soreness. Patient feels better by bathing with vinegar. An important concomitant symptom is perspiration on parts laid on with itching.

Chronic Urticaria

Anacardium : Urticaria with itching, burning and swelling, ending in desquamation; intense redness of skin, with eruption of little blisters and unbearable itching which is worse in the evening and when in bed.

Calc-carb : Chronic urticaria which always disappears in the fresh air. There are elevated red strips on the tibia which itch and burn severely on being rubbed. Urticaria with unhealthy skin; every little injury tends to suppurate. Urticaria in patients with scrofulous diathesis. Suppression of urticaria and other eruptions leads to other physical troubles like epilepsy, asthma and nervous palpitation.

Conium : Urticaria from violent bodily exercise. There is erratic itching of all parts of the body, as from fleas. Itching is worse from scratching. Urticaria of old people and in person with scrofulous diathesis.

Kali carb : The skin of *Kali carb* patient is extremely sensitive and dry. The attacks of urticaria come, especially during menses. There is a sensation of burning as if plaster of mustard is applied on affected part. Urticaria in patients of tubercular and scrofulous diathesis. Ill effects of suppressed urticaria and other skin eruptions.

Lycopodium : *Lycopodium* has an unhealthy skin which is dry, hot skin which burns and itches when warm. It is more suited to the chronic type of urticaria, which are characterised by severe itching and burning, worse by warm application and worse by exercise. Urticaria in patients with liver, gastric and renal disorders. Urticaria in patients with scrofulous and uric acid diathesis.

Nat. Mur : The skin of *Nat-mur* is characteristically dirty, unhealthy and greasy, with a yellowish colour. There is great rawness and soreness of the skin, beginning at the feet and gradually ascending. Urticaria around joints with great itching, especially above the ankles. Eruptions itch, smart and burn after exposure to cold damp air, near the seashore and in intermitent fever. Itching is particularly worse from physical exercise. Urticaria may even be over the whole body with large red intensely itching blotches.

Nitric Acid : Chronic urticaria with itching which is markedly worse in cold open air and after scratching.

Sepia : Chronic urticaria with burning, stitching, and itching which gets worse on exposure to open air. The urticaria first appears on face, neck and forearms and then gradually spreads over the whole body. The attacks are preceded by nausea and pressing headache with face swollen as in erysipelas. Urticaria on upper body breaks out in cold air and disappears in a warm room. Eruption in the form of wheals as if due to blows with a whip or rod.

Sulphur : The urticaria of sulphur is found on the face, arms, on back of hand, neck and lower extremities. Urticaria with fever. Itching urticaria over the whole body, hands and feet. Eruptions alternate with other complaints. There is voluptuous itching which is worse at night, worse when in bed and worse after scratching and washing. Scratching is followed by burning.

ANGIONEUROTIC OEDEMA

Since it is a variety of urticaria, thereby, one gets giant oedematous lesion, chiefly involving eyelids, tongue, lips and genitals.

It is usually a self-limiting disease, hence, treatment should be aimed at quick palliation also it is known to recur. Hence deep acting constitutional remedies should be given between the attacks.

The homoeopathic approach remain the same as that of urticaria. Only care should be taken, that if it involves the glottis, then the prognosis is quite serious. However, death can occur, if, the oedema interferes with the respiration. Hence one should not hesitate to put tracheostomy tube as an emergency measure.

The dietetic regime also remains the same as that of urticaria.

Over and above the drugs mentioned in the chapter for urticaria the following drugs are also useful.

Agaricus : The angioneurotic oedema of *Agaricus* is characterised by sudden swelling with redness, especially affecting face, nose, extremities, genitals. There is sensation of burning and itching in the affected part. The attacks come especially when the person is exposed to cold weather. The Angioneurotic Oedema also becomes worse after consumption of alcohol, in the morning and when exposed to sun.

Antipyrinum : *Antipyrinum* has a special affinity to skin and produces a scarlet red rash with oedema. The oedema chiefly affects face, arms and legs. There is presence of excessive itching in affected part. The symptoms come suddenly and disappear suddenly.

Helleborus : *Helleborus* has a tendency to develop oedematous swelling. In cases of angioneurotic oedema, the appearance of the lesion is multiple pale swellings with practically no redness or itching. There are lots of conditions of the Helleborus patient where angioneurotic oedema is a concomitant,e.g., angioneurotic oedema with severe debility; angioneurotic oedema after scarletina. Angioneurotic oedema with fever, pain diarrhoea and suppressed urine. I would like to specially mention two remedies which have time in and time out helped me to save patients from critical conditions. They are :

Thyroidinum : This drug is indicated in cases of angioneurotic oedema because the thyroid gland in its disturbed state produces dropsy and anasarca. There is extreme dryness of the skin, the skin is cold to touch, the affected part is cold to touch. The angioneurotic oedema tends to become worse at night. It is indicated when the well selected remedy fails to act curatively.

Prunus Spinosa : In *Prunus spinosa*, the angioneurotic oedema comes whenever a person is exposed to sun. Tendency to develop angioneurotic oedema in person with cardiac illness. It typically affects the skin around the eyes and the face. The right side is more affected than the left.

THE HAHNEMANNIAN GLEANINGS

Vol. XXVIII - No. 2 (1961)
Page No. 77

Urticaria Appearing Annually

Mrs. S. about forty years old, wife of a prominent clergyman in the city, consulted me for annually appearing paroxysms of urticaria, or whatever you may be pleased to call it. On the thirteenth day of May every year for seven years she had been seized with a burning and itching of the skin that would nearly drive her to distraction. I saw her in bed with one of these attacks with her entire surface and here eyes closed with oedema of the lids. The hives were so confluent that not a spot of healthy integument could be seen. The whole paroxysm lasted twenty-four hours. She seemed to be in terrible distress and exclaimed every moment, "I shall die this time, surely." She seemed suffocating and was throwing off the covers. It seemed from her movements and speech that her skin felt as if on fire. There was no perceptible thirst and time was precious, and I am satisfied that I made waste by my haste in giving her dose of *Apis* 200 which has no effect. But the paroxysm passed off and another year rolled by, when she called on me, as I requested her to do, a month before the expected paroxysm. I then learned more of her symptoms. I learned that when the eruption was out distinctly in nearly all of the attacks she had found that heat calmed her terrible distress and ameliorated the itching and burning. While she craved cold and had even thrown the covers off she was made worse by it, but when she had retained presence of mind and covered herself warmly with clothing she soon became quiet and the paroxysm terminated with less suffering. This being the case *Apis* could not be her similimum, and I could now understand clearly why I had failed to interrupt the paroxysm and bring about a feeling of contentment so usual in such cases. I have quieted such patient very frequently in an hour, and plainly as a result of a Homoeopathic remedy, but this case furnished me with no evidence of curative action of my selected remedy. With the symptoms as given and the new modality I gave her one dose of *Rhus rad.* 200 bided my time ten days before the expected paroxysm. Within a few hours after taking the remedy she declared that her 'spell' was coming on; but it was only the shadow, the paroxysm never appeared again. She missed it two years and she is in better health than ever. She remarked to me one day, "Doctor, your powders have made a new woman of me." She had been treated allopathically, physiologically, electrically, pathologically, and with all very badly. This may not have been urticaria. Some of the wise heads of the old school told her it was from eating strawberries, and she refrained from these luxurious fellows and still did not miss the paroxysm. One told her one thing and another disputed his. What was it? I don't know, neither do I care. Perhaps some pathologist could inform me as to the scientificity of my prescription, I simply know that when comparing the pathogenesis found in the Symptomen Codex I found a picture of the disease to be cured, and that is enough for me. The highest potency at hand was administered and never repeated. The slight aggravation usual to such work followed, and then I was contented to await results. I am contented with such results, and so will any man who knows how to apply the law — the simillimum, the smallest dose, the dynamized drug. In this way shall we become the most useful to our patrons.

A girl, aged 20, having urticaria. Pressure urticaria, since many years. Has taken many medicines, allopathic, ayurvedic. They did not help much. After stopping of the medicines urticaria comes up again.

The symptoms were such that, she could have urticaria whenever she wanted; i.e., by scratching with a pointed thing like a nail or a pencil, eruption would come up. If a straight line is drawn eruption would come up in a straight line; if a circle is drawn, eruption would come up in a circle form. If the wrist-watch is tight on the wrist, eruption round the wrist would come up, elevated and itching around the wrist. That would remain for a few minutes to an hour or two. Even without pressure, urticaria would come up, mostly in the evening or night, and would come in different parts of the body each time. She was about to be married and that made me joke with her, "When you go to your husband's home, we will write on your hand 'To Kamlesh, with Love'." That comment of mine brought tears in her eyes, and she started weeping. I was embarrassed, I said sorry, but she would not stop weeping. The parents who accompanied her told me that she had, of late, become very sensitive and cries often, without any reason; especially when anyone jokes about her or with her.

P.H. : of measles, strong attack, but no after effects. The age at that time was 17. After measles, the first menses came up.

Hot patient, always better in cold weather. Wants to wear thin clothes; Thirst — less, takes only two glasses of fruit juices, water intake, almost nil; even in summer. Appetite good, but can't have steaming hot food, even would take tea when it gets cold. Would prefer cold dishes than hot dishes.

Menses — very irregular; sometimes early, sometimes late. Flow also, sometimes profuse, sometimes scanty.

Repertorisation — *Kent's Repertory* :

Offended easily	:	p. 69
Weeping, causeless	:	p. 93
Weeping, involuntary	:	p. 93.
Desires cold food	:	p. 485
Desires refreshing things	:	p. 486
Desires sour, acids,etc.	:	p. 486

Referring to Allen's *Key Notes* : On Pulsatilla

1. The first serious impairment of health is referred to puberty age.

2. Menses — Derangement at puberty. Irregular, intermittent flow. Delayed first menses.

3. Symptoms ever changing; no two attacks alike.

Treatment was started with *Puls.* 1m every week, three doses for 1½ months; and S.L. in between days t.d.s. Then *Puls.* 10m. and S.L. in identical way for another one month.

No more urticaria. Completely alright.

INDIAN JOURNAL OF HOMOEOPATHIC MEDICINE
Page No. 50

A Little Known Remedy 'Bombyx'

I met with a case of urticaria which I am sending to you for publication in your esteemed Journal.

Nearly two months back (on August 21) my grandson, about one and half years of age, suffered from urticaria, caused by a particular type of mosquito bite (type not known) with the following symptoms :

"Intense irritation of the whole body, hard, large red spots on the whole body, very thick, hardly leaving any space, starting from the buttocks, the whole body swollen, burning heat of the skin. Temp. 103° F, accompanied by severe yawning, no thirst, appetite diminished. He slept only in the lap of the mother; frequent urination." I administered him *Rhus-tox* 6, every two hours, but no relief. On 22nd I referred the case to another homoeopath of my locality, who also tried 4 or 5 remedies (names not known), but no improvement. Since there was no improvement, the other members of the family thought to change to allopathy, but I boldly resisted the move and consulted Therapeutic Index in *Pocket Manual of Homoeopathic Materia Medica.* Meanwhile, I noticed one more symptom, viz., very acute constipation.

From Therapeutic Index I selected *Bombyx* (after studying it in the *Dictionary of Practical Materia Medica.* I decided on it).

I got *Bombyx* 30 from the market after a great search and with only two powders at 5 hours interval the boy became normal.

Urticaria

Acon, Agar, All-c, Am-c, Am-m, Anac, Ananth, Ant-c, Ant-t, Anthrak, Antipyr, Apium gr, Apis, Arn, Ars, Ars-i, Arum-t, Asim, Astac, Aur, Bapt, Bar-c, Bar-m, Bell, Benz-ac, Berb-v, Bombyx, Bov, Bry, Bufo, Calad, Calc, Calc-s, Camph, Carb-an, Carb-s, Carb-v, Caust, Cham, Chin, Chin-a, Chin-s, Chlol, Chlor, Cic, Cimic, Clem, Coca, Cocc, Cocl, Condur, Con, Cop, Corn, Crot-h, Crot-t, Cub, Cupr, Dolich, Dulc, Elat, Fagop, Ferr-i, Form, Fragar, Guarana, Hep, Homar-fl, Ichth, Ign, Iod, Ip, Kali-ar, Kali-br, Kali-c, Kali-chl, Kali-i, Kali-m, Kali-p, Kali-s, Kreos, Lach, Led, Lyc, Lycps, Mag-c, Medusa, Merc, Mez, Nat-a, Nat-c, Nat-m, Nat-p, Nat-s, Nit-ac, Nux-v, Op, Pall, Petr, Phos, Ph-ac, Pic-ac, Pip-n, Psor, Puls, Rhus-t, Rhus-v, Rob, Rumx, Ruta, Sabin, Sal-ac, Sanic, Sec, Sel, Sep, Sil, Stann, Staph, Stram, Stroph, Strych-p, Sulph, Ter, Tetradyn, Triost, Thuj, Til, Urt-u, Valer, Verat, Vesp, Zinc.

Morning — *Bell*
Awakening on — *Bov*
Afternoon — *Chlol*
4 P.M. and evening — *Hyper*
Evening — *Kreos, Nux-v.*
Night — *Apis, Ant-c, Ars, Bov, Chlol, Cop, Hydr, Nux-v, Puls.*
Air open from — *Nit-ac, Rumx, Sep.*
Air open from amel — *Calc*
Alternating with asthma — *Calad*
  with rheumatism — *Urt-u*
Ascarides with — *Urt-u*
Asthmatic troubles in — *Apis*

Bathing after — *Bov, Phos, Urt-u.*
Burning — *Cop, Sep, Urt-u.*
Catarrh with — *Cepa, Dulc.*
Change of air and weather — *Apis*
Chill before — *Hep*
  during — *Apis, Ars, Ign, Nat-m, Rhus-t.*
  after — *Elat, Hep.*
Children in — *Cop*
Chronic — *Anac, Ant-c, Antipyr, Ars, Astac, Bov, Calc, Chloral, Condur, Cop, Dulc, Hep, Ichth, Lyc, Nat-m, Rhus-t, Sep, Stram, Sulph, Urt-u, Ver.*
Recurring — *Hep*
Climacteric at — *Morph, Ustil.*
Cold air in — *Ars, Caust, Dulc, Kali-br, Nat-s, Nit-ac, Rhus-t, Rumx, Sep.*
Amel — *Calc, Dulc.*
Colds agg — *Dulc*
Cold bath after — *Calc-p*
  amel — *Apis, Dulc.*
  from taking — *Dulc*
Constipation, fever with — *Cop*
Croup : alternating — *Ars*
Drinking cold water agg — *Bell*
Drinks : spirituous from— *Chloral*
Drinks hot amel — *Chloral*
Diarrhoea with — *Ars, Apis, Bov, Puls.*
Emotion from — *Anac, Bov, Ign, Kali-br.*
Erysipelatous eruption or petechial disturbance with — *Asthac, Fragar.*
Exercise violent after — *Apis, Calc, Con, Hep, Nat-m, Psor, Sanic, Urt-u.*
Exercise warmth of amel — *Hep, Sep.*
Exposure from — *Chloral, Dulc, Rhus-t.*
Flat, plaques in — *Form, Hob.*
Fish agg — *Ars*
Shell fish agg — *Terb, Urt-u.*
Fever during — *Amyg, Apis, Chlor, Cop, Cub, Ign, Rhus-t, Rhus-v, Sulph.*
Fruit, pork, buck wheat from — *Puls*
Gastric derangement from — *Ant-c, Ars, Carb-v, Cop, Dulc, Nux-v, Puls, Robin, Trios*

Giant — *Ap, Kali-i.*
Itching, burning, after scratching, no fever — *Dulc*
Itching without — *Uva*
Livid — *Apis*
Liver disturbance with — *Astac, Calc-fl, Myr, Ptel.*
Lying amel — *Urt-u*
Intense — *Chloral*
Itching — *Dulc, Sep, Sulph, Urt-u.*
Itching in open air — *Nit-ac*
Itching blotches — *Phos*
Meat after — *Ant-c*
Menses after — *Kreos*
  before — *Dulc, Kali-c.*
  during — *Bell, Cim, Dulc, Kali-c, Puls, Mag-c, Sec.*
  delayed — *Puls*
  profuse with — *Bov*
Nausea before the — *Sang*
Nodular — *Agar, Alum, Am-c, Am-m, Anac, Ant-c, Ant-t, Apis, Arn, Ars, Aur, Bar-c, Bar-m, Bell, Bry, Calc, Cann-s, Canth, Caps, Carb-an, Carb-s, Carb-v, Caust, Chel, Chin, Chlol, Chlor, Cic, Cocc, Con, Cop, Dig, Dros, Dulc, Graph, Hell, Hep, Ign, Iod, Ip, Jug-c, Kali-ar, Kali-br, Kali-c, Kali-i, Kali-n, Kali-s, Kreos, Lach, Led, Lyc, Mag-c, Mag-m, Mang, Merc, Mez, Mur-ac, Nat-a, Nat-c, Nat-m, Nat-p, Nit-ac, Nux-v, Olnd, Op, Pall, Petr, Ph-ac, Phos, Puls, Rhus-t, Rhus-v, Ruta, Sabin, Sec, Sel, Sep, Sil, Spig, Spong, Squil, Stann, Staph, Stram, Sulph, Sul-ac, Tarax, Thuj, Urt-u, Valer, Verat, Verb, Viol-t, Zinc.*
Rosy (erythema) — *Bell, Bry, Chlol, Chlor, Coca, Cop, Crot-t, Gels, Jug-c, Kali-br, Kali-i, Merc, Nat-c, Petr, Phos, Phyt, Rhus-t, Sil, Stram, Ter.*
Nodosa — *Bov, Urt.*
Oedema with — *Apis, Vespa.*
Palpitation with — *Bov*
Periodically : every year same season — *Urt-u*
Perspiration during — *Apis, Rhus-t.*
Pinworm with — *Urt*
Pressure where skin in — *Med*
Purple — *Chin-s*
Receding — *Stroph*
Respiration : difficult : with — *Apis*
Rheumatism during — *Rhus-t, Urt-u.*

Rheumatic lameness, palpitation, diarrhoea — *Bov, Dulc.*
Rubbing amel — *Elat*
Scratching after — *Agar, Alum, Am-c, Am-m, Ant-c, Ars, Bar-c, Bry, Calc, Carb-an, Carb-s, Carb-v, Caust, Chin, Chin-a, Cic, Cocc, Con, Dulc, Graph, Hell, Hep, Ip, Lach, Led, Lyc, Mag-c, Mag-m, Mang, Merc, Mez, Nat-c, Nat-m, Nit-ac, Nux-v, Olnd, Petr, Puls, Rhus-t, Ruta, Sel, Sep, Sil, Spig, Staph, Sulph, Thuj, Verat, Zinc.*
Sequelae from suppressed hives — *Apis, Urt-u.*
Seashore at — *Ars, Mag-m*
Shell-fish : roe — *Camph*
Shuddering with — *Ap-g*
Spring every — *Rhus-t*
Sudden coming and going — *Antipyr*
Suppressed malaria — *Elat*
Sweat — *Apis*
Syncope with — *Camph*
Tubersa — *Anac, Bolet-lur.*
Tar from — *Bov*
Undressing agg — *Puls*
Uterine trouble from — *Apis, Bell, Kali-c, Nat-m, Puls, Sep.*
Walking in cold air while — *Sep*
Warmth and exercise — *Apis, Bov, Con, Dulc, Kali-c, Kali-i, Led, Lyc, Nat-m, Nit-ac, Psor, Puls, Sulph, Urt-u .*
amel — Ars, Chloral, Hep, Lyc, Sep.
Wet, becoming from — *Rhus-t*
White lumps, red areolae, itch, worse after meal — *Ant-c*
White — *Nat-m*
White apex — *Ant-c, Puls.*
Wine, from — *Chlol*
Head — *Agar*
Face — *Aran, Am-c, Apis, Ars, Bell, Calc, Chel, Chin-s, Chlol, Cop, Crot-t, Gels, Hep, Hydr, Kali-i, Lach, Led, Mez, Nat-m, Rhus-t, Sep, Sil, Sulph, Urt-u.*
morning — *Chin*
disappearing in open air — *Calc*
winter in — *Kali-i*
External throat — *Bry, Kali-i.*
Abdomen — *Merc, Nat-c.*
Genitalia — *Clem, Cop, Merc, Nat-c.*
Chest — *Calad, Hydrc, Sars, Sulph, Urt-u.*

Back — *Apis, Lach, Lac-ac, Sulph.*
Scratching after — *Lyc*
Extremities — *Acon, Ant-c, Apis, Bell, Berb, Calc, Chin-s, Chlol, Cop, Hep, Hydrc, Hyper, Indg, Kali-i, Lach, Lyc, Merc, Nat-c, Nat-m, Nat-s, Phos, Rhus-v, Sulph, Thuj, Urt-u.*
Shoulder — *Lach*
Elbow — *Aran*
Forearm — *Am-c, Calad, Chin, Clem, Lyc, Nat-m, Sil.*
  morning — *Chin*
  evening — *Lyc*
Heat during — *Calad*
Scratching after — *Calad, Calc, Chin.*
Hand — *Apis, Berb, Bufo, Carb-v, Hep, Hyper, Nat-c, Nat-m, Nat-s, Sars, Sulph, Urt-u.*
  morning — *Chin*
Spots in — *Apis*
Whitish — *Nat-m*
Hand back of — *Acon, Apis, Berb, Cop, Hyper, Indg, Sulph, Thuj.*
When hands become cool — *Thuj*
Palms — *Rhus-v*
  between the fingers — *Hyper Merc.*
Fingers — *Hep, Thuj, Urt-u.*
  on becoming cold — *Thuj*
Lower Limbs — *Apis, Calc, Chlol, Clem, Kali-i, Merc, Plan, Sulph, Zinc.*
  after scratching — *Clem, Zinc.*
Nates — *Hydr, Lyc.*
Thigh — *All-c, Clem, Iod, Merc, Zinc.*
  after scratching — *Clem, Zinc.*
Knee — *Zinc*
Hollow of knee — *Zinc*
Leg — *Calc, Chlor, Rhus-t, Sulph.*
Calf — *Carb-v*
Foot - *Calc, Sulph.*

HERPES

The term 'Herpes' signifies a group of vesicles on an inflammatory base like a bunch of grapes. Clinically, herpetic lesions are typical and are seen in two main herpetic conditions — simplex and zoster.

Herpes Simplex

It can occur anywhere on the body, but the common sites are mainly the body orifices — lips, nose, mouth and genitalia. It is not unilateral like herpes zoster : mid-line may be crossed by the eruption.

There are two distinct antigenic types of herpes simplex viruse : HSV-1 and HSV-2. While HSV-2 is responsible for genital herpes simplex, all other clinical varieties are due to HSV-1. Development of carcinoma may be related to HSV-2 infection of the cervix.

It occurs after a stress, for instance, a psychogenic stress : injury; fever, particularly malaria, pneumonia, meningitis; general illness; debility, etc. Recurrent herpes implies the relapsing type of herpes simplex occurring on the same site. The local cutaneous resistance is low in such cases. The virus of herpes is ubiquitous; it is more prevalent in the temperate climate and the cold season. This accounts for the layman's name of "Cold Spots."

Herpes hominis virus is thought to remain dormant in sensory root ganglion (like H-Z) to be activated intermittently by various stress factors. Passively transferred maternal antibodies usually confer protection on the infant during the first 3 months of life.

Clinical features : Herpes starts with a sensation of burning or itching after there has been an exposure to the cold wind, sun, etc. Erythematous macules appear, on which grouped, pinhead sized, superficial vesicles rapidly develop : their contents soon become opaque. They may rupture and become crusted, or dry up to leave faint reddish stains. There are usually negligible constitutional symptoms. The course of herpes is about 7 to 14 days. There is usually no scarring except when secondary infection occurs. Occasionally, hyperpigmentation or depigmentation may follow.

Besides the common herpes simplex affection, primary infection may manifest in the following three ways :

(i) Gingivo-stomatitis or vulvo-vaginitis or kerato-conjunctivitis associated with fever, malaise, regional lymphadenopathy.

(ii) Herpetic whitlow-painful vesiculo-pustular eruption around the nailfold, often associated with regional lymphadenopathy.

(iii) Eczema herpeticum type or Kaposi's varicelliform eruption.

Recurrent herpes implies relapsing type of herpes simplex occuring on the same site — usually perioral and genitalia. Local resistance is low : emotional stress, exposure to cold and lack of personal hygiene tend to bring on an attack.

Erythema multiforme may be a complication at times.

Herpes progenitalis implies herpes simplex lesions on the genitalia. It is transmitted sexually. In the male, the lesions are on the glans, prepuce or body of the penis : in the female, on the labia, vaginal wall and cervix. The eruption on the genitalia is painful, and may cause a constitutional upset. Genital herpetic lesions rupture early producing erosions, which at times, are in a circinate pattern. The common predisposing causes of recurrent genital herpes are phimosis, lack of personal hygiene, discharge per vaginum and sexual neurosis. Furthermore, recurrent herpes progenitalis is responsible for syphilophobia in some cases.

Buccal herpes is rare in adults but common in infants as aphthous stomatitis which involves the mucous membrane of the palate, cheeks and tongue. Because of moisture and friction, the vesicles get rapidly eroded producing painful, superficial erosions on erythematous bases accompanied by constitutional upset.

Diagnosis : Herpes simplex of the face is so characteristic that it can be diagnosed without any difficulty. Herpes zoster is unilateral : the lesions appear along the nerve distribution : they are painful and non-recurrent.

Herpes progenitalis should be differentiated from syphilitic chancre by the presence of multiple, superficial lesions and the absence of induration, shotty regional lymph glands and spirochaetes in the dark-field examination. Moreover, herpes develops within a few days of exposure while syphilitic chancre develops much later (about 4 weeks).

Chancroid is characterized by painful ulcers which are deeper than the superficial erosions of herpes : suppurating bubo, and the presence of B. ducrey in the smear.

Very rarely can scabies of the penis, monilial balanitis, lichen planus and fixed drug eruption be confused. If their respective features are remembered, there will be no difficulty at all.

Prognosis : In an individual attack of herpes the prognosis is good, in the sense that lesions heal up nicely and no scarring results. Only in recurrent herpes is the treatment rather unsatisfactory, and the malady can become a nuisance, especially in the variety termed herpes progenitalis.

In recurrent herpes which is a knotty problem, an attempt must be made to raise the general resistance and to eliminate the precipitating causes like chronic rhinitis, phimosis, debility, anxiety, stress etc.

Herpes Zoster

Synonym : Shingles.

Varicella-zoster virus (VZV) is the causative organism, and the site of its pathology is the posterior root ganglion : the skin is only secondarily affected. One or several posterior root ganglia may be involved. The inflammation, sometimes, though rarely, spreads to the posterior horn and then to the anterior horn and even the meninges. Besides the virus, the diminished resistance of the skin and the body is essential for the development of an attack. Physical injuries, mental trauma, febrile illnesses and drugs are also known to act as triggers as well as predisposing factors.

Shingles may occur at any age, though of course, adults are more often affected. Occasionally, herpes zoster may take an epidemic form.

Herpes zoster is closely related to chickenpox on microbiological, serological and epidemiological basis. While varicella is primary exogenous VZV infection, herpes zoster is thought to represent activation of an endogenous infection that has persisted in latent phase following an earlier infection by varicella. Patients are infectious : in the first week virus can be isolated from the vesicles.

Clinical features : An attack starts with neuralgic pain, local increased sensitivity of the skin (hyperaesthesia) and fever with a range of 102° to 103° F. Cutaneous lesions develop three days after the onset of the attack. Sometimes, the rash may develop suddenly without any premonitory symptom. The rash develops in the segmental distribution of the affected nerve roots, and consists of typical herpetic lesions, e.g., groups of vesicles on inflammatory bases in several patches with intervening areas of normal skin. The contents of the vesicles soon turn opaque. The vesicles may become confluent to form flat bullae. The lesions develop in several crops, each crop lasting a week or so. Towards the end of this period, the lesions rupture or dry up to form crusts. When the crust separates in about a week's time, there is temporary pigmentation and faint scarring. The latter is marked when there is secondary infection and ulceration. The regional glands may be enlarged and painful. An attack lasts for 2 to 3 weeks. The sites of predilection are the trunk (intercostal nerves), neck (cervical) and the face (trigeminal distribution). Involvement of the first root of the trigeminal nerve gives rise to lesions on the eye-herpes opthalmicus. The rash is mainly unilateral; very rarely it affects both sides. Immunity in herpes is lifelong; second attack is rare. Important sequelae are the post-herpetic neuralgia and rarely muscular paralysis. The former is seen in middle age and old persons having severe attack of the disease. Pain is along the course of nerve; it can be very severe and excruciating. It may interfere with work and sleep. Neuralgic pain lasts for months to years.

Diagnosis : It is based upon the sudden onset of a unilateral, herpetic eruption along the distribution of one or more nerve roots accompanied by pain and hyperaesthesia. In the initial stage of sudden pain, before the rash develops, confusion may occur with other local causes of pain like mastoiditis, pleurisy, appendicitis, cholecystitis, pyelitis, etc.

Prognosis.: It is good as far as the cutaneous lesions are concerned. An individual attack subsides nicely, leaving faint scars.

The troublesome sequelae may be the annoying post-herpectic neuralgia and muscular paralysis due to extension of inflammation to anterior horn of the spinal cord. Viraemia and meningo-encephalitis may rarely occur in susceptible patients or patients under immunosuppressive drugs.

Herpes — Homoeopathic Approach

Herpes is primarily a virus infection. That is why it should be classified under the tubercular miasm. However, if one closely observes a complete evolutionary pattern of herpes, then one can appreciate its multi-miasmatic nature,viz :

(a) Burning sensation prior to development of eruptions — psoric stage. .
(b) Formation of vesicle — sycotic stage.
(c) Transformation of vesicles to pustules — tubercular stage.
(d) Rupture of pustules forming thick scabs with ulceration — syphilitic stage.

It is extremely essential on the part of a homoeopath to clearly state in history, at what stage the patient presented initially.

Herpes is known to occur with many systemic conditions and hence during history taking, detailed inquiry should be made for the following :

(a) fever — malaria, pneumonia, meningitis
(b) injury
(c) psychogenic stress.

I would like to lay importance on the psychogenic stress as this is one of the most common exciting factors known to initiate the herpes infection, exposure to cold and lack of personal hygiene are also to be considered in the history.

In cases where herpes progenitalis is suspected, one should enquire confidently about history of having indulged themselves in either fornication or adultery. They should be advised to keep proper personal hygiene of the genitals.

Recurrent herpes is one of the most tricky problems to tackle in private practice. An attempt must be made to increase the gen-

HERPES ZOSTER TREATED WITH VARIOLINUM

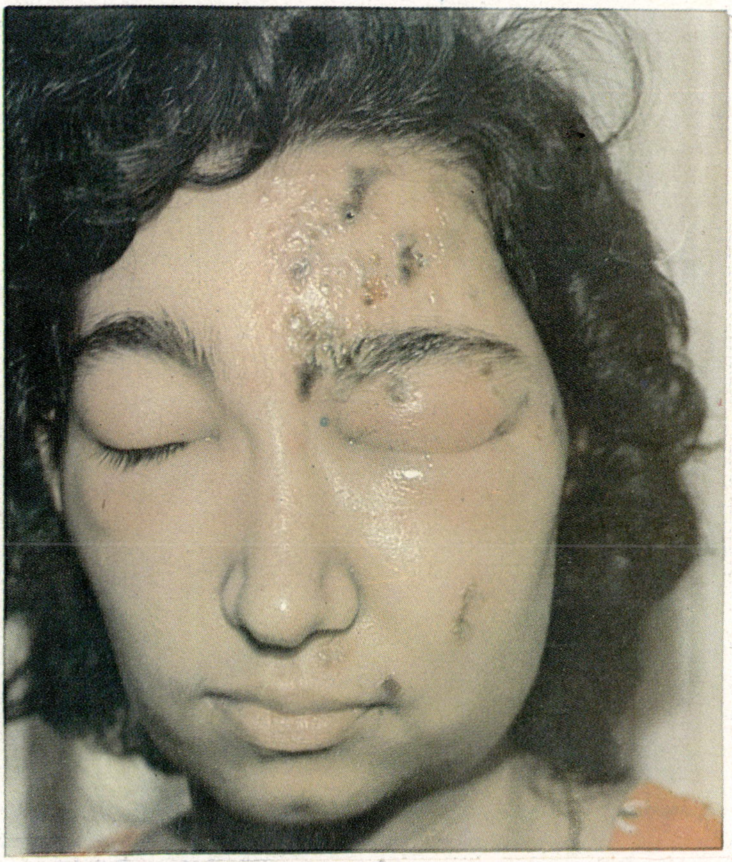

BEFORE

HERPES ZOSTER TREATED WITH VARIOLINUM

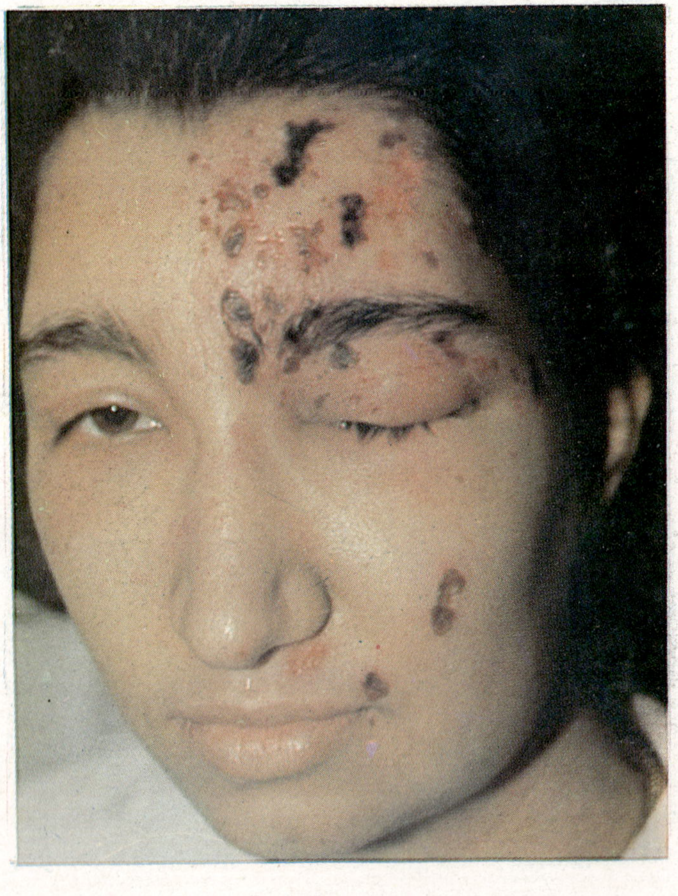

DURING

HERPES ZOSTER TREATED WITH VARIOLINUM

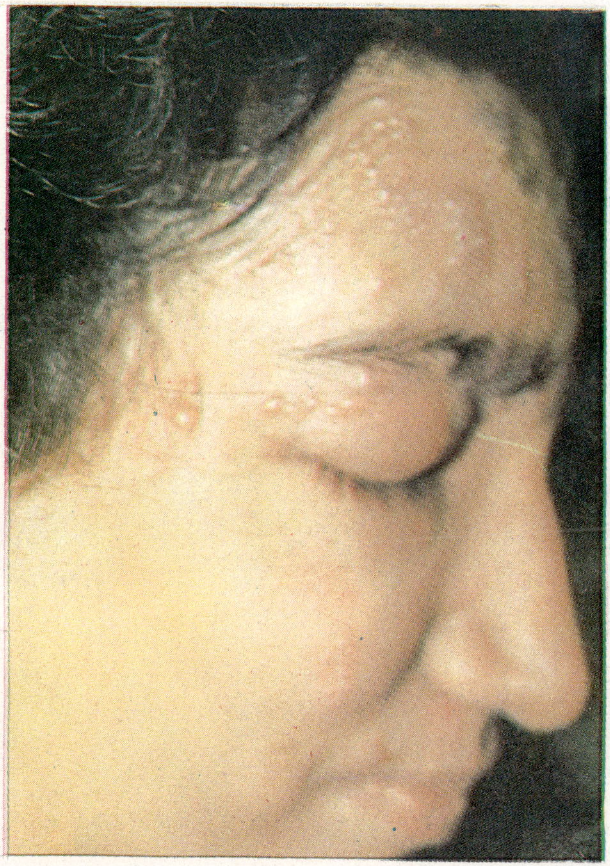

AFTER

HERPES ZOSTER TREATED WITH VARIOLINUM

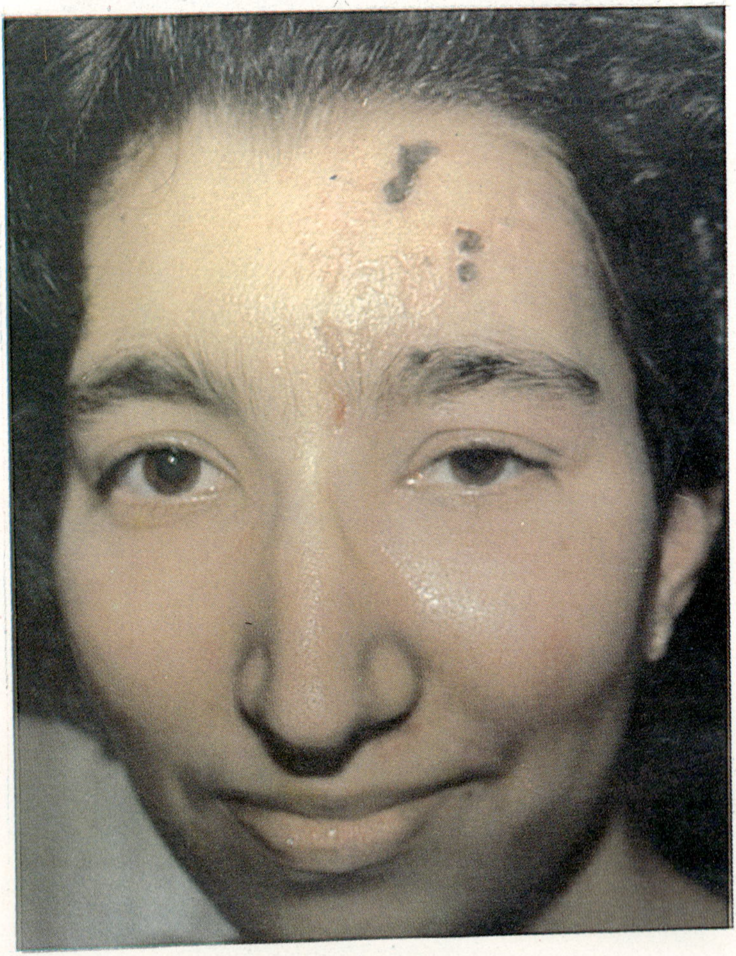

CURED

HERPES ZOSTER TREATED WITH MEZEREUM

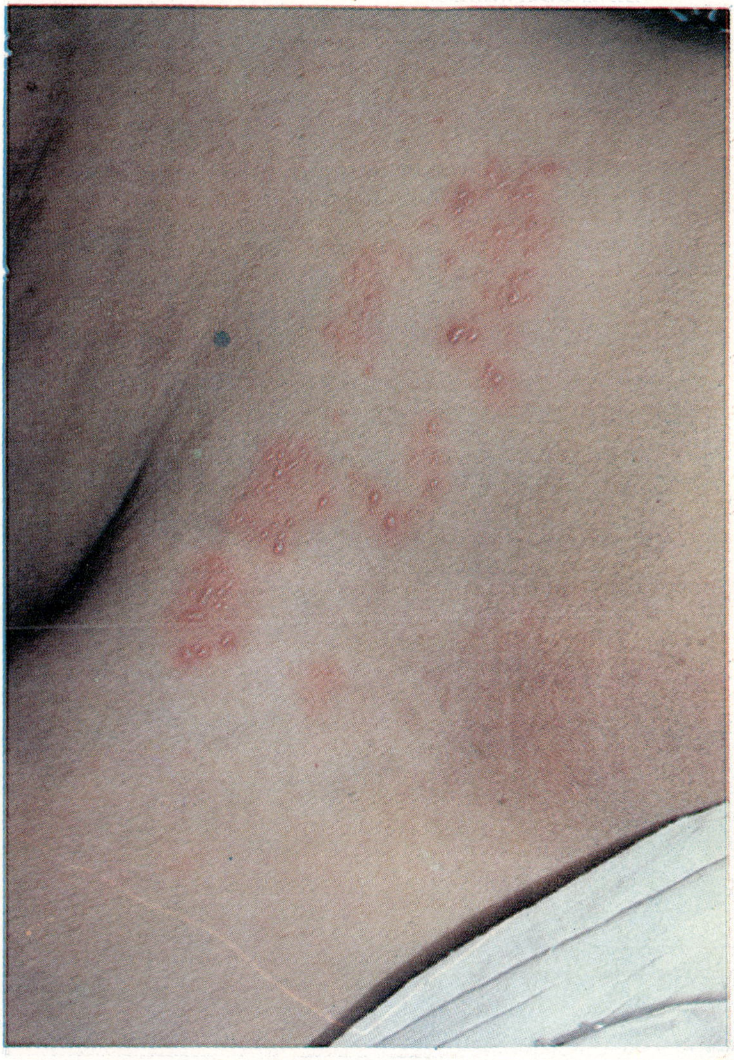

HERPES ZOSTER TREATED WITH MEZEREUM

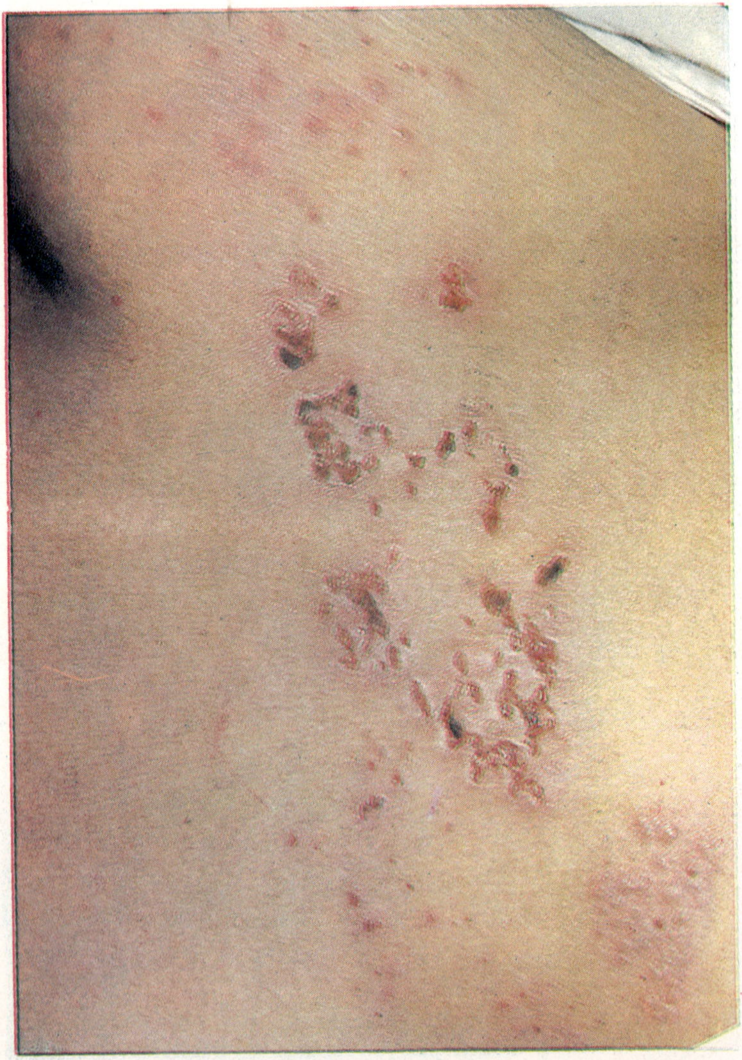

AFTER 4 DAYS

HERPES ZOSTER TREATED WITH MEZEREUM

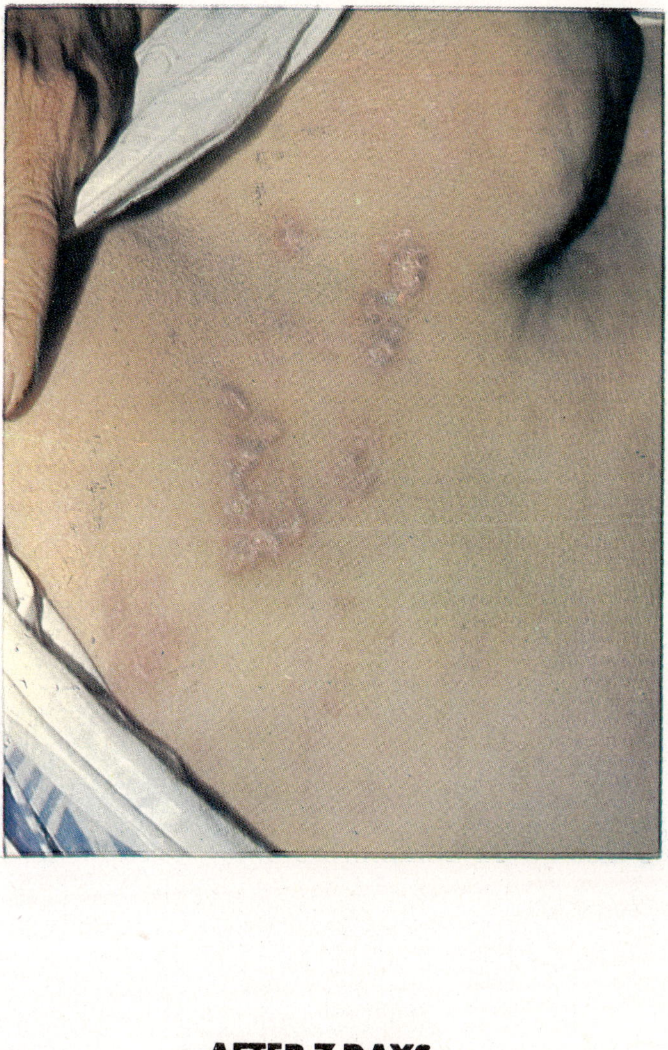

AFTER 7 DAYS

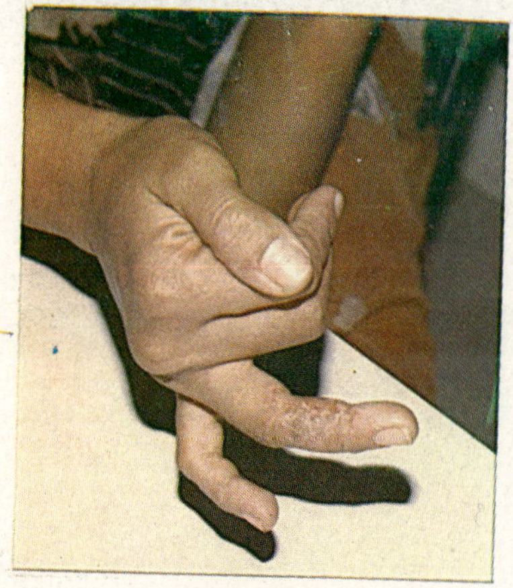

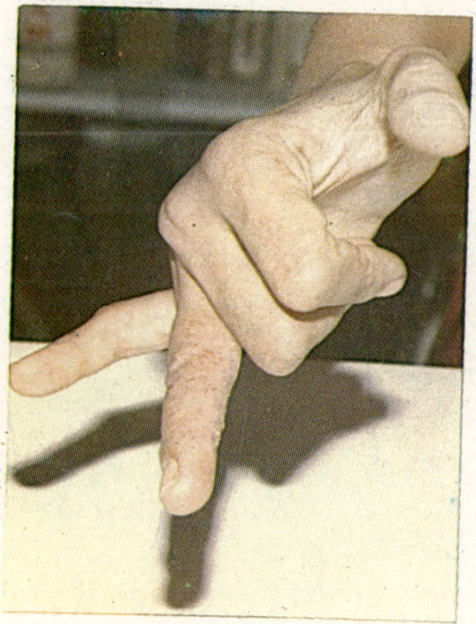

HERPES TREATED WITH RHUS VEN

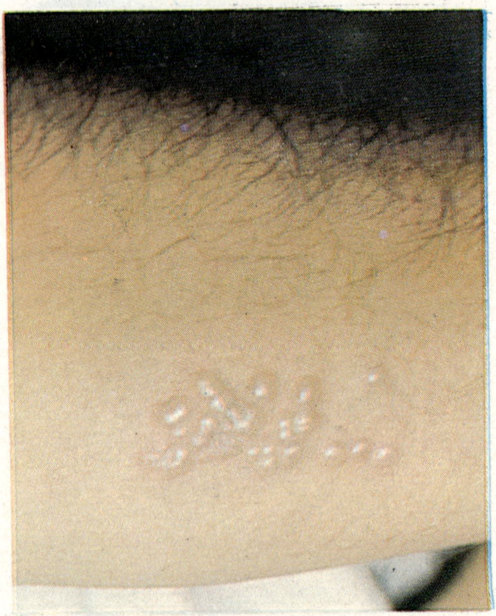

BEFORE

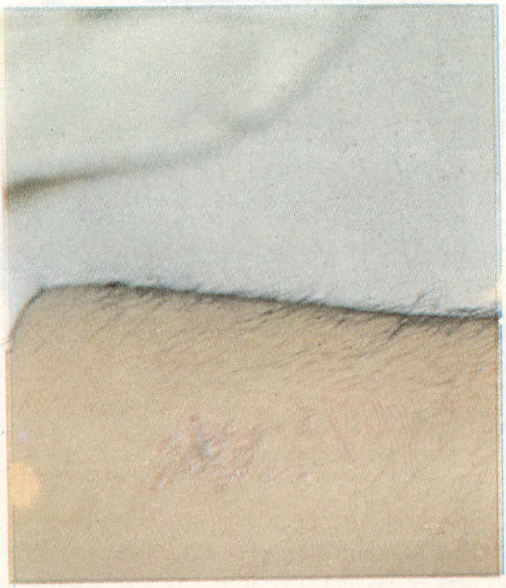

AFTER

eral resistance of the patient by giving indicated constitutional medicine preferably nosode. At the same time, to eliminate the precipitating causes like chronic rhinitis, phimosis, debility, anxiety, stress, etc.

I have found encouraging results with the use of D.N.A. and R.N.A. potentised and used in cases of recurrent herpes infection. The reader is advised to read the provings in detail before prescribing, from a scientific paper written by Dr. Maurice Jenaer.

In a case of herpes zoster, one has to be extra cautious because under rare circumstances, patient may develop meningo-encephalitis. For post-herpetic neuralgia, drugs like Variolinum, D.N.A., should be thought of.

The pattern of deciding or arriving at the prescription remains the same as in the case of eczema,viz. :

(a) location,
(b) sensations — e.g., burning, pricking, cutting;
(c) pattern of eruptions — vesicles, pustules, crusts;
(d) nature of discharge;
(e) thermal and time modalities;
(f) exciting and causating factors if any;
(g) past and family history to decide the fundamental cause;
(h) patient as a person that is general and mental symptoms.

Locally on the lesions, mixture consisting of calendula and water in the ratio of 1:2 should be applied as it reduces the irritation as well as prevents secondary bacterial infection. At the site of post-herpetic neuralgia, *Hypericum* mother tincture should be applied to give a soothing sensation to the patient.

HERPES

Aethiops : Especially adapted to person with scrofulous and syphilitic diathesis, who are prone to easy suppuration.
Herpes after abuse of Mercury.

Agaricus : Herpetic eruptions are characterised by burning, itching and redness with swelling. The burning pain is worse whenever the patient is exposed to cold application or cold air.

Alnus : It is suited in cases of chronic Herpes. The fingers are covered with pustules which cause formation of a crust.
Eruption on the skin alternating with disease condition of mucous membrane.

Arsenic Alb : Herpes typically affects the lips, the face and intercostal region. The eruptions are confluent with intense burning sensation in the blister. Patient is worse after midnight and from cold in any form. Patient feels better by warmth. Associated with herpes, patient feels very thirsty and gets prostrated very easily. Herpetic eruptions alternate with internal affections.

Borax : Herpetic eruptions on the cheeks, around chin and on nates. Tiny vesicles which when ruptured exude hot, excoriating, watery fluid. The burning sensation is worse in warm room and better in cold air and fan. Post herpetically, the skin becomes wrinkled and wilted.

Bovista : The vesicles of *Bovista* are moist like small red pimples. Hard lentil sized on chest and foot. There is itching and burning sensation on getting warm; there is aggravation after scratching; in hot weather, at full moon and on washing. The discharge from the eruption is sticky and watery forming thick crusts or scabs with pus underneath.

Calc-C : Adapted to persons with impaired nutrition scrofulous diathesis who have a tendency to grow fat; herpes with burning and jerking pains which are worse in the cold at night. Herpes with thick corrosive scabs which have yellow pus beneath them. Suppressed herpes causes central nervous system disorders.

Capsicum : The herpetic eruption of *Capsicum* are usually found on the face, forehead and breasts. There is stinging, burning pain as if cayenne pepper spread on the affected part which is worse from scratching; from uncovering and changing position. Intense itching on the scalp as if due to vermin, which causes great restlessness and is worse from scratching.

Carbo-Veg : Moist herpetic eruptions on face, chin, about lips and mouth and on the knees. Fugitive itching hen getting warm in bed. The itching changes to burning when patient scratches. The itching is worse after eating pork or butter; patients have a tendency to hot perspiration.

Carbon Oxygenatum : Vesication along the course of nerves associated with anaesthesia.

Carbon Sulph : Especially useful in the chronic form of herpes has a special affinity for dorsum of left hand. Herpes phylyctenoides with vesicles on a red inflamed and swollen base. Vesicles contain an opaque yellowish fluid which either forms thick scabs or discharges, excoriates and causes violent itching which is better in open air and worse on bathing and in warm damp weather.

Causticum : Herpetic eruptions on shoulders, neck, around nipples and chin, face. Herpes preputialis. Herpes zoster. There is itching burning pain which is worse in open air, in clear fine weather and is better in damp weather and from walking.

Chrysarobinum : Vesicular lesions which are associated with a foul smelling discharge and crust formation. The lesions tend to coalesce and give the appearance of a single large scab. *Chrysarobinum* particularly affects the thighs, legs, ears and skin around the eyes and ears.

Cistus Can : Herpes on face, ears and various parts of the body. Patient has an itching sensation as if ants are running through the whole body which is worse at night. Herpes on a mercurio-syphilitic base. Zoster like eruptions on the back.

Clematis Erecta : Herpetic eruptions which are moist during increasing and dry during decreasing moon. Herpetic eruptions coming up after suppression of gonorrhoea. Chronic constitutional herpes. Scaly herpes with yellow, corrosive, watery discharge. There is a tendency of the vesicles to rupture and ulcerate. Gnawing, itching sensation in the skin which is not better by scratching and is worse from washing in cold water, from warmth of bed at night and from wet poultices.

Comocladia Dentata : Herpes zoster affecting face, arms and legs with tormenting itching and burning which is better in open air, by scratching and worse by warmth, touch and at night.

Conium Mac : Herpetic eruptions forming scabs as large as the hand on various parts of the body. Herpes which appears suddenly, beginning as a small spot and spreading over the whole part,e.g., the arm. The skin is red, swollen, corrugated and oozes blood or lymph from broken places. These form crusts under which the exudation still continues. There is intense itching and an irresistible desire to scratch especially in the evening. Adapted to persons of a scrofulous and cancerous diathesis with induration of glands. Patient complains of stinging like flea bites but always a single sting at a time.

Croton Tig : Herpes alternating with summer diarrhoea. Vesicular and pustular herpes with redness of skin, burning, stinging which is worse after eating; from touch and is better by rubbing gently. Herpes of face, genitals and abdomen. The vesicles become confluent and form large brown scabs. Itching followed by painful burning which is better by very gentle scratching.

Dolichos : Dry herpetic eruptions on arms, legs and axilla. The eruptions on axilla spreads forward to the sternum and backward to the spine. There is much itching, burning which is worse on scratching and at night preventing sleep. Dolichos is especially useful in post herpetic neuralgia.

Dulcamara : Herpes of the hands, arms, face, genitals in persons who are always worse in the cold season. Moist suppurating herpes with red areolae which bleed when scratched. Herpes zoster coming on after exposure to cold. The eruptions are associated with foetid perspiration. Itching, tearing pains which are aggravated by application of cold water; at night; damp cold weather around menstrual period and is better by moving about. Adapted to persons of a rheumatic diathesis. Herpes with glandular enlargement.

Eucalyptus : Herpetic eruptions which are associated with glandular enlargement and later develops foul indolent ulcers.

Graphites : *Graphites* has a special affinity for folds of skin, e.g., joints, behind ears, groins, neck. Herpes in obese females with delayed and scanty menses. Herpes appearing at climateric. Large blisters from umbilicus to the spine, mainly affecting left side. Itching spots on various parts of the body which oozes a watery sticky fluid. Itching as though foreign matter would pass out through the skin. Circular herpes, feels hard to touch and is wrinkled. The itching is worse at night, during and after menstruation and is better from wrapping up.

***Hepar Sulph*:** Face, hands, genitals and bends of knees and elbows are the commonly affected regions. Herpes after abuse of mercury. Adapted to persons with unhealthy skin which suppurates easily. Patients are highly sensitive to cold. Herpes zoster from spine forwards, especially the left side. The eruption is the seat of acute neuralgic pains which are worse at night; vesicles on an inflamed base associated with splinter like pains, severe itching and scratching. There is marked aggravation at night, from cold; touch and the patient feels better in damp weather and from wrapping up warmly. Especially suited to persons with a sour body odour. Herpes circinatus.

***Iris Versicolor*:** Herpes zoster associated with gastric derangements. Herpes zoster especially affecting the right side of the body. There is itching pain which is worse at night.

***Kali Bichromicum*:** Herpes after exposure to cold; herpes with respiratory disorders. At first there is violent itching over the whole surface, then there is pustule formation, mostly over the extremities. The scabs smart and burn; there is aggravation in hot weather and when undressing and patient feels better in cold weather.

***Kali-Carb*:** Herpetic eruptions in persons with dry sensitive skin where there is burning stitching pain as if from a mustard plaster associated with itching which is better after scratching. Herpetic spots on face. The eruption is dry at first but when scratched exudes moisture, itching is worse from cold air and better when getting warm. Adapted to persons of a tubercular diathesis and who have had eruptions suppressed in childhood.

Kalmia : Especially suited to cases of post herpetic neuralgias. Pains shift rapidly, shooting outwards along the course of the nerves. The skin is stiff, dry adapted to person of a rheumatic diathesis.

Kreosote : The sites of affection are both the dorsal and palmar surfaces of the hands, fingers, joints; on the ears, elbows, knuckles and malleoli. Herpes is moist and itches violently. The itching is better by warmth and is aggravated in evening and in open air to such an extent as to drive the patient wild.

Lachesis : The eruption consists of large vesicles, at first yellow in colour, then turning dark with much pain. The vesicles later break and leave on excoriated surface which burns when touched. The eruptions come on every spring and fall and are worse from acids old reddish herpes with thick scurf affecting the whiskers. Herpes of the face which reappears after suppression. Herpes zoster after external application of *Rhus tox* characterized by haemorrhagic pustules in groups near the spine and spreading to the mid axillary line.

Ledum Pal : Typically affects the face and forehead. Violently itching dry herpes which is worse in the evenings, before midnight and in open air and is better from cold applications and rest. Adapted to persons of rheumatic diathesis who have a lack of internal heat yet is intolerant of external heat.

Lithium Carb : Herpes of hands. Rough, harsh, dry skin with much itching and burning.

Lycopodium : Herpes which affects the nape of neck, the axillae, arms, thighs, tibiae and calves of legs.

Scaly, furfuraceous herpes which is yellow at the base in persons with unhealthy humid skin. Insensible yellow brown shrivelled herpes or moist, suppurating herpes full of deep rhagades with violent itching as from lice. The itching is worse from pressure; touch, eating cabbage, oysters, drinking wine and is better from uncovering. Herpes associated with urinary gastric or hepatic disorders.

Mag. Carb : Small, red, slightly elevated, smooth herpes found mainly in chest, calves of legs and about mouth. There is violent itching over the whole body which is better by scratching. Patient gets a sensation of formication at night.

Manganum : Herpes of the forearm in persons with unhealthy skin. Patient suffers from lancinating pains which are worse from touch and while lying on a feather bed. There is itching which is worse when sweating but better by scratching.

Mercurius : *Mercurius* has a marked affinity for right side. Herpes of right forearm, wrist and hand. Herpes prepucialis of the right side extending across the abdomen. There is itching which changes to burning on scratching and shooting pains which are worse at night and in cold damp weather. Herpetic eruptions which are surrounded by small pimples. Herpes with a tendency to suppurate especially in persons with profuse sweat.

Mezereum : Herpes zoster following the intercostal or supraorbital nerves with severe neuralgia; itching after scratching turns into burning. Itching worse in bed and from touch. Post herpetic neuralgia and burning with great coldness of the body. Herpes tends to ulcerate and forms thick scabs under which purulent matter exudes; tearing off these scabs causes great pain and retards healing. Herpes after suppressed eruptions; vaccination and abuse of mercury.

Nat-Carb : Herpes circinatus; herpes iris spreading and suppurating herpes on outside of hands, around nose and mouth; on tips. Herpes with yellow rings. Vesicles with shooting pains and itching which is better by rubbing the parts gently chronic ailments after sunstroke.

Nat-Mur : *Nat-mur* has a special predilection for skin about the mouth; on arms and eyes, chest, nape of neck; genitals and bends of elbows and knees; knuckles. Adapted to persons with greasy unhealthy skin. Herpes circinatus with burning spots. Gnawing, itching, shooting pains which are worse from heat; worse at seashore and from eating too much salt and are better in open air and while sweating. Herpes labialis during fever. Herpes zoster.

Nat-sulph : Herpes associated with bilious complaints. Vesicles with watery, yellow fluid with itching which is worse while undressing. Barber's itch with vesicular eruptions around mouth and chin. Itching and swelling of the fingers in bakers. There is marked aggravation from living in damp houses, basement; eating plants or fruits grown near water.

Nitric Acid : Herpetic eruptions develop in whiskers, between fingers, on alae nasi, on outer side of the thigh. There is presence of itching which is worse on undressing, worse in open air, at change of weather, from contact. Associated with itching, the overall appearance of the skin is dry, cracked and fissured with blackish discoloration. The skin is cracked practically at all angles. It is also useful in post herpetic neuralgia where the pain is sticking like a splinter.

Petroleum : Herpes on nape of neck, chest, scrotum, inner side of thigh, perineum knees and ankles. The vesicles are itching with a tendency to form crusts and cracks. Itching is so violent that the patient scratches till the skin bleeds. The skin becomes cold after scratching. Itching is worse in open air, while perspiring better from warmth and in warm air.

Psorinum : Eruption affects the bends of joints, especially of elbows and knees. The eruptions itch intolerably, when getting warm before midnight and in open air. Herpetic eruptions develop after suppression of itch. The skin of the *Psorinum* patient has a dirty look and an offensive carrion like odour, despite the most careful washing.

Ranunculus Bulbosus : Herpes zoster affecting the supra orbital and intercostal nerves. There are sharp stitching pains which are worse from touch, motion, change of temperature and on entering a cold place. The vesicles are filled with a thin, acrid fluid and are found in clusters. Herpetic eruption over fingers and palms of hands which finally spreads over the whole body. Herpes in drunkards.

Rhus Tox : Herpes zoster with a marked predeliction for the right side and hairy parts. Herpes of the face. The itching is worse in winter and while sweating. Itching alternates with pains in the chest and dysenteric stools.

Sarsaparilla: Herpes affecting the genitals, upper lip, hands, left leg, calves. The herpetic ulcers extend in circular fashion but do not form crusts; the ulcers show red granulated bases with white margins. The lesion oozes red serous fluid. Herpes which follows hot weather and vaccinations.

Sepia : Herpes circinatus especially when found in isolated spots. Herpetic eruption on lips, about mouth and nose, on neck behind ears in the bends of elbows and knees. Dry scaly desquamation after drying up of vesicles. Intolerable itching which turns to burning when scratched. Itching is worse during menses, pregnancy and lactation. Especially adapted to females with yellow complexion and uterine complaints.

Silicea : Dry herpes affecting the chin. Eruptions are inclined to suppurate. Suited to malnourished persons with unhealthy easily suppurating skin.

Staphysagria : The areas usually affected by herpes are bends of joints; hands, thighs and legs. Dry, crusty herpes in patients with easily suppurating skin. Itching is relieved by scratching but reappears at a different location. Itching associated with tingling as from insects. Chilly creeping feeling in affected parts which is worse by rubbing and by contact.

Sulphur : Herpes miliaris, phlyctenoides, circinatus and squamosus. Dry scaly herpes on nape of neck and ankles. Moist herpes with small white vesicles in groups, forming scabs over the whole face, especially above nose and about the eyes. There is burning pain after scratching. The patient is always worse from washing, bathing and getting warm in bed. Herpes after suppressed.

Tellurium : Herpes circinatus in intersecting rings. Minute itching vesicles on lower limbs or on single parts. Example scrotum, perineum. There is itching and pricking as from bugs, which is worse at night, in cool air and on sweating. The vesicles are filled with a watery, excoriating fluid smelling like fish brine.

Thuja : Herpes zoster. Herpes all over the body with violent itching and burning. White, scaly, dry, mealy herpes after suppression of gonorrhoea. Eruptions only on covered parts, burning violently when scratched and are worse from cold water, heat of bed and at night. The itching is relieved by gentle rubbing. Adapted to persons of hydrogenoid or lymphatic constitution. Herpes after vaccination.

Variolinum : Herpes zoster with sensation of bugs crawling under the skin. Neuralgia persisting after disappearance of herpes. It is an excellent remedy for post herpetic neuralgia.

Xerophyllum: Herpes affecting the flexures of the knees. There is vesication and intense itching associated with stinging and burning.

Zincum Met : Herpes on back and on hands with burning pains. Herpes with formication and tingling felt as if between skin and flesh. Dry herpes over the whole body, with herpetic ulcers. Neuralgia following herpes zoster with burning, jerking and itching, worse in the evenings and better by touch.

THE HOMOEOPATHIC HERITAGE, JULY 1983
Page No. 328 - Case No. 1023

A Herpes Cure

Dr. Burnett once wrote in regard to herpes that he 'wiped it out, pain and all', with *Variolinum.* Here is such a case within the last few days.

Mrs. A.H. 58, came to out-patients on June 1st 1937. The 'bad rash' she complained of proved to be a pustular form of (we decided) herpes, over the sacrum, down between the nates, and on edges of the labia. It itched badly; and the pain was so severe that she said, she 'would faint if she stood'. And 'she couldn't lie on it.'

The eruption was, as said, pustular. She had been vaccinated three or four times; the last time it did not take. She was given a dose of *Variolinum* 200.

She returned in a week — on the 8th — 'I' m better !' and she was ! 'Eruption better; comfortable now.' She had first come on Tuesday, and 'was surprised on Thursday night' — two days later — 'because the pain suddenly went and she could sleep'. 'The medicine was wonderful,' she said, 'It was like a miracle!'

On examination one found the pustules dry and dead, just isolated scabs : no inflammation now, and no pain.

THE HOMOEOPATHIC HERITAGE
No. 6 - June 1983

Page No. 271 - Case No. 1005

An interesting case a few years ago, was that of an elderly lady, a very severe case, involving the breast, with ulceration and great pain. She was away from home, and ordinary local treatment failed to give relief, while painting with colloidion "only made the matter worse". She wrote for homoeopathic treatment, and was very quickly well (the remedy being Ranunculus). And here the pain which in elderly people may go on indefinitely (one patient I know was even told that he would keep it as long as he lived) was promptly and permanently wiped out.

One has seen again and again the failure (even to the loss of an eye in one bad case) with ordinary treatment for herpes and the blessed relief that Homoeopathy can give provided that the remedy is well chosen. It is a tragedy that when the means of healing are so simple, they should not be within reach of all.

Dr. Burnett's great remedy for shingles was *Variolinum* (a medicine made from small-pox pus of course sterilized and potentized with this remedy, he said that he "wiped it out, pain and all."

And one has seen its very rapid action (even in a few hours) in an elderly lady who was giving little cries with the sharp pains, which were positively terrifying. The rash was 'gone practically and all'. This is the more interesting as it has now been demonstrated that herpes is allied to chicken-pox; that the one may be caught, apparently, from the other. Variolinum is one of the remedies to be thought of for chicken-pox.

JOURNAL OF THE
AMERICAN INSTITUTE OF HOMOEOPATHY
Vol. 74 — No. 4 (1981)
Page No. 21

Homoeopathic Treatment

When considering homoeopathic treatment, one must be well acquainted with the basic philosophy behind classical homoeopathy. In classical homoeopathy the whole person — mental, emotional and physical symptoms — must be evaluated in each case. There are a number of different natural medicines which can cause, and therefore cure eruptions similar to herpes simplex; that is, through the principle of 'like cures like'. Upon examining the First Memorandum of International Bibliography about Scientific Studies in the Field of Homoeopathy in 1977 and the Index Medicus, 1958 and 1959, by James Stevenson, M.D., no papers have been done on herpes simplex or zoster as such. All information on herpes virus has been done through 'provings' that is, giving the medicine to humans and observing a symptom picture similar to HSV, or from clinical experience.

One of the most frequently indicated medicines in the *Materia Medica* from many sources is *Sepia.* Farrington states, 'We know that when the vaso-motor nerves are inactive the skin is more liable to the effects of irritation and particularly to herpetic eruptions which *Sepia* cures.' *Sepia* is well known for venous congestion and frequently has a sensation of 'bearing down' in the pelvic area which might be associated with herpetic eruptions. The mental-emotional picture of Sepia is often one of indifference to those loved best; irritability and sadness with anxiety toward evening. It is particularly adapted to delicate females with rather fine skin, sensitive to all impressions, usually with dark hair; the face is apt to be sallow, and the eyes surrounded by dark rings. In *Kent's Repertory*, *Sepia* is in bold print under the rubrics 'Eruptions, herpes about the lips', and 'Eruptions, herpetic' in female genitalia.

One of the most dramatic cures of herpes genitalis was seen in September 1979 in a 33-year old dark haired, slim woman, gravida 2, para 0, with miscarriages at 6 weeks and 3 months. She complained of having herpes genitalis involving the labiae every 2 months for many years. The herpes eruption occurred mostly before and after her period. She also related that she has a yellowish white pruritic vaginal discharge intermittently for years. She also stated that her menarche was at 19 and that her menstrual periods were every 40 days with the last period being about three months ago. She was quite concerned about being sterile and also afraid that if she did become pregnant the herpes might have a deleterious effect. This patient was easily irritated, depressed and often found herself avoiding conversation. She had a strong desire for pickles, lemons and sauerkraut.

Her routine blood studies were normal and a vaginal wet mount was negative for pathogens. She was given *Sepia* 200 and approximately two weeks later she had a menstrual period, followed by two more periods every month thereafter. Her herpes erupted on two more occasions at intervals of a month and were much less severe. Her vaginal discharge disappeared after three weeks. In January 1980 she became pregnant and had no more herpes at that time. Her pregnancy was normal with delivery of a healthy child.

It is important to note that Nahmias from the Emory School of Medicine states that if the HSV is present at delivery the risk of neonatal herpes is at least 40% if the infant is not delivered abdominally before or within 4 hours of membrane rupture. It is very opportune that this situation was not encountered in this patient.

Another important medicine in the treatment of HSV is *Natrum mur*. As mentioned previously, stress and psychic disturbances are often associated with the outbreak of herpes. *Natrum mur* is well known for its relationship to this etiology. Like *Sepia*, it also is listed in bold print in Kent's Repertory under the rubric 'Eruptions, herpes about the lips'. It is in common type in female and male genitalia under the rubric 'Eruptions, herpetic'. Farrington stated that herpes labialis with accompanying chills (which are worse around 10 a.m.) and fever are particularly characteristic of *Natrum mur*. Mentally and emotionally, *Natrum mur* often has difficulties with memory, irritability, and depression which is quite similar to *Sepia*. There is frequently an associated anaemia with yellowish skin, moderate to mild emaciation, and a desire for salt and acidic. foods.

One interesting case of chronic herpes labialis occurred in an 18-year old girl who had eruptions associated with fever and chills about every 2-4 months for about two years. She had many of the constitutional symptoms of *Natrum mur*, such as chronic grief because of boy-friend and family problems; also there was a pronounced desire for salty and spicy foods. She was given *Natrum mur* 200 in May 1979 which caused a slight aggravation of her herpes followed by only one minor case since that time.

Mercurius vivus is another frequently indicated medicine for HSV especially involving the male, and less so, the female genitalia. In *Kent's Repertory* it is in italics for herpes affecting the face, but not present for herpes labialis. It is also in italics in male genitalia and common print for female genitalia. Mental — emotional, there is a weakened memory and at times a feeling as if 'I am losing my reason'. In general there is a tendency to free perspiration and sensitivity to both cold and heat.

A 43-year old man was seen in April 1977 with 4-5 year history of recurrent herpetic lesions of the glans penis occurring every 2-3 months. There was no strong mental picture but there was a tendency to free perspiration and sensitivity to cold and heat. He was given *Merc Viv* 1M. Without any definite aggravation, the patient had two minor eruptions over the next three months and no more lesions have been reported since that time.

Another case of probable *Merc viv* was a 28 year old woman seen in January 1980 with primary herpetic eruptions in the vagina and external genitalia for three days. There was an excessive amount of foul smelling perspiration with a subsequent pruritic ulceration. her RPR was negative. There was no strong mental or emotional picture, so *Merc viv* 30C was given on the physical symptomatology.

There was quick improvement of the pain and itching with a disappearance of lesions in about five days. This, of course, is not a dramatic improvement from the normal course, but the patient had relief and had no recurrence reported since that time.

There are many other medicines which should be considered, but cannot be done in much detail in this small article. Some of these are mentioned by Douglass in his book, *Skin Diseases*.

Aconite : In the earlier stages with catarrhal fever.

Apis Mel : Large confluent vesicles; burning, stinging pains; vesicular eruptions on the lips; cold sores.

Ars. Alb. : Red herpetic skin around the mouth, with burning, worse from scratching and after midnight. Herpes iris.

Clematis : Itching blisters on the lower lip. Gnawing itching not relieved by scratching. Worse during increasing moon, better during decreasing moon.

Graphites : Herpes in females with scanty menstruation; burning blisters on the lower side and tip of the tongue; dryness of the skin.

Hepar : Herpes which tend to recur; on the prepuce, exceedingly sensitive to the touch; small ulcers form around the large one; unhealthy suppurating skin, after mercurial poisoning.

Petroleum : Herpes on the perineum and genitals; itching worse in the open air.

Rhus Tox : Herpes upon the hairy parts with burning and stinging; itching worse after scratching; rheumatic pains with great weariness.

Sulphur : Herpes about the mouth and nose with itching and burning, aggravated by warmth. Hot palms and soles.

HERPES

Acon, Acet-ac, Aethiops, Agar, Alnus, All-s, Alum, Ambr, Am-c, Anac, Anan, Anthrak, Apis, Arn, Ars, Ars-i, Aster, Aur, Bacill, Bar-c, Bar-m, Bell, Berb, Bor, Bov, Bry, Bufo, Cadm, Calad, Calc, Calc-s, Canth, Caps, Carb-an, Carb-s, Carb-v, Caust, Chel, Chrysarob, Cic, Cist, Clem, Cocc, Cod, Com, Con, Crot-h, Crot-t, Cupr, Cycl, Dol, Dulc, Eucal, Fl-ac, Graph, Grat, Hell, Hep, Hyos, Iod, Iris, Kali-ar, Kali-bi, Kali-c, Kali-chl, Kali-i, Kali-n, Kali-p, Kali-s, Kalm, Kreos, Lac-c, Lach, Led, Lith-c, Lyc, Mag-c, Mag-m, Manc, Mang, Mar, Merc, Mez, Mosch, Mur-ac, Nat-a, Nat-c, Nat-m, Nat-p, Nat-s, Nit-ac, Nux-v, Olnd, Op, Par, Petr, Ph-ac, Phos, Plb, Psor, Puls, Ran-b, Ran-s, Rob, Rhus-t, Rumx, Ruta, Sabad, Sars, Scil, Sep, Sit, Spig, Spong, Squil, Stann, Staph, Sulph, Sul-ac, Tarax, Tell, Teucr, Thuj, Valer, Variol, Valer, Viol-t, Xerophyl, Zinc.

Alternating chest affections and dysenteric stools — *Rhus-t.*
Barber's itch — *Nat-m, Nat-s.*
Biting itching — *Psor*
Bleeding — *Aeth, Anac, Dulc, Lyc.*
Blotches red after scratching — *Ipec.*
Body all over — *Dulc, Psor, Ran-b.*
Branlike — *Psor*
Brown thick, red border — *Dulc*
Burning — *Amb, Anac, Ars, Calc, Con, Kali-c.*
Burning after scratching — *Staph*
Burning when touched — *Merc*
Burning — *Agar, Alum, Ambr, Am-c, Anac, Ars, Aur, Bar-c, Bell, Bor, Bry, Calad, Calc, Caps, Carb-an, Carb-v, Caust, Cic, Clem, Cocc, Con, Dulc, Hell, Hep, Kali-c, Kali-n, Kreos, Lach,*

Led, Lyc, Mang, Merc, Mez, Nat-c, Nat-m, Olnd, Par, Petr, Ph-ac, Phos, Plb , Psor, Puls, Ran-b, Rhus-t, Sabad, Sars, Sep, Sil, Spig, Spong, Squil, Staph, Stram, Sulph, Teucr, Thuj, Verat, Viol-t, Zinc.

Burning excessive — *Mosch*

Chapping — *Alum, Aur, Bry, Cadm, Calc, Cycl, Graph, Hep, Kali-c, Kreos, Lach, Lyc, Mag-c, Mang, Merc, Nat-c, Nat-m, Nit-ac, Petr, Puls, Rhus-t, Ruta, Sars, Sep, Sil, Sulph, Viol-t, Zinc.*

Chronic — *Agnus, Anthrak, Clem.*

Chronic : constitutional — *Clem*

Chronic, with nightly twitching — *Staph*

Circinatus : suppressed — *Ars.*

Circinate — *Anac, Anag, Ars-s-fl, Bar-c, Calc, Chlora Chrysar, Clem, Dulc, Equis-a, Eup-per, Graph, Hell, Hep, Iod Mag-c, Nat-c, Nat-m, Phos, Phyt, Sep, Spong, Sulph, Tell, Thuj, Tub.*

— in isolated spots — *Sep*

Circinatus on back — *All sat*

— spring every — *Sep*

Circinatus pustular — *Hippoz*

Circinatus on single parts — *Tell*

Clusters in — *Dulc*

Circumscriptus — *Anthrak*

Constipation with — *Carbol ac*

Cracking — *Cadm-s*

Corroding — *Anac, Con.*

Cold water agg — *Clem, Dulc, Sulph.*

Corrosive — *Alum, Am-c, Bar-c, Calc, Carb-v, Caust, Chel, Clem, Con, Graph, Hell, Hep, Kali-c, Lach, Lyc, Mag-c, Mang, Merc, Mur-ac, Nat-c, Nit-ac, Nux-v, Olnd, Par, Petr, Ph-ac, Phos, Plb, Rhus-t, Sep, Sil, Squil, Staph, Sulph, Tarax, Viol-t.*

Crusty — *Alum, Ambr, Am-c, Anac, Ars, Aur, Aur-m, Bar-c, Bell, Bov, Bry, Calc, Caps, Carb-an, Carb-v, Cic, Clem, Con, Cupr, Dulc, Graph, Hell, Hep, Kali-c, Kreos, Lach, Led, Lyc, Mag-c, Merc, Mez, Mur-ac, nat-m, Nit-ac, Nux-v, Olnd, Par, Petr, Ph-ac, Phos, Plb, Puls, Ran-b, Rhus-t, Sars, Sep, Sil, Squil, Staph, Sulph, Thuj, Verat, Viol-t, Zinc.*

Crusty, itching, burning — *Rhus*

Thick crusts — *Clem, Lyc, Sulph.*

Dry — *Alum, Anac, Ars, Bar-c, Bov, Bry, Cact, Calc, Carb-v, Caust, Clem, Cocc, Cupr, Dol, Dulc, Fl-ac, Graph, Hep, Hyos, Kali-i,*

Kreos, Led, Lyc, Mang, Mag-c, Med, Merc, Nat-c, Nat-m, Nit-ac, Par, Petr, Phos, Ph-ac, Psor, Rhus-t, Sars, Sep, Sil, Stann, Staph, Sulph, Teucr, Thuj, Valer, Verat, Viol-t, Zinc.

Dry especially in bends of knees — *Psor*
Dry over whole body — *Zinc*
Dry violently itching, burning in open air — *Led*
Dry with scabs on joints — *Staph*
Dry with white scales on and behind ears — *Mar-v*
Dry, scaly, without itching — *Cact*
Dyscrasia — *Carb-s*
Excoriating — *Caps, Clem, Grat, Nat-m.*
Worse evening and in open air, better by warmth — *Kreos*
Fevers in — *Carb-v, Nat-m, Rhus-t.*
Exudate — *Sil*
Exedens, acrid purulent fluid — *Clem*
Exedens of lupus — *Kali-bi*
Exuding sticky matter — *Graph*
Favinosus all over body except head — *Bar-m*
Furfuraceous — *Calc, Dulc, Merc-s, Mur-ac, Phos.*
Glands covered with — *Dulc, Graph.*
Glandular swelling with — *Dulc*
Gray — *Ars*
Heat worse from, which causes burning — *Con.*
Impetiginous — *Ars, Bapt, Cinch, Merc, Psor, Rhus-t.*
Indent — *Lyc, Mag-c, Psor.*
Itching, burning — *Ars, Psor.*
Itching, burning, after scratching — *Lac-def*
Itching, crusty — *Thuja*
Itching in hollows of knees — *Ars*
Itching of old, at time of menses — *Carb-v*
Itching pain — *Nit-ac*
Itching prevents sleep till late — *Staph*
Itching from warmth of bed and after washing — *Clem*
Itching — *Agar, Alum, Ambr, Am-c, Anac, Ant-t, Ars, Bar-c, Bell, Bor, Bry, Calad, Calc, Caps, Carb-an, Carb-s, Carb-v, Caust, Chel , Cic, Clem, Cocc, Con, Cupr, Dulc, Elaps, Graph, Guarea, Hep, Jug-r, Kali-c, Kali-i, Kreos, Lach, Led, Lyc, Mag-c, Mag-m, Mang. Merc, Mez, Nat-c, Nat-m, Nit-ac, Nux-v, Olnd, Par, Petr, Ph-ac, Phos, Plb, Puls, Ran-b, Ran-s, Rhus-t, Sabad, Sars, Sep, Sil, Spig, Spong, Squil, Stann, Staph, Sulph, Tarax, Thuj, Valer, Verat, Viol-t, Zinc.*

Jerking pain with — *Calc, Caust, Cupr, Lyc, Puls, Rhus-t, Sep, Sil, Staph.*

Jerking and itching burning — *Rhus*

— with mealdust, humid — *Psor*

Ear — *Am-m, Caust, Cist, Graph, Kreos, Mag-m, Olnd, Phos, Sep, Teucr.*

— behind ear — *Am-m*

— lobule on — *Mar*

Face — *Agar, Alum, Am-c, Am-m, Anac, Anan, Apis, Ars, Bar-c, Bell, Bov, Bry, Bufo, Calc, Calc-f, Calc-s, Caps, Carb-an, Carb-s, Carb-v, Caust, Chel, Cic, Clem, Colo, Con, Crot-t, Dulc, Elaps, Graph, Hep, Kali-ar, Kali-bi, Kali-c, Kali-i, Kali-s, Kreos, Lach, Led, Limulus, Lyc, Merc, Nat-a, Nat-c, Nat-m, Nat-s, Nicc, Nit-ac, Petr, Ph-ac, Phos, Psor, Ran-b, Rhus-t, Sabad, Sars, Sep, Sil, Spong, Sulph, Tarent, Thuj.*

Cracks with oozing — *Lach*

Circinatus — *Anag, Bar-c, Calc, Cinnb, Clem, Dulc, Graph, Hell, Kali-chl, Kali-m, Lith, Lyc, Nat-c, Nat-m, Phos, Puls, Sep, Sulph, Tarent, Tell, Tub.*

Dry scaly burning in open air — *Led*

Humid — *Hep*

Itching — *Kali-i*

Moist and spreading — *Con*

Extending to side of neck — *Psor*

Mealy — *Ars, Bry, Cic, Kreos, Lyc, Merc, Nit-ac, Sulph, Thuj.*

Scaby — *Colo, Phos.*

Scurfy — *Anac, Anan, Calc, Graph, Kreos, Led, Lyc, Phos, Rhus-t, Sarrac, Sep, Sulph.*

Spots — *Kali-c.*

Reappearance of suppressed — *Lach.*

Cheeks — *Ambr, Alum, Am-c, Anac, Ant-t, Bar-c, Bov, Bry, Caust, Chel, Con, Dulc, Graph, Hep, Kali-i, Kreos, Lach, Merc, Nat-m, Nicc, Ph-ac, Sars, Sil, Spong, Staph, Stront, Thuj.*

- on right cheek with disposition to break out on left — *Lyc.*

— size of a dime on cheek — *Kali-i*

Chin — *Ars, Am-c, Bov, Carb-v, Caust, Chel, Dulc, Graph, Mez, Nat-m, Nux-v, Ph-ac, Sars, Sil.*

Forehead — *Bad, Bar-c, Bov, Caps, Dulc, Tarent.*

Lips about — *Agar, Anac, Ars, Asc-t, Bov, Brom, Calc-f, Canth, Carb-v, Caust, Chel, Crot-t, Dulc, Graph, Hep, Ip, Kali-p, Lac-c, Lach, Med, Nat-a, Nat-c, Nat-m, Nicc, Par, Ph-ac, Rhus-t, Sars, Sep, Sil, Spong, Sulph, Tub, Urt-u.*

Upper — *Agar, Sars*
White scaly near upper lip — *Anac.*
Cold sores, herpes, hydroa — *Agar, Ars, Calc-f, Caps, Dulc, Frax-am, Hep, Med, Nat-m, Rhus-t, Rhus-v, Sep, Sul-i, Upas.*
Mouth around — *Am-c, Anac, Ars, Bor, Cic, Con, Hep, Kreos, Mag-c, Med, Nat-c, Nat-m, Par, Phos, Rhus-t, Sep, Sulph.*
— below — *Calc-f, Nat-m.*
Nose — *Aeth, Aloe, Aur, Calc, Chel, Graph, Grin , Iod, Lyc, Nat-c, Nat-m, Nit-ac, Ph-ac, Rhus-t, Sep, Sil, Spig, Sulph.*
— across nose — *Sep, Sulph.*
Old reddish, with thick scurf in region of whiskers — *Lach.*
Whiskers — *Agar, Calc, Lach, Nat-m, Nit-ac, Sil.*
Wing of nose — *Nit-ac*
Temples — *Alum*
Tonsorans — *Calc, Cic, Graph, Sep, Sulph-i.*
Tongue, on — *Nat-m, Zinc.*
Mouth, Ulcers herpetic — *Ars-s-f*
External throat — *Lac-d, Psor, Sars, Sep.*
Abdomen — *Sep.*
Zona — *Ars, Graph, Merc, Rhus-t. Sulph, Thuj.*
Across abdomen from right side — *Merc*
Right side — *Iris*
Warmth of bed agg — *Merc*
Iliac region — *Tell*
Inguinal region — *Graph*
Rectum — *Berb, Graph, Ipec, Lyc, Nat-m, Petr.*
Perineum — *Kali-c, Petr, Tell.*
Genitalia — *Anac, Aur-m, Calc, Caust, Crot-h, Crot-t, Dulc, Graph, Hep, Jug-r, Merc, Nat-m, Nit-ac, Petr, Ph-ac, Sars, Sep, Sil, Tell, Tereb.*
— between thighs — *Nat-m, Petr.*
Scrotum — *Dulc, Petr.*
Female genitalia — *Bufo, Carb-v, Caust, Cench, Dulc, Kali-c, Kreos, Merc, Nat-m, Nux-v, Petr, Sep, Thuj.*
— from every cold — *Dulc*
Chest — *Ars, Graph, Hep, Lyc, Mag-c, Petr, Staph, Syph.*
Zona — *Graph, Lach, Mez, Rhus-t.*
Zoster, on left side of chest — *Graph*
— on chest, nape of neck — *Nat-m, Petr.*
— mammae — *Dulc*
Back — *All-s, Ars, Lach, Nat-c, Sep, Zinc.*

Zoster — *Cist, Lach, Merc, Rhus-t.*
Zoster like a girdle from back around abdomen — *Merc*
Zoster from spine around left side to median line — *Hep*
  — dry — *Sep*
Nape — *Caust, Hyos.*
Extremities — *Dulc, Kreos, Staph.*
Herpes — *Alum, Bor, Caust, Com, Con, Cupr, Dulc, Graph, Led, Lyc, Manc, Mang, Merc, Mur-ac, Nat-m, Nicc, Nux-v, Petr, Psor, Sars, Sec, Sep, Staph, Thuj, Zinc.*
Upper limbs — *Alum, Bor, Bov, Calc, Caust, Con, Cupr, Dol, Dulc, Graph, Kali-c, Kreos, Lyc, Mag-s, Manc, Mang, Merc, Nat-c, Nat-m, Nux-v, Phos, Psor, San, Sec, Sep, Sil.*
Crusty — *Con, Thuj.*
Furfuraceous — *Merc, Phos.*
Joints on the — *Calc, Merc.*
Shoulder — *Kali-ar*
Upper arm — *Kali-c, Mang, Nat-m, Sulph.*
Elbow — *Bov, Cact, Cupr, Hep, Kreos, Phos, Psor, Sep, Staph, Thuj.*
Ringworm — *Cupr*
Bend of elbow — *Cupr, Graph, Kreos, Nat-m, Sep, Thuj.*
Forearm — *Alum, Con, Mang, Mag-s, Marc, Nat-m, Sulph.*
Wrist — *Jug-ac, Mez, Psor.*
Hand — *Bor, Bov, Calc, Cist, Con, Dulc, Graph, Kreos, Linul, Lith, Merc, Mez, Nat-c, Nat-m, Nit-ac, Ran-b, Sars, Sep, Staph, Verat, Zinc.*
  — back of — *Carb-s, Graph, Lyc, Nat-c, Petr, Sep, Thuj.*
  — palm — *Aur, Kreops, Psor, Ran-b, Sep.*
  — between the fingers — *Ambr, Graph, Merc, Nit-ac.*
  — between Index finger and thumb — *Ambr*
Fingers — *Ambr, Caust, Cist, Graph, Kreos, Merc, Nit-ac, Psor, Ran-b, Thuj, Zinc.*
White, Scabby on dorsum of hand and fingers — *Thuj*
Lower limbs — *Alum, Bov, Caust, Clem, Com, Graph, Kali-c, Lach, Led, Lyc, Merc, Mur-ac, Nat-m, Nicc, Petr, Sars, Sep, Sil, Staph, Tell, Zinc.*
Nates — *Bor, Caust, Kreos, Nat-c, Nicc.*
Hip — *Nat-c, Nicc, Sep.*
Thigh — *Clem, Graph, Kali-c, Lyc, Merc, Mur-ac, Nat-m, Nit-ac, Petr, Sars, Sep, Staph, Zinc.*

Itching — *Agar, Carb-v, Fago, Merc, Nat-m, Sep, Til.*

Knee — *Ars, Carb-v, Dulc, Graph, Kreos, Merc, Nat-c, Nat-m, Petr, Phos, Sulph.*

Flexures of knees — *Graph, Hep, Nat-m, Sep, Xero.*

Hollow of — *Ars, Calc, Con, Graph, Kreos, Led, Nat-c, Nat-m, Petr, Phos, Psor, Sulph.*

Leg — *Ars, Calc, Calc-p, Con, Graph, Kali-c, Lach, Lyc, Lyss, Mag-c, Merc, Nat-m, Petr, Sars, Sep, Staph, Zinc.*

Calf — *Cycl, Lyc, Sars.*

Ankle — *Cact, Cycl, Kreos, Nat-c, Nat-m, Petr, Sulph.*

Foot — *Alum, Mez, Nat-m, Petr, Sulph.*

Toes — *Alum*

Toes between — *Alum, Graph.*

Ulcers : herpetic — *Sars*

Mealy — *Am-c, Ars, Aur, Bov, Bry, Calc, Cic, Culx, Graph, Kreos, Led, Lyc, Merc, Mur-ac, Phos, Sep, Sil, Sulph, Thuj, Verat.*

Mercurial — *Aur, Mosch, Nit-ac.*

Moist — *Alum, Am-c, Anan, Ars, Bar-ac, Bell, Bov, Bry, Cact, Cadm, Calc, Carb-an, Carb-v, Caust, Cic, Cist, Clem, Con, Dulc, Graph, Grat, Hell, Hep, Kali-c, Kreos, Lach, Led, Lyc, Merc, Mez, Nat-c, Nat-m, Nit-ac, Olnd, Petr, Ph-ac, Phos, Psor, Ran-b, Rhus-t, Ruta, Sep, Sil, Squil,, Staph, Sulph, Sul-ac, Tarax, Tell, Thuj, Viol-t.*

Moist, red — *Clem*

Moist with large scales on edges — *Merc*

Old, tettery itch, when menses should appear — *Carb-v*

Moist after scratching — *Kali-c*

Neuralgia after — *Kalm, Mez, Ran-b, Still, Variol.*

Preceding neuralgia costalis — *Ran-b*

Painful, small, red, scaling off — *Mag-c*

Patches — *Anat-c, Caust, Con, Crot-h, Graph, Hyos, Lyc, Merc, Mur-ac, Nat-c, Nat-m, Nit-ac, Petr, Phos, Sabad, Sars, Sep, Sil, Sulph, Zinc.*

— brown — *Sep*

Phlyctenoides — *Acon, Ars, Bov, Calc, Canth, Carb-s, Clem, Merc, Phos, Ran-s , Rhus-t, Sar, Sil, Sulph, Tell.*

Phlyctenoides over dorsal surface of hand — *Carb-s*

Prickling — *Nit-ac*

Pale - red — *Dulc*

Pimples or pustules surrounding, spreads by coalescing — *Hep*

Red — *An-c, Ars, Bry, Cic, Clem, Dulc, Kreos, Lach, Led, Lyc, Mag-c, Mag-s, Merc, Olnd, Petr, Ph-ac, Staph, Tax, Tell.*

Round, scaly, small — *Dulc*
Scabby — *Sulph*
— forming scabs as large as hand — *Con*
Scaly — *Agar, Anac, Anan, Ars, Aur, Bell, Bov, Cact, Cadm, Calc, Cic, Clem, Con, Cupr, Dulc, Graph, Hep, Hyos, Kali-c, Kreos, Lach, Led, Lyc, Mag-c, Merc, Nat-m, Olnd, Ph-ac, Phos, Plb, Psor, Ran-b, Rhus-t, Sep, Sil, Staph. Sulph, Teucr, Thuj.*
— white — *Anac, Ars, Graph, Lyc, Thuj, Zinc.*
— dry mealy — *Ars, Calc, Dulc, Lyc, Sep, Sil, Thuj.*
— yellow scabs — *Cub*
Scaly, furfuraceous, yellow at base — *Lyc*
Fish scales, burning, worse at night — *Ars*
Scarlet, shining under, worse scratching, odour, offensive — *Lach*
Minged with scorbutic spots over whole body — *Merc-c*
Spreading — *Alum, Caps, Carb-s, Dulc, Merc.*
Scrofulous persons in after a cold, with dry croupy cough — *Spong*
Scurfy — *Sulph*
Scurfy, itching — *Lyc*
Sero-purulent, itching violent towards evening — *Kreos*
Spring every — *Sep*
Sore pain — *Nit-ac*
Spots — *Hyos, Kali-c.*
Spots, inflammation and suppuration — *Ferr*
— round spots — *Nat-m*
Spots, white scaling — *Anac*
Spreading — *Nat-c*
Spring and Fall — *Lach*
Stinging — *Alum, Anac, Ars, Bar-c, Bell, Bry, Calc, Caps, Carb-v, Caust, Clem, Cocc, Con, Cycl, Graph, Hell, Hep, Kali-c, Kreos, Led, Lyc, Mag-c, Mez, Mur-ac, Nat-c, Nat-m, Nit-ac, Nux-v, Petr, Phos, Puls, Ran-b, Ran-s, Rhus-t, Sabad, Sep, Sil, Spong, Squil, Staph, Sulph, Thuj, Viol-t, Zinc.*
Suppressed (Palpitation) — *Ars*
Suppressed — *Alum, Ambr, Calc, Lach, Lyc, Nat-c, Sep, Sulph.*
Suppurating — *Ars, Bell, Cadm, Cic, Clem, Cocc, Con, Cycl, Dulc, Hep, Jug-c, Led, Lyc, Mag-c, Merc, Nat-c, Nat-m, Petr, Plb, Puls, Rhus-t, Sars, Sep, Sit, Spig, Staph, Sulph, Tarax, Thuj, Verat, Viol-t, Zinc.*
Suppurating, lancinating — *Zinc*
Suppurating, yellow — *Dulc*

— with Fetid sweat — *Dulc*
Syphilitic — *Osm*
Secondary Syphilis — *Lyc, Syph.*
— hypertrophy of testicle — *Bar-m*
Tearing — *Ars, Bell, Bry, Calc, Carb-v, Caust, Clem, Cocc, Dulc, Graph, Kali-c, Lyc, Merc, Mez, Nat-c, Nit-ac, Nux-v, Phos, Puls, Rhus-t, Sep, Sil, Staph, Sulph, Zinc.*
Venereal — *Mosch*
— first vesicular then pustular, surface red and swollen, around margin of each patch after external application of Rhus — *Lach*
Washing after - red and smooth — *Bry*
Whitish — *Anac, Thuj, Zinc.*
White, Scabby, on dorsum of hand and fingers — *Thuj.*
Yellowish — *Agar, Ars, Carb-s, Cic, Cocc, Cupr, Dulc, Hell, Kreos, Led, Lyc, Merc, Nat-c, Nit-ac, Par, Sep, Sulph.*
Yellow with brown scabs — *Carb-s*
— brown — *Carb-s, Cupr, Dulc, Lyc, Nat-c.*
— resembles zona — *Dol*
Zoster, zona — *Agar, Apis, Arg-n, Arn, Ars, Aster, Bry, Bufo, Canth, Carb-s, Caust, Cedr, Cham, Cist, Clem, Com, Crot-h, Crot-t, Dol, Dulc, Euph, Graph, Grind, Hep, Hyper, Iod, Iris, Kali-ars, Kali-bi, Kali-chl, Kali-i, Kali-m, Kalm, Lach, Merc, Mez, Merph, Nat-c, Nat-m, Petr, Phyt, Pip-m, Prun, Puls, Ran-b, Ran-s, Rhus-t, Sal-ac, Sel, Semperv-t, Sep, Sil, Staph, Strych-Ars, Sulph, Thuj, Variol, Zinc, Zinc-p, Zinc-v.*
Chronic — *Ars, Semperv-t.*
Zoster burning — *Graph, Mez.*
Zoster burning with gastric disturbance — *Merc*
Zoster burning and neuralgic pains — *Rhus*
Zoster, itching — *Merc.*
Zoster, neuralgia — *Ars, Dol, Kalm, Hep, Mez, Ran-b, Still, Zinc.*
Zoster with facial neuralgia — *Kalm*
Zoster intercostal neuralgia following — *Mez*
Zoster on lt side of body — *Iris*
Zoster tendency to suppurate — *Merc*
Zoster stitching — *Ran-b*
Head, eruption, herpes — *Agar, Alu, Anan, Bad, Bar-c, Caps, Cupr, Graph, Kali-c, Lyc, Mag-c, Mag-m, Petr, Psor, Ran-b, Rhus-t, Thuj.*
Circinatus — *Calc, Dulc, Phyt, Sep, Tell, Tub.*
Occiput — *Arg-n, Petr.*

Temples — Alum, Cadm, Psor.
Eyes — *Alum, Bry, Caust, Con, Kreos, Lach, Olnd, Spong, Sulph.*
Cornea — *Graph, Hep, Ign.*
Eyelids — *Bry, Rhus-t, Sep.*

CHAPTER 9

Dermatitis And Eczema

Introduction

Dermatitis and eczema are a common problem all over the world. Their incidence is 2-3 per cent of all medical problems seen in practice (about 30 per cent of all the dermatoses).

In the practice of dermatology, the first step is to establish the clinical diagnosis of dermatitis and eczema. Then decide the clinico-morphological pattern, viz. Contact, Atopic, Neurodermatitis, Gravitational Endogenous or Seborrhoeic. The final and most important step is to make an etiological diagnosis i.e. establishing the role of the different causes or cause responsible for the dermatitis.

Definition: Dermtitis and eczema are non-contagious inflammation of the skin, characterized by erythema, scaling, oedema, vesiculation and oozing. Dermatitis literally means inflammation of the skin and as such can include all inflammations of the skin except by specific infections. The term 'Eczema' is a Greek word (Ec : means out, and zeo means boil). The whole word implies 'boil out'. The Hindustani name for eczema is *chambal*. Eczema is a specific type of allergic cutaneous manifestation of antigen-antibody reaction. It is characterized by superficial inflammatory oedema of the epidermis associated with vesicle formation.

Itching varies from mild to severe paroxysms which may even interfere with work and sleep. The natural history of eczema is diagrammatically represented as follows :

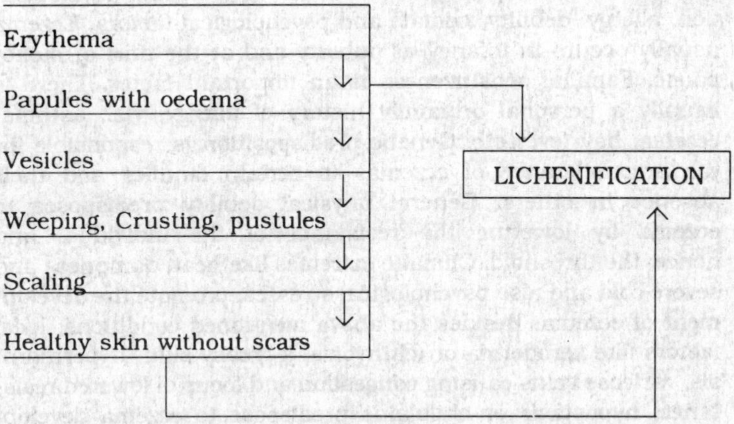

The morpho-clinical classification into acute, sub-acute, and chronic stages, helps us to decide about the prognosis and line of symptomatic treatment. The acute stage is characterized by itchy erythema followed by oedema, papules, vesicles, oozing and crusting. Most of the typical eczemas of moderate intensity start with these morphological features. This stage does not last long. In about a couple of weeks the lesions start to heal. If the cause persists, and the eczema lasts over months or years, it becomes chronic. In such cases, the integument appears thickened and pigmented with prominent criss-cross markings (Lichenification). This is the end result of all types of long standing eczemas. In between the acute and chronic stages, is the sub-acute stage, characterized by papules and scaling with moderate oedema and erythema. Acute eczema may pass through this stage before it heals completely or becomes chronic.

Histopathology : Characteristic features are intercellular oedema (spongiosis) and vesicle formation. There may be mild to moderate dermal reaction. In chronic cases, hyperkeratosis, acanthosis and infiltration of upper dermis with lymphocytes are seen.

Etiology : Basically, two factors cause dermatitis and eczema. Firstly, an allergic or a sensitive skin; and secondly, exposure to an allergen or an irritant. Darier had correctly said that, "there is no eczema but an eczematous patient."

The general predisposing causes are : Age, familial predisposition, allergy, debility, climate and psychological factors. Eczema usually occurs in infancy, at puberty and at the time of menopause. Familial sensitiveness is an important factor. There is usually a personal or family history of allergy, viz., asthma, eczema, hay fever, etc. Genetic predisposition is responsible for the preponderance of eczemas in certain families and their absence in others. General physical debility predisposes to eczema by lowering the resistance of the individual and hence, the threshold. Climatic extremes like heat, dampness and severe cold and also psychological stresses, promote the development of eczema. Besides the above mentioned conditions, local factors like xeroderma or ichthyosis, a greasy skin, hyperhidrosis, varicose veins causing congestion and focus of lowered resistance, hypostasis or chilblains predispose to eczema development. In the dry winters of Northern India, cracking of the integument of exposed parts may result in eczematization — "Eczema crackle."

There is no eczema but an eczematous patient. Establish the cause/causative factors. While managing eczema, treat the patient and respect the skin.

It is still controversial whether the endogenous factors like diet, emotional strain and stress, focal sepsis, state of digestion, nutrition and metabolism, etc., are more important than exogenous factors like infections, irritants and sensitizers or vice versa.

In practice, mixed eczemas are much more common than pure entities. History and clinicial observation are helpful in establishing the exact etiological diagnosis. The case of an eczematous patient, therefore, must be studied from all angles, attention being given to multiple precipitating, exciting and aggravating factors which may be summarized as follows :

1. Irritants — Physical, chemical or electrical.

2. Sensitizers — Plants, cosmetics, clothing, medicaments and occupational hazards.

3. External infections—Streptococci, staphylococci, fungus etc.

4. Mental and emotional conflicts, strains and stresses.

5. Internal septic focus shedding toxins or causing bacteraemia.

6. Diet and state of digestion.

7. Diathesis — Allergic, xerodermic, hyperhidrotic or seborrhoeic.

8. Drugs — given for the disease, or otherwise.

9. State of local or general nutrition.

10. Climate — temperature and humidity.

Eczemas which appear resistant to treatment and do not correspond to the known picture, must make one suspect conditions like reticuloses and drug eruptions.

Immunology
Sensitization develops when a different clone of T-lymphocytes is activated. The sensitized T-lymphocytes yield two subpopulations of lymphocytes, viz., memory cells that are responsible for the persistence of contact allergy, and the effector cells that initiate the allergic response when appropriately challenged.

Reaction time is the time taken by a sensitized individual to manifest a clinical reaction following contact with a known sensitizer. It is usually 12-24 hours but may vary from one hour to 120 hours. The reaction time is inversely proportional to the severity of the allergy.

Dissemination reaction is a fleeting, erythematous, macular reaction, involving the face and flexures, seen in some cases of contact dermatitis. There is some evidence that dissemination reaction is caused by the escape of lymphokines in the circulation resulting in vasodilatation at a distant site.

Flare reaction, another clinical feature of contact dermatitis, reaction or a positive patch test reaction following renewed challenge or exposure to the same allergen at another site. This is because of persistence of sensitized lymphocytes at the site of earlier reaction, which react to minute amounts of antigen that sometimes escape in the circulation from the new site and find its way to the old site.

Photodermatitis

Dermatitis is the condition, confined to the exposed parts of the body,viz., face, neck, 'V' of the chest, hands and external surfaces of the forearms and dorsa of feet and the adjoining parts of legs. Because of different clothing patterns prevalent in India, different parts of the body may be exposed producing different pictures. The integument is sensitive to sunlight and ultra-violet rays. Eruption develops, or becomes aggravated on exposure to light. Seasonal variations are an important consideration, particularly, more so, in countries with extremes of climate.

The common causes of photodermatitis are : (i) drugs like sulphonamides, chlorpromazine, promethazine, declamycin, terramycin, chlorthiazide, diuretic different hypotensive and antidiabetic drugs, quindexin in animal feeding stuff, (ii) foods like figs, buckwheat, (iii) external application of (a) Chemicals like sulphonamides, acridine dyes, tar, soaps containing bithionol, tetrachlorsalicylanilide, etc., (b) plants and their products like parsnips, cow parsnips, meadow grass, mustards, lime oil, psoralea, celery, bur clover, bergamot oil,etc., Vit B Complex deficiency, porphyrinuria, seborrhoeic diathesis and liver disorders predispose to photodermatitis.

Phytophotodermatitis means photo-sensitization of the skin after contact with plants which have either phototoxic or photo allergic action. Clinically the lesions consist of a linear erythematous, bullous rash which heals in a week or two. On healing, pigmentation is left behind which takes several months to disappear. The rash develops after contact with the plant during, or followed by, exposure to sunlight.

Photodermatitis must be differentiated from contact dermatitis due to pollens, particularly congress grass. Both occur on the exposed parts. While the former is seen in winter, the latter is seen at least to begin with, in the pollinating season, in parthenium growing areas. Both get aggravated by exposure to sun, the former more than the latter. In some cases, it is difficult to distinguish the two.

Diagnosis of photodermatitis is based upon : (i) Affection of exposed parts, (ii) Worsening by exposure to sun, (iii) Seasonal variation, (iv) Eruption is followed by hyperpigmentation. Photodermatitis is a clinical diagnosis, and a search should be made to establish the cause.

Contact Dermatitis

Synonym : Chemical eczema

With industrialization and increasing use of chemicals and synthetics, the incidence of contact dermatitis is on the increase everywhere. Contact dermatitis develops within a few hours after contact with the offending agent (allergen to which the patient is potentially hypersensitive). The erutpion develops briskly, spreading far beyond original point of contact. It has an ill-defined margin, fading at the periphery. Brisk oedema and uniform versiculation are the features that dominate the eruption. Distribution depends upon the offending agent. Hence the localization of dermatitis helps in establishing the cause.

An unprejudiced history and patch tests are of considerable help in finding out the exact allergen. Failure to discover the cause results in chronic eczema and lichenification, It has been appropriately said that, especially in the diagnosis of contact dermatitis and eczema, the homoeopath should be a good "detective" with powers of observation and deduction almost like those of Sherlock Holmes. Patch tests may be done to confirm the diagnosis. Contact dermatitis is usually caused by chemical agents in plants, cosmetics, external medicaments, clothing and occupational chemicals. Here are a few important examples from each group :

1. **Plants** : Phytodermatitis is fairly common in practice. Irritant and sensitizing properties of plants have long been known to Indian homoeopaths. Mechanical, chemical and physical irritants should be separated from true sensitizers. Primary irritants set up, on contact dermatitis in the form of redness, blisters or even ulcers. Common examples are marking nut,

cashew nut, euphorbias, buttercups, anemones, delpheniums, mustards, radish, lobelia and podophyllum. Turpentine is also a primary chemical irritant. In allergic contact dermatitis the skin reaction consists of typical eczematous lesions varying from erythema to violent vesiculation, pustulation, oozing and crusting accompanied by marked itching. The sticky sap of plants containing phenolic oily resins or like substances is usually responsible. Handling of bulbs (tulips and hyacinths) causes dryness and fissuring of finger tips.

The plants responsible for sensitization dermatitis are many and the etiological diagnosis can be difficult indeed unless this fact is borne in mind. Contact dermatitis usually occurs on the exposed parts, particularly the face and hands. Well-known examples of such plants : Anacardiaceae (marking nut, cashew nut, mango, rhus, holigarna); Euphorbiaceae (blinding tree, castor oil plant, puring nut, euphorbias); Asclikiadaceae (Ak), Compositae (ragweed, chrysanthemums); Primulaceas (Primulaceae primulas); Liliaceae (tulip); Amaryllidaceae (daffodil, narcissus); celery, hops, peel of oranges and lemons; garlic and onions; chewing of plants like buttercup stalks causes severe cheilitis.

Cutting of vegetables especially garlic, onion, tomatoes, ladies fingers produces dermatitis on the tips of thumb and index fingers of left hand and right thumb. Peeling of oranges affects the thumb and index finger of right hand. The eruption develops briskly, spreading far beyond the original point of contact. It has an ill-defined margin, fading at the periphery.

Sometimes, allergic dermatitis is produced by inhalant allergies from pollens and moulds. Acute recurrences of dermatitis are observed on the head, neck, limbs, and hands which do not correspond to direct external contact; even parts covered by clothes may be affected by inhalant allergies. Occasionally, generalized erythroderma-like picture may be produced.

Common example is congress grass (Air-borne contact Dermatitis)

Dermatitis due apparently to plants, but really due to adventitious factors associated with plants are conveniently labelled pseudo-phyto-dermatitis (Wood). These adventitious factors are parasites, smuts and rusts, insecticides, fertilizers, fungicides (particularly those containing thiuram). Latter is also used in rubber industry and is related to disulfirm — antabuse.

The diagnosis of contact dermatitis due to plants is based on the following criteria : (i) seasonal incidence, (ii) distribution on exposed parts, (iii) eruption, (iv) marked itching and burning sensation after exposure to contact, (v) history of previous attacks of sensitization. Diagnosis is confirmed by patch testing.

2. **Cosmetics** :Incidence of contact dermatitis due to cosmetics is on the increase all over the world, particularly in urban areas. Hair dyes, particularly the derivatives of paraphenylenediamine and 'kumkum' are the common culprits; less so are lipstick, red sandal paste, eau de cologne, powders — particularly medicated or perfumed face cream, nail polish and remover, eye-brow pencil, perfumes, depilatories, deodorants and hair oil. Selective distribution of dermatitis is very typical. Common ingredients in cosmetics responsible for dermatitis are the perfumes, parabens, dyes and anti-microbial agents.

Lipstick dermatitis is confined to the vermilion of the lips, the lower lip more than the upper. The presenting features are swelling and oozing or dryness and cracking. The cause is mainly the eosin dye. Such patients should be recommended a hypo-allergenic lipstick containing some other colouring agents.

Nail polish dermatitis is usually seen on the cheeks, eyelids, and neck because of accidental contact depending upon the individual's habits.

Hair dye and hair oil dermatitis are common problems. Mustard and Brahmi oil (an indigenous herbal preparation) contact dermatitis should be distinguished from oil acne produced by it on the face and scalp. Dermatitis due to oil and dyes is usually severe; it affects the forehead, eyes and ears more than the scalp. A prior patch testing is essential in the prevention of hair dye dermatitis. Dermatitis of the scalp and face may also be seen following the use of shampoos, hair sprays and "wave lotions".

Deodorants and depilatories cause dermatitis in the axillae. Kumkum (Bindi) dermatitis is seen on the forehead. Sindhur (Mercuric sulphide) causes dermatitis on the scalp at the site of parting of the hair. Henna dermatitis is uncommon. Perfumes commonly produce dermatitis behind the ears and upper part of breast. After shave lotions and Eau de Cologne cause dermatitis on the face, neck and hands. Feminine hygiene sprays produce eczematous reaction in the vulval region and groins.

3. **Clothing** : The common offending substances are : Rubber chappals and footwear, spectacle frames, watch straps, furs, suspenders, artificial jewellery, clothes. The basic substances commonly responsible for contact dermatitis are rubber, nickel, dyes, synthetic finishing chemicals, resins etc. The distribution of eczema produced by clothing is typical; a knowledge of regional dermatology is very helpful.

Rubber contact dermatitis is a common problem in practice. Distribution of footwear dermatitis is typical; dorsum of the feet are more involved than the soles. It is not the natural rubber but the additives like T.M.T., M.B.E.H., resins, oil etc., which are responsible for sensitization. Dermatitis is more common in summer than in winter because of increased sweating and the leaching effect of sweat. Rubber is used in footwear particularly Hawai chappals, also in rubber suspenders, condoms, gloves etc.

Incidence of nickel dermatitis is markedly on the increases. Nickel in ear rings, artificial jewellery, suspenders, corsets and brassiere hooks causes nickel sensitization. It takes a long time before dermatitis develops; it may extend beyond the site of contact. Car ignition key is another culprit.

Nylon dermatitis is not so common as tinea and dyshidrosis produced in individuals who wear nylon. Synthetic dyes and resins are potent sensitizers. Nylon hairnets cause dermatitis on the scalp margins, ears and back of the head.

Textile dermatitis is characterized by severe itching and purpuric dermatitis on the body. The trunk is involved in Khaki uniform dermatitis and the legs in trouser or pyjama dermatitis. I have seen cases of dermatitis in children who wear terycot toy horses.

Hands	:	Occupational — primary irritants and sensitisers. Hobbies — gardening, photography, painting etc. Cutting vegetables like garlic, onions, tomatoes, ladies fingers; drivers steering wheel, ignition key, detergents, cigarette paper, etc.
Wrists	:	Watch and its strap, bracelet and bangles.
Thighs	:	Clothing, things in pockets particularly matchboxes, and suspenders (rubber or nickel).
Feet	:	Footwear, shoes (chrome dyes and rubber). The dorsum and sides of the feet are selectively involved, interdigital spaces are spared (comparison, tinea pedis). Coloured socks (dyes and nylon), elastic show strap.

Ten common Allergens come across in practice :

1. Paraphenylene diamine.
2. Nickel sulphate.
3. Potassium dichromate.
4. Parthenium hysterophorus.
5. Nitrofurazone ointment.
6. Neomicin sulphate.
7. Formaldehyde.
8. Turpentine.
9. Garlic.
10. Epoxy resin.

Contact dermatitis sometimes fails to respond to treatment because of certain complicating factors like super-added infections, emotional stresses, focal sepsis, additional sensitizations arising from the patient's hobbies, friction, scratching, etc. An attempt must be made to eliminate these complicating causes too, in addition, to the basic offending agent.

Infectious Eczematoid Dermatitis

Synonym : Infective eczema

This results from sensitization to certain organisms like streptococci, staphylococci, dermatophytes and yeast organisms. Infective eczemas are very common in tropical countries; about three-fourths of hospital eczema cases fit into this category. Clinically, they are characterized by their slow development; so no vesiculation is usually evident, a crust is formed instead. The patch or patches are sharply defined, and there is no erythematous halo; they take the form of circles which by union become polycyclic. The lesions spread not only by direct contiguity but also to the other body folds, parts and hair follicles. These eczemas respond to mild antiseptic astringents. They become notoriously recurrent in some cases. A trivial itch is sufficient to reproduce it; the genetic susceptibility for sensitization seems operative. Infectious eczematoid dermatitis is commoner in the monsoon and summer than in the winter.

Infective eczemas can be divided further into three sub-types according to their distribution :

Post-traumatic Infective Eczema : The history is usually very typical. It starts with a crack in the integrity of the skin brought on by an injury, a blister, an insect bite or exposure to a severe cold wind etc. This gets infected; sensitization results in eczematization and a well-defined circular or oval patch of eczema consisting of erythema, oozing and crusting is formed. If there are several patches, the intervening skin is completely clear. Similarly, prickly heat can become eczematized.

Eczematization, secondary to acute tinea, particularly tinea pedis, is frequently seen. It starts from the interdigital spaces and spreads to the dorsum of the feet or the soles. Treatment has to be skilful; the condition must first be treated like eczema. Only when the eczematization process has been controlled completely, must fungicidal agents be employed.

Follicular Infective Eczema : It involves hairy regions, like the scalp, beard and legs. When it occurs on the scalp, it is often labelled as seborrhoeic dermatitis. It starts, usually with pityriasis capitis which gets complicated by one on several itchy patches of oozing, pits and crusting. These patches become confluent. The eczema spreads to the forehead, retro-auricular folds and cheeks, streptococci, staphylococci and less so, pityrosporon organisms are the causative organisms. If accompanied by seborrhoeic diathesis, both the infective eczema and seborrhoeic background should be treated at the same time. Infective eczematides may develop later, on the back, sternal region, pubic region, arms and legs, if the disease is not properly controlled. On the beard region, it must always be differentiated from ordinary folliculitis. The latter is a chronic disease, spreads slowly, and there is no oozing or itching in contrast with infective eczema. In infants, cradle cap may get complicated by infective or seborrhoeic dermatitis. True constitutional infantile eczema should be excluded in such cases.

Flexural Infective Eczema : The flexures (body folds) are the sites of predilection. Common examples are : the retro-auricular folds, the eyelids, the neck folds, the axillae, the bends of elbows, the groins and the popliteal fossae. It starts with a crack in the depth of the fold, and the two opposing surfaces are equally affected like the leaves of a book. The inner part looks moist and red; only at the periphery crusting is clearly evident. In the groins, it usually complicates simple intertrigo; oozing and crusting are added to the redness and maceration of intertrigo. Tinea cruris can be eliminated by the fact that it affects the inner surfaces of the thighs, but spares the inguinal fold; the peripheral border is most inflammed consisting of vesicles and pustules; the scraping for fungus is positive.

Causative Agents of Occupational Dermatitis

Occupation		*Causative Agents and Dermatitis*
Agriculturists and gardeners.	:	Plants, weeds, insecticides, fertilizers and oils — mechanical injuries and contact dermatitis.
Automobile workers.	:	Oils, petrol, solvents, grease, paints, thinner, acne and dermatitis.
Building workers	:	Cement, lime, insecticides, fungicides, wood, paints, kerosene oil, turpentine oil, etc.
Chemical and Pharmaceutical	:	Different dyes, chemicals, pharmaceuticals, explosives,solvents, oils, disinfectants, detergents etc — contact dermatitis.

Coal miners	: Mechanical injuries.
Dentists	: Cocaine and its derivatives — Contact dermatitis.
Engineering industries	: Cutting oils, solvents, detergents, etc. — oil acne and dermatitis.
Housewives	: Soaps and detergents, vegetables and fruits, nickel, polishes, paraphenylene diamene, keys, kerosene oil, wooden cutlery, flowers, rubber gloves, and sensitisers added to foods like sodium bisulphide in salads, artificial flavours parabens, dyes, fluorescent whitening agents in laundry products.
Nurses and Doctors	: Iodine, Streptomycin, chlorpromazine, sulphonamide, tinct, benzoin, cocaine derivatives — Contact dermatitis.
Painters	: Turpentine, paints, detergents — Contact dermatitis.
Photographers.	: Metol, bichromate — Contact dermatitis.
Plastic factory workers	: Resins, hardeners, solvents, glues, cellulose esters, etc. — Contact dermatitis.
Printers.	: Dyes, acrylic plates and inks causing dermatitis rarely lichenoid rash.
Rubber workers	: M.B.E.H., T.M.T., M.B.T., dyes glues, oils etc., Contact dermatitis and depigmentation.
Tannery workers	: Chromate, formaldehyde, dyes, arsenic, alkalies, acids, etc. — dermatitis and depigmentation.
Tar workers	: Dermatitis and tar acne.
Textile workers	: Formaldehyde, solvents, dyes, bleaches, etc. — Contact dermatitis.

Exfoliative Dermatitis

Synonym : Erythroderma

The above terms imply dermatosis with generalized and universal inflammatory erythema of the skin accompanied by continuous scaling. The skin is thickened and feels hot. The patient becomes extremely sensitive to cold because heat is being continuously lost through the inflammed skin. The hair and nails may fall, Pruritus is constant, hence the patient's movements are restricted. He is extremely uncomfortable and irritable, develops insomnia, grows weak and later, becomes emaciated. Emaciation is brought on by irritability, the loss of heat and loss of proteins through the continuous shedding of scales. Secondary pyoderma, diarrhoea and pneumoia ar the usual complications.

Causes and Classification Based Upon Etiology

(A) **Primary :**

New Born and Infants :

(a) Dermatitis exfoliativa neonatorum (Ritter).
(b) Erythroderma desquamativum (Leiner).
(c) Congenital ichthyosiform erythroderma.

Adults :

(a) Exfoliative dermatitis (Wilson).
(b) Exfoliative dermatitis (Hebra).
(c) Epidemic exfoliative dermatitis (Savill).
(d) Recurrent scarlatiniform erythroderma.

(B) **Secondary**

1. Drugs — arsenic, gold, sulphonamides, butazolidine, brufen, tegretal, anti-tubercular drugs.
2. Reticuloses — mycosis fungoides, leukaemia and Hodgkin's disease.
3. Psoriasis.
4. Pemphigus.
5. Eczema.
6. Pityriasis rubra pilaris.

(3–6: Conditions which may progress into erythroderma)

In practice, secondary erythrodermas are much more common than primary ones and, since the causes can be tackled, the prognosis is generally speaking better.

Dermatitis Exfoliativa Neonatorum (Ritter)

It is a rare exfoliative dermatitis of the new-born. It begins within the first few days of life as a red scaly patch, and soon becomes generalized, spreading rapidly over the entire body to produce erythema and exfoliation; occasionally, vesicles, pustules and bullae may develop. The cutaneous lesions are accompanied by mild to severe constitutional symptoms. The course extends over a few weeks. The outlook is fair in mild cases, but bad in severe ones. The etiology is unknown but the general feeling is, that infection with staphylococcus aureus or drugs used by mother (antenatal or at the time of delivery), may be responsible for the condition.

Erythroderma Desquamativum (Leiner)

It is a rare condition resembling Ritter's dermatitis exfoliativa neonatorum but with the following differences : (1) It starts later, i.e., between 3 to 8 weeks after birth. (2) There is erythema and scaling as in seborrhoeic dermatitis but no vesiculation. (3) The course is protracted. The etiology is unknown. Gastro-enteritis accompanies the disease or precedes it.

Congenital Ichthyosiform Erythroderma

It is a rare heredo-familial, epidermal nevoid condition resembling ichthyosis noticed at birth or some time after. The characteristic features are : (1) Involvement of the whole integument, especially over the flexures (cubital and popliteal fossae, axillae and the neck), the face, the scalp and the palms of the hands. (2) Redness and dryness of the integument. It may be complicated by bullous formation. The condition may or may not improve with puberty. It is considered by some as a severe inflammatory form of ichthyosis vulgaris. Use of drugs during pregnancy may be an exciting or aggravating factor.

Primary Exfoliative Dermatitis (Wilson)

Its etiology is unknown; hence it is called primary or idiopathic. It is a rare disease of middle and old age; males are affected more commonly than females. The onset is subacute in the form of a red, scaly plaque on the trunk which spreads to become generalized in a couple of weeks' time. The whole integument is dry, red, inflammed and thickened, accompanied by exfoliation in the form of large scales. The palms of the hands, the soles of the feet, and the scalp are equally involved; nails and hair may be shed. There is pruritus. The erythrodermic skin feels uncomfortable and restricts the movements of the joints. Constitutional complications like pyoderma, pneumonia and gastro-intestinal upsets may develop and prove fatal. The course extends over months and years, marked by ups and downs; eventually, most cases recover.

Exfoliative Dermatitis (Hebra)

It differs from Wilson's variety in the following respects : (1) The onset is slow and insidious; it takes months, even longer, for the disease to become generalized. (2) It begins in the flexures. (3) The skin is not too greatly thickened; on the contrary, it may become atrophic. (4) The scaling is finer. (5) The course is chronic, and most cases end fatally. Often, it is difficult to distinguish between the two — Wilson and Hebra's primary exfoliative dermatitis.

Epidemic Exfoliative Dermatitis (Savill)

It is a rare kind of erythroderma occurring in an epidermic form. The cause is, presumably, an infection. One such epidemic occurred in London in 1891; a few others have also been reported.

Recurrent Scarlatiniform Erythroderma

It is an uncommon, scarlet fever-like eruption recurring from time to time, and is presumably, caused by toxins from a septic focus or drugs. The constitutional symptoms are mild, and the rash subsides within about four to eight weeks. The eruption consists of bright-red erythema involving the whole integument, especially the trunk, arms and thighs; when desquamation starts within a day or two of the onset of the eruption, the skin peels off in flakes, and the redness begins to subside.

Endogenous Eczemas

There is no evidence of external irritants or allergens in endogenous eczemas; parts of the body become sensitized to internal body products — toxins from focal sepsis, metabolites i.e. products of digestion or elements of diet and drugs — with or without familial predisposition. To this list, should be added psychosomatic influences. In most cases, the cause is hypothetical, big names often boil down to nothing in practical dermatology. For this reason, the treatment of endogenous eczemas is rather unsatisfactory, and will remain so, till more light is shed on their exact etiology and pathogenesis.

There are three common patterns produced according to their distribution. (1) Atopic — involving the eyelids, the sides of neck, the bends of elbows and the popliteal fossae. (2) Nummular pattern affecting the dorsum of fingers and hands, the feet, the arms and the thighs; in short, the extremities. (3) Centripetal pattern affecting the trunk, particularly, the upper chest, the scapular and gluteal regions. Then, there is the sympathetic variety in which the corresponding site on the other extremity is affected through endogenous distribution from a patch of eczema on the extremity. This sympathetic dermatitis is comparable with sympathetic opthalmia seen in eye lesions. Occasionally, unilateral dissemination of eczema from the right foot to the right hand, and the left foot to the left hand is seen. How nature brings about these selective affections and disseminations is difficult to explain. The common sub-varieties of endogenous eczemas are : infantile eczema, atopic eczema, nummular eczema, disseminated eczema and cheiropompholyx.

Infantile Eczema

This occurs in children between the ages of three months and two years. It usually starts on the cheeks, spreading slowly to the forehead, chin, scalp, arms, trunk and legs. On the buttocks and in the groins, napkin rash-like dermatitis may develop. The typical lesions are characterized by erythema, vesicles, exudation, and crusting. Pruritus is a prominent symptom; it comes in spasms. The progress is marked by spontaneous remissions and exacerbations. Teething, digestive upsets, change of season, dietitic indiscretions and tantrums affect the condition adversely, and may even cause flare-ups. To start with, the infants are usually plump. They soon go off food, have restless days and nights resulting in debility, misery and fretfulness. The general belief is that there are two types of infantile eczemas :

1. With high familial predisposition to an allergic disease — the atopic variety. These are rather resistant to

treatment. The infant becomes restless and fatigued, very irritable and pruritic. The condition develops later, into typical atopic dermatitis.

2. Without familial predisposition — the simple variety. The infants are plump and good natured. Itching is moderate. These do well with treatment, and the child recovers completely by the age of two.

Parents must be told that infantile eczemas are not infectious, and they heal completely without scarring unless a secondary infection occurs. Contact eczemas are rare in infancy for two reasons : Firstly, sensitivity is extremely uncommon before puberty, and secondly, chemical contacts are few. But one does see infective or seborrhoeic eczema in infancy (see Table below). This type of eczema starts as scruff or cradle cap on the scalp which develops into slight exudation and thick crusting; eczema spreads from the scalp to the auricular region, the periphery of the face and neck, sparing the centre of the face in comparison with true constitutional infantile eczema. Similarly, infective eczema in infancy may develop as a complication of suppurative otitis media, conjunctivitis, rhinitis or neglected boils and impetigo. The response to mild antiseptics is good in this infective variety.

Distinguishing Features of True Infantile and Seborrhoeic Eczema

Infantile eczema	*Seborrhoeic eczema*
1. Disease develops at 3-6 months after birth, sometimes earlier.	1. Cradle cup at the time of birth, seborrhoeic dermatitis afterwards.
2. Child is irritable and weak.	2. Child is usually healthy and happy otherwise.
3. Starts from cheeks and extends to forearms and legs.	3. Starts from scalp, posterior auricular folds, and involves neck and trunk. On the trunk flat macular erythematous or hypopig-

	mented and scaly rash. In some cases, it manifests as diaper dermatitis.
4. Oozing more areas look clean.	4. Crusting more and the areas have a dirty appearance.
5. Family history of atopic disorders except in simple variety.	5. Family history of seborrhoeic disorders.
6. Itching is severe and spasmodic.	6. Itching, mild to moderate.
7. Recurrences — frequent and usually independent of season.	7. Recurrences mostly seasonal, i.e., summer and monsoon; at times in winter also.
8. On the whole, poor response to treatment.	8. Comparatively better response.

Etiology: The exact causation of infantile eczema is not well-established but the following factors must be kept in mind. Dietetic allergies may play an important role in the causation. Infants who are overfed, and are too rapidly introduced to adult foodstuffs, frequently suffer from infantile eczema. In the author's experience infantile eczema is rather uncommon amongst Indian infants who are fed the conservative way, namely they are given mainly milk only for the first year; eggs, bread, fruit and vegetables being added slowly in second year.

Atopic Eczema

Synonym : Besnier's Prurigo

It is also called Asthma — Eczema Syndrome. There is a strong familial predisposition to allergic diseases like asthma, eczema and hay fever: frequently, a personal history of collateral allergies is present. The eczema is characterized by a selective flexural

CONTACT DERMATITIS TREATED WITH PULSATILLA AND NAT MUR

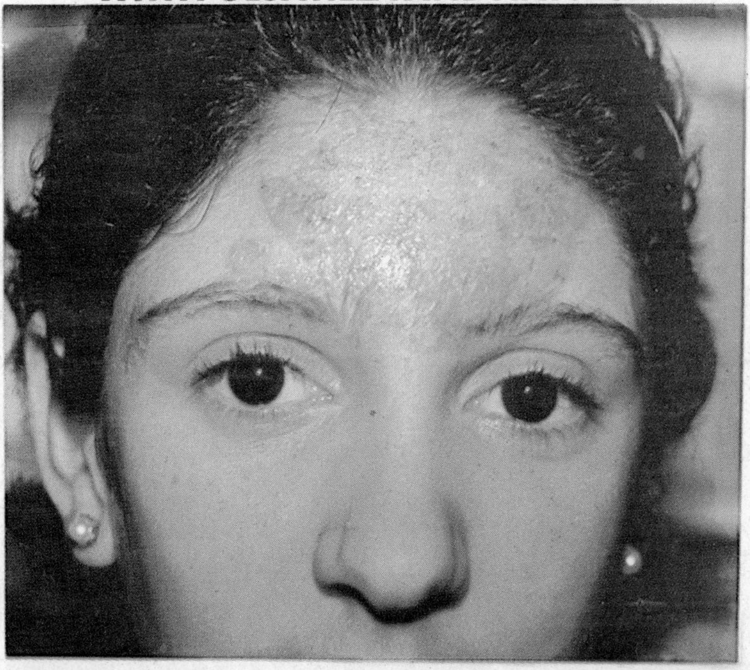

BEFORE

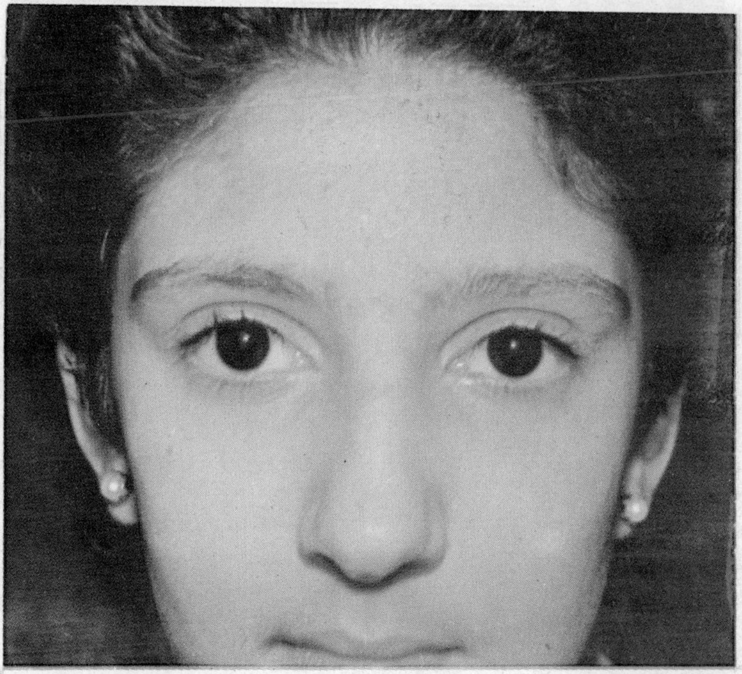

AFTER

ALLERGIC DERMATITIS TREATED WITH GRAPHITES

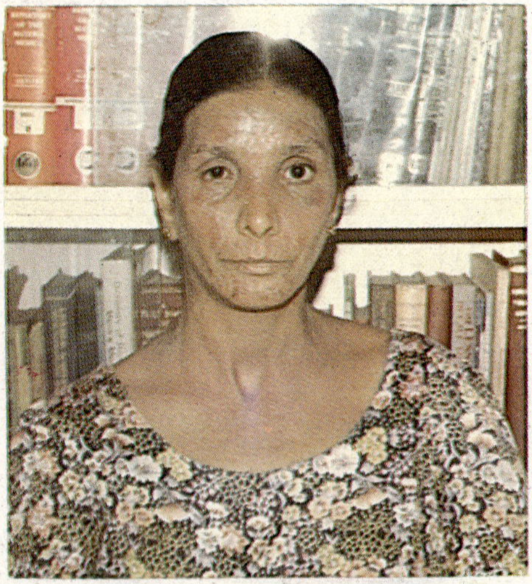

BEFORE

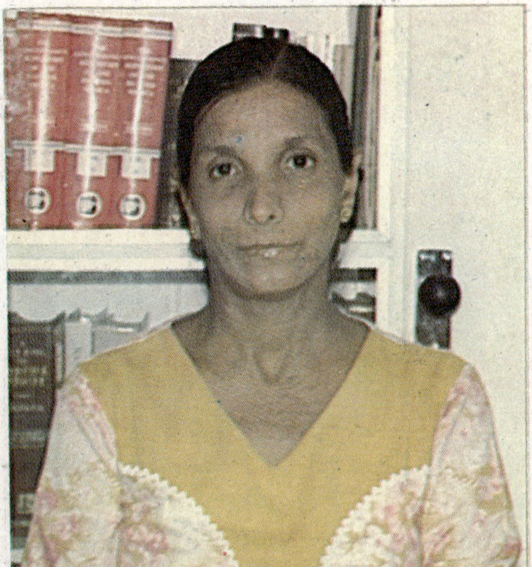

AFTER

distribution, extreme chronicity with acute exacerbations from time to time, a familial and personal allergic predisposition and a very sensitive emotional nature. The eczematous process is usually the result of endogenous sensitization, but exogenous allergies may also play a part. The latter can be proved by patch tests, and the former, by scratch tests, which show allergy to multiple agents. There is more than normal susceptibility to develop passive transfer antibodies in the blood serum (Prausnitz Kustner reaction). Besides allergens, emotional stresses and parental attitudes can also cause this condition. The parents are usually the anxious type, and the patient is usually very sensitive and highly strung but often very intelligent. The atopic patient is also very sensitive to physical stresses like heat, cold and humidity and also infections. There is also vasomotor sensitivity.

Clinical features : They are rather characteristic. The integument is generally dry and rough with a definite tendency to dermographism. The eyelids, the sides of the neck, the popliteal and cubital fossae are the sites predominantly affected. Itching is a predominant symptom; it usually occurs in spasms. Clinically, there are three stages of atopic eczema : (1) Infantile stage, described above. (2) Childhood type, in which the main lesions are lichenoid and succulent, polyhedral papules. The eczema may become generalized on the face, trunk and upper part of the extremities. It starts at about the age of five, either as such, or as a continuation of infantile eczema; this goes on till the age of about twelve. (3) Adult type is marked by ill-defined, lichenoid patches, scratch marks and blood crusts with exacerbations of acute eczema from time to time. The skin is dry and injures easily. This stage is most marked till the age of 25, and may last through life.

There may be associated cataract. Intolerance to high temperatures and humidity is fairly common.

Diagnosis : It is not difficult in a typical case. In an atypical case, differentiation is from lichen simplex chronicus, endogenous dermatitis, seborrhoeic dermatitis and prurigo. In every case, an attempt should be made to establish the specific etiology and assess the personality of the individual.

Prognosis : The course of atopic eczema through all stages is marked by spontaneous cures, remissions and exacerbations. Seasonal variation is autumn and spring, by pollens; summer and monsoons, by heat and high humidity. Besides eczema, asthma, hay fever and other allergies may be present at the same time or may alternate with eczema. Lately attention has been drawn to ophthalmic changes in connection with atopic dermatitis; they are conjunctivitis, keratitis, and juvenile cataracts. The pathogenesis of these is not understood. It may also be associated with other ectodermal defects. There is a constitutional susceptibility to different stresses the blood count shows eosinophilia.

Etiology : In every case, an attempt should be made to discover the cause or causes : (1) Emotional — by psychiatric evaluation of the patient's home, parent's occupation and other environments. (2) Allergic by a search into his diet, external contacts and inhalants, if any.

A detailed history will help considerably; also the patient's own ideas as to the cause, an eliminative diet or diet diary, along with scratch and patch tests. As a general rule, it should be impresed upon the patient that he has an inborn weakness of the skin, and an unstable, emotionally sensitive nature, and that he should learn to live with these weaknesses, avoiding stresses as far as possible.

Nummular Eczema

Synonym : Discoid eczema

It is characterized by circular coin-shaped plaques of papules, vesicles and crusting, distributed bilaterally and symmetrically on the dorsum of fingers, the hands, the forearms, the arms, the legs and the thighs. These plaques may enlarge slowly with a tendency to clear at the centre. The condition is chronic and recurrent.

Etiology and Pathogenesis : These are not definitely established; psychogenic stresses, focal sepsis, food allergies, alcohol, debility and drugs are usually held responsible. A dry skin and cold weather may be associated with it.

Nummular eczema should be distinguished from circular patches of infective eczema and tinea circinata. Both of these are asymmetrical, acute and non-recurring conditions. Focal sepsis may produce bilaterally symmetrical patches of infective eczematoid dermatitis resembling discoid dermatitis.

Dermatitis papulosa alba (Sugarthan) and miliarial dermatitis (Behl) are seen in the hot summer, on forearms; sweat retention may be the exciting cause. Sometimes, discoid dermatitis may be associated with dyshidrosis of palms and soles, and discoid patches of keratoderma.

Treatment :This consists of reassuring the patient, correcting the known etiological factors. Dry skins are massaged with oil and the nutritional status of the patient must be improved.

Disseminated Eczema

Synonym : Eczematides

It is characterized by tiny papular, vesicular and occasionally, bullous crusted lesions occurring singly or in small patches resulting from sensitization to the products of primary active eczema being conveyed by the blood stream to distant sites producing dissemination of the eczematous process. This process is called auto-sensitization, brought on particularly by the use of strong medicaments (irritants of sensitizers, or both) applied to the primary eczematous site. When primary eczema is infective, the eczematides are termed infective eczematides.

Sympathetic dermatitis from one foot to another, and unilateral eczematides from one foot to the hand on the same side, are further examples of dissemination. Primary active eczemas on the feet usually disseminate to the palms, producing an eruption resembling cheiropompholyx; primary eczemas on the hands disseminate to the ears, face and trunk. If the process is widespread, bilaterally symmetrical and generalized eczema may develop, which may involve even the face accompanied by swelling of the eyelids.

Constitutional symptoms like fever, headache, pains and malaise, are produced by toxaemia during dissemination. The patient looks ill and weak. Disseminated eczemas should not be treated lightly. Firstly, they take a long time to heal, and even after the condition clears up, the integument is left in a weak and hypersensitive state, and is, for some time, prone to pyoderma. Secondly, patients suffering from this kind of eczema are very sensitive to local medication. Therefore, the medication employed should be as simple as possible. In underdeveloped Asiatic countries, disseminated eczemas are a common problem because of the ill-treatment of primary eczemas by the laxity and the presence of quacks. If scientific treatment is delayed, recurrences are common and eczema becomes chronic.

Eczematides must be distinguished from other identical eruptions, namely :

1. Dermatophytides. Ide-eruption from a primary active fungus infection. When it is due to trichophyton, it is called trichophytide; when due to epidermophyton, it is called epidermophytide.

2. Seborrhoeides from seborrhoeic dermatitis of the scalp.

3. Bacterides from a primary bacterial septic focus. They are found on the soles and palms when there is a septic focus in the nose, throat, lungs and abdomen.

4. Tuberculides from a primary active tuberculous focus.

Varicose Dermatitis or Eczema

This is simply traumatic, chemical or infective eczema, complicating varicose veins or ulcers of the legs. The predisposing factors are chronic congestion and stasis which lower the local resistance. A similar situation is created by hypostasis following white leg in pregnancy, and fracture in the lower extremities. The dorsum of the foot and lower part of the leg show telangiectasis, oedema and pigmentation produced by varicose veins. Itching in varicose legs may start eczema by excoriation, secondary infection and by the use of medicaments. The eczema has the features of the exciting cause which may be traumatic, chemical or infective.

VARICOSE ULCER
TREATED WITH SECALE COR

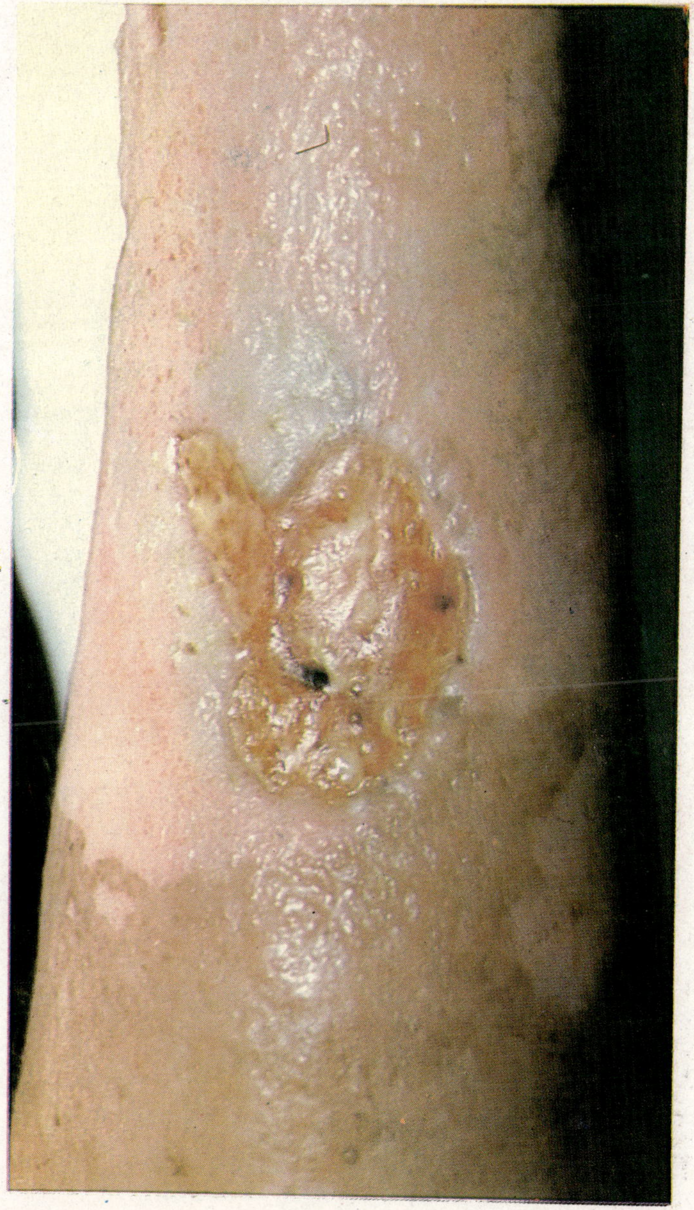

BEFORE

VARICOSE ULCER
TREATED WITH SECALE COR

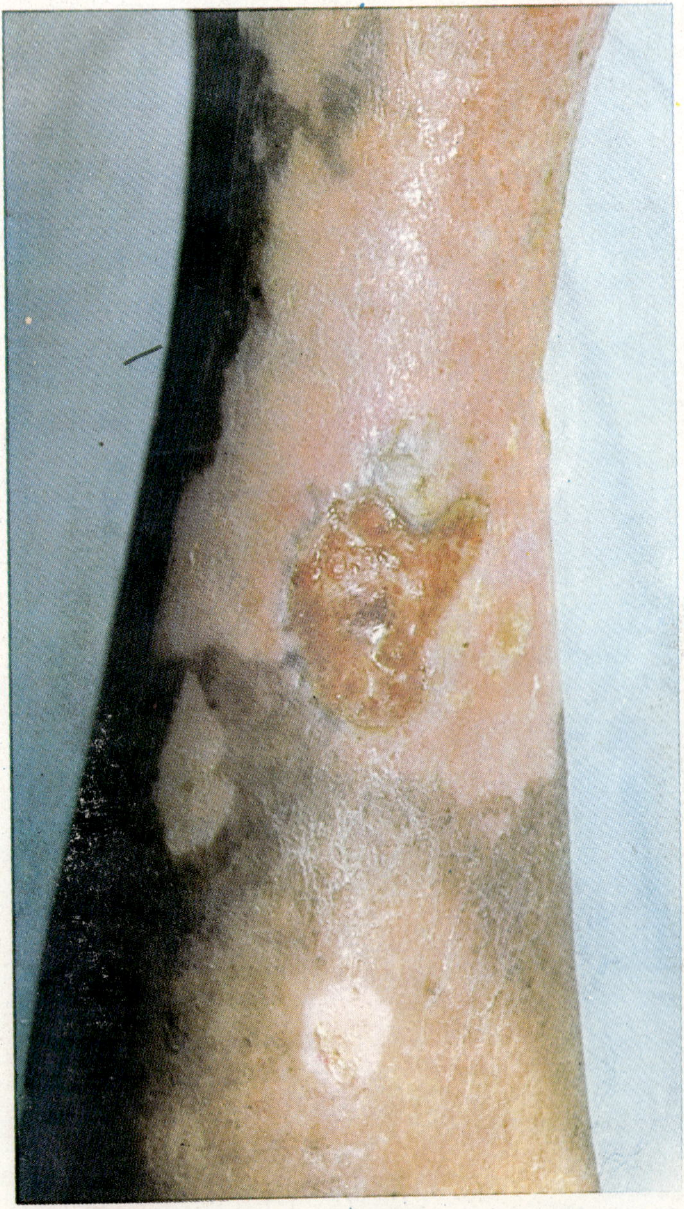

AFTER

Varicose eczema may become disseminated due to auto-sensitization. Because of the indolent nature of the basic condition — varicose veins and hypostasis — varicose dermatitis is a very chronic and persistent condition. Secondary complications like thrombophlebitis are common.

Treatment : It consists of (1) Controlling the congestion and stasis by avoiding long hours of standing, elevating the legs while resting, foot exercises. (2) Crepe bandages or elastic stockings. (3) Surgery for the varicose veins. (4) Symptomatic treatment of eczema.

Neurodermatitis

Synonym : Lichen Simplex Chronicus.

It more commonly affects neurotic people. . This condition may be defined as the lichenification process resulting from chronic scratching and rubbing of the skin under stress and anxiety. The condition is common amongst young people and menopausal women. These patients tend to tear off their skin when they cannot get at others for social reasons. Any emotional conflicts particularly those arising from sex, financial and social problems, may initiate itching; scratching produces further irritation, and a vicious cycle is established resulting in lichenification.

The integument becomes thickened, infiltrated and pigmented; the crisscross markings become more prominent. Margins are irregular but usually well-defined. There may be one or several localized patches. Occasionally, an extensive disseminated variety of neurodermatitis may be seen with multiple disseminated lesions of lichenified integument. The sites commonly affected are : the nape of neck, arms, ano-genital area, scrotum, backs of knees, legs and ankles.

Chronic eczemas may become lichenified through constant scratching, lichenification is a prominent feature of atopic eczema. In the dark Indian skin, lichenification occurs early. Neurodermatitis should be distinguished from lichenified eczemas, atopic, dermatitis, lichen planus hypertrophicus and lichen sclerosus et atrophicus.

Prognosis : This is good if the primary emotional conflict can be resolved satisfactorily.

Treatment consists of psycho-therapy.

Radio-Dermatitis

It implies dermatitis produced by excessive doses of X-rays received by the skin. This was common in the past when X-ray machines were crude and people inexperienced. Acute radio-dermatitis is rarely seen; what one usually comes across in practice is the chronic type. The features of acute radio-dermatitis depend upon the degree of burn, and hence, vary from erythema, scaling, vesicular or bullous reaction to ulceration; in chronic cases, there is long latent period of months and years, followed by redness, telangiectasis, pigmentation and atrophy. In severe cases, however, ulceration and even epitheliomas may develop. Plastic surgery gives the best results in chronic localized X-ray burns with ulcer and a tendency to neoplasms. Epitheliomas caused by X-ray burns, should, under no circumstances, be treated with further X-ray therapy. Complete excision and Z-plasty/skin flap are the answer.

Dermatitis Medicamentosa

It comprises all cutaneous eruptions resulting from the internal (by mouth or injections) use of drugs.

Dermatitis Autophytica

Synonym: Dermatitis artefacta

It implies self-produced dermatitis brought on with strong physical agents or acids by hysterical individuals. Young single girls are the usual victims; sympathy is the motive. The sites of affection are the commonly accessible regions. Lesions have the features of dermatitis, but are usually, bizarre and do not conform to any known picture. The use of liquid irritants by the patient produces trickle lines.

Dyshidrosis

Synonym : Cheiropompholyx

It consists of bilaterally symmetrical eruption affecting the palms of hands, and less frequently, the sides and soles of feet. Lesions consist of deeply-set vesicles, looking like embedded sago grains, accompanied by tingling, burning and itching. The interdigital spaces, the sides of fingers and the palms are the typical sites. The dorsum of the hands is rarely affected. The vesicles dry up in 10 to 14 days, leaving behind slight scaling. Sometimes they become infected with pyogenic organisms, or complicated by infective eczema. To begin with, the condition is acute and occurs in attacks. If the attacks become frequent, and the condition becomes chronic, the clinical picture shows a thick hyperkeratotic skin accompanied by deeply set vesicles. At times it takes a dry and hyperkeratotic form from the very beginning, then it is called Dyshidrosis sicca.

Etiology : The disease usually affects neurotic individuals with hyperhidrosis of the hands. Psychogenic stresses and active focal sepsis are the important causes. The disease usually occurs at the change of seasons, particularly in spring and summer, and may develop every year at the same time.

Differential diagnosis : Cheiropompholyx has nothing to do with the obstruction of the sweat glands. It must be distinguished from ide-eruption, in which a similar clinical picture is produced by active fungus infection in the feet; eczematides; contact dermatitis and drugs eruptions. History and physical examination help in establishing the diagnosis.

In contact dermatitis, lesions are confined to specific fingers, thumb and index fingers due to cutting vegetables and flower bulbs, middle and ring fingers to cigarette paper and dorsum of fingers due to soaps and detergents. Condition is usually asymmetrical. If the primary lesion is pustular from the beginning, pustular bacteride should be suspected, and a search made for a septic focus. The hyperkeratotic form should be distinguished from other types of keratoderma.

Treatment : It consists of correcting the causative psychological factors and focal sepsis. In resistant cases, X-ray therapy in small doses.

Perioral Dermatitis

Dermatitis is seen on the lower part of the face, mainly chin and around the mouth. Erythema is more evident and is accompanied by slight crusting or scaling and itching. Oozing is little.

Presumable causes are seborrhoea, emotional stress, gastro-intestinal disturbances, photosensitivity, hormonal contraceptives and use of fluorinated steroids. Course is chronic, slow and insiduous with occasional exacerbations. Treatment consists of correction of the underlying causes, local use of calamine lotion.

Prognosis : Dermatitis and Eczema

The outlook rests mainly on correct elicitation and the complete eradication of the cause or causes. It is regrettable that potential sensitizers are sold so freely in the market and advertised as panaceas in the lay press. The skin is a superficial subject and so it is easily accessible to over-treatment and ill-treatment.

Dermatitis and eczema are, as a rule, curable conditions. Eczemas are non-infective except when they are impetiginized and of the infective variety. They do not leave scars. The patient needs reassurance on these points.

It must be remembered that epidermis is an ectodermal structure, and so, takes time to heal. Patience must be the watchword; energetic treatment is to be strongly discouraged. Once warned, the patient will readily co-operate.

Acute eczema heal readily, in about 1 to 4 weeks, with treatment. Chronic eczema, in which anatomical and functional changes set in, take time to disappear. Disseminated and generalized eczemas are not only slow to heal, but are accompanied by ill-health. Infantile and atopic eczemas are troublesome and uncomfortable. The former lasts till the age of two unless it develops into atopic eczema which may continue till the age of twenty five or even through life. Its course is marked by spontaneous remissions and exacerbations. Climatic extremes, psychogenic stresses and poor health, aggravate dermatitis and eczema. The cure of these conditions is retarded in tropical countries, by heat, humidity and the prevalent unhygienic conditions.

Treatment

It consists of :

1. Reasurring the patient and his relatives about the disease being curable, non-infectious and non-scarring. A patient with chronic eczema naturally worries about the chronic nature of his illness, the expense of treatment and the loss

FUNGAL ECZEMA TREATED WITH CALC SULPH

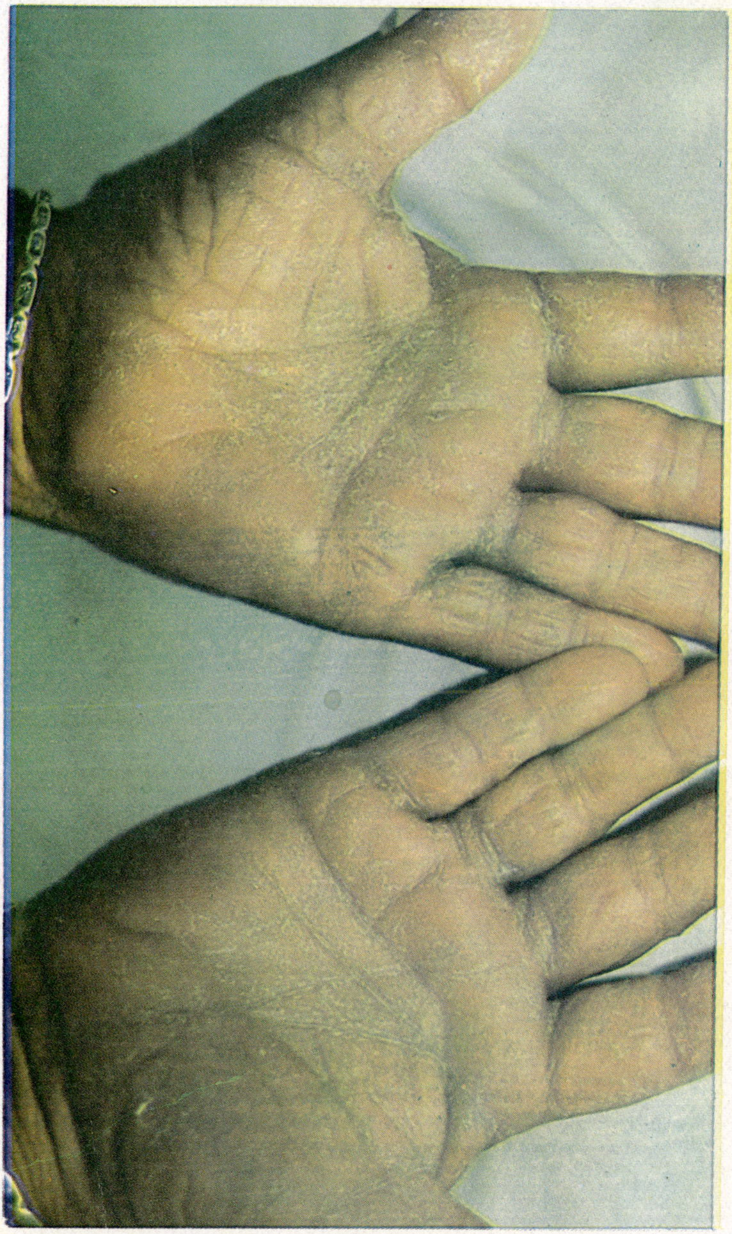

BEFORE

FUNGAL ECZEMA TREATED WITH CALC SULPH

AFTER

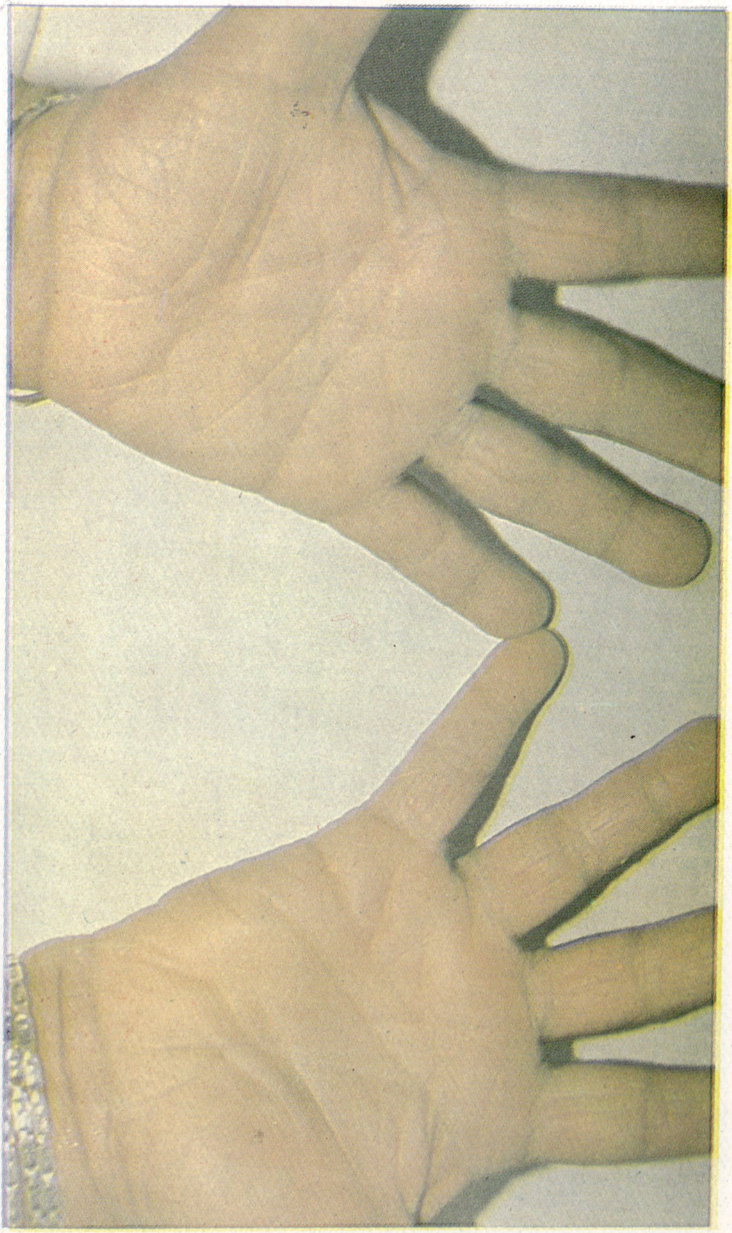

ECZEMA TREATED WITH CHELIDONIUM

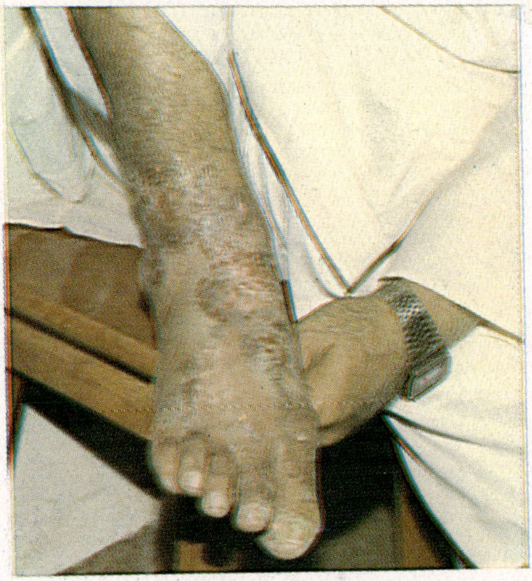

BEFORE

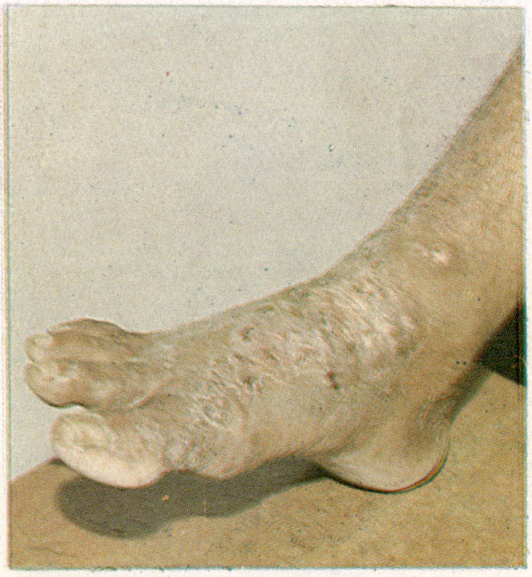

ECZEMA TREATED WITH CHELIDONIUM

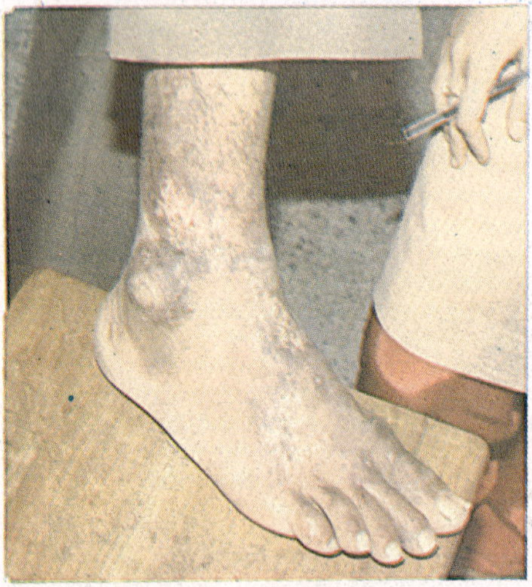

AFTER THE TREATMENT

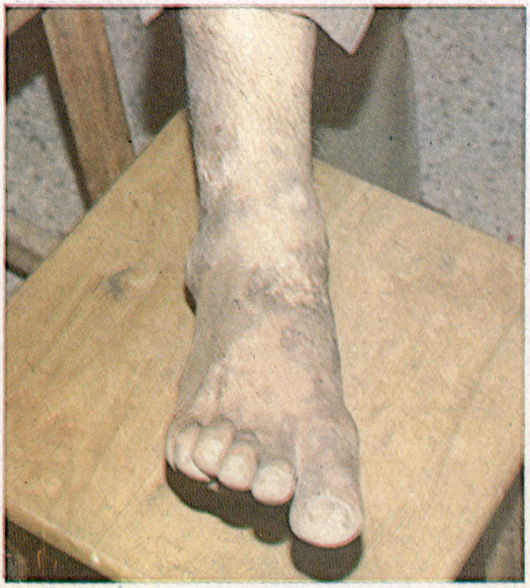

CHRONIC ECZEMA TREATED WITH IGNATIA

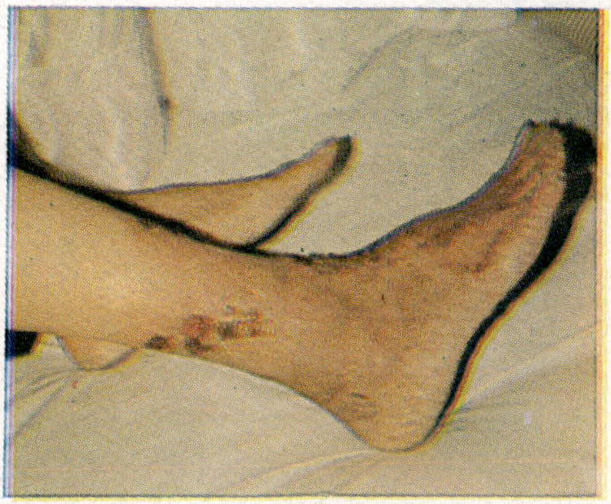

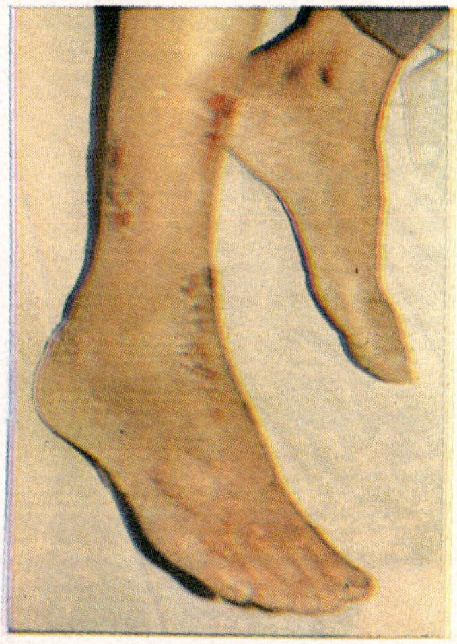

BEFORE

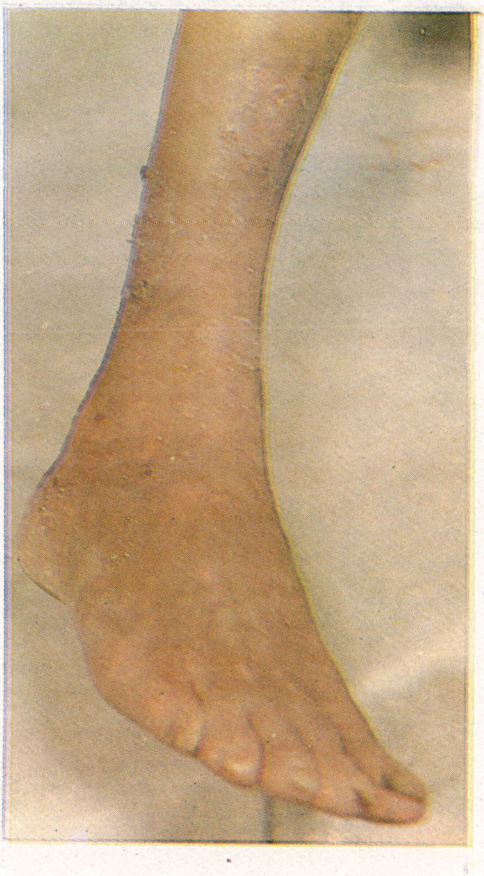

AFTER

ECZEMA OF SOLE TREATED WITH SILICEA

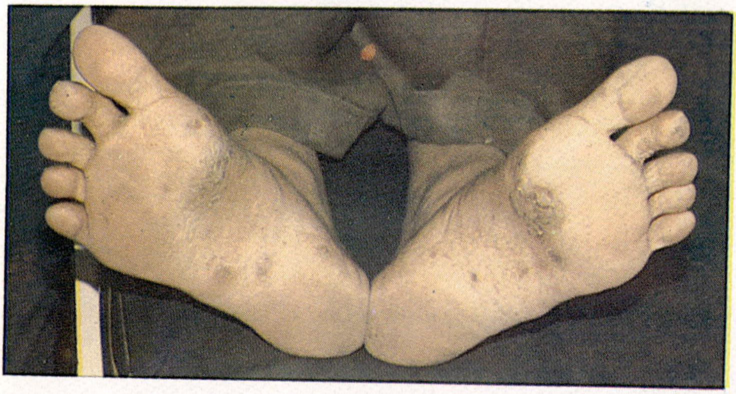

BEFORE

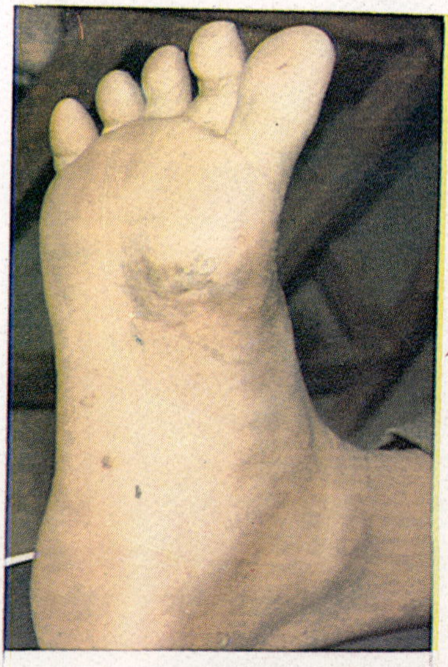

AFTER

ALLERGIC ECZEMA TREATED WITH NAT. SULPH.

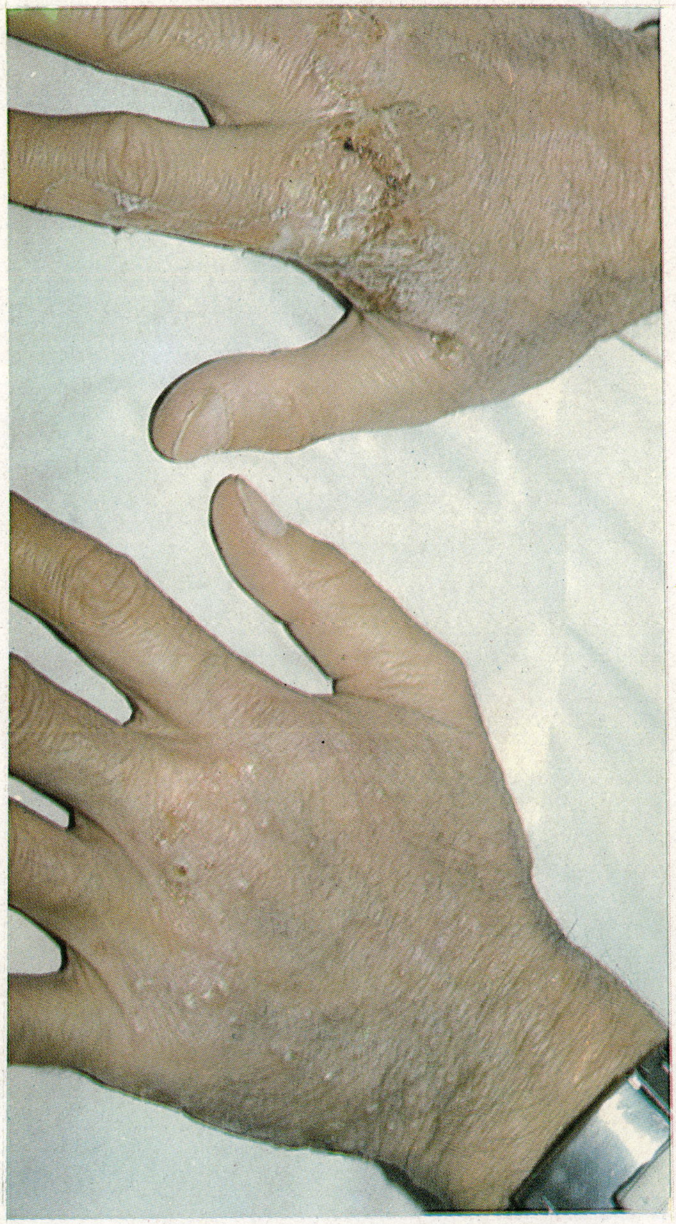

B E F O R E

ALLERGIC ECZEMA TREATED WITH NAT. SULPH.

AFTER

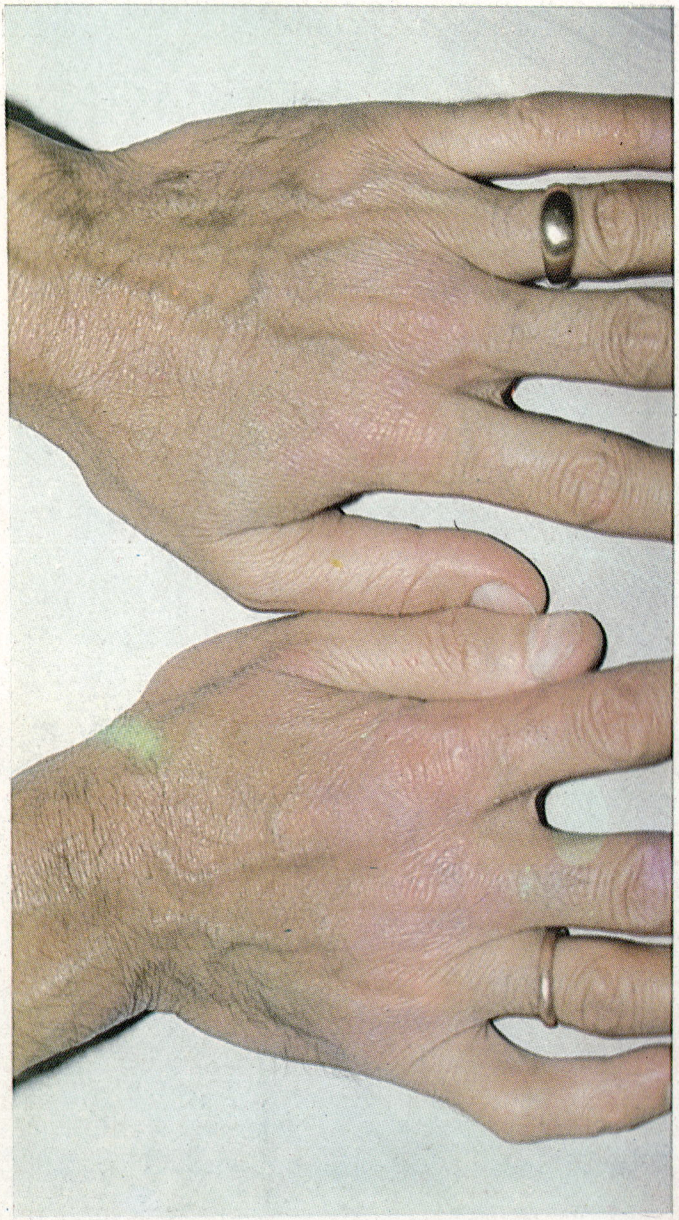

ECZEMA TREATED WITH ANAGALLIS

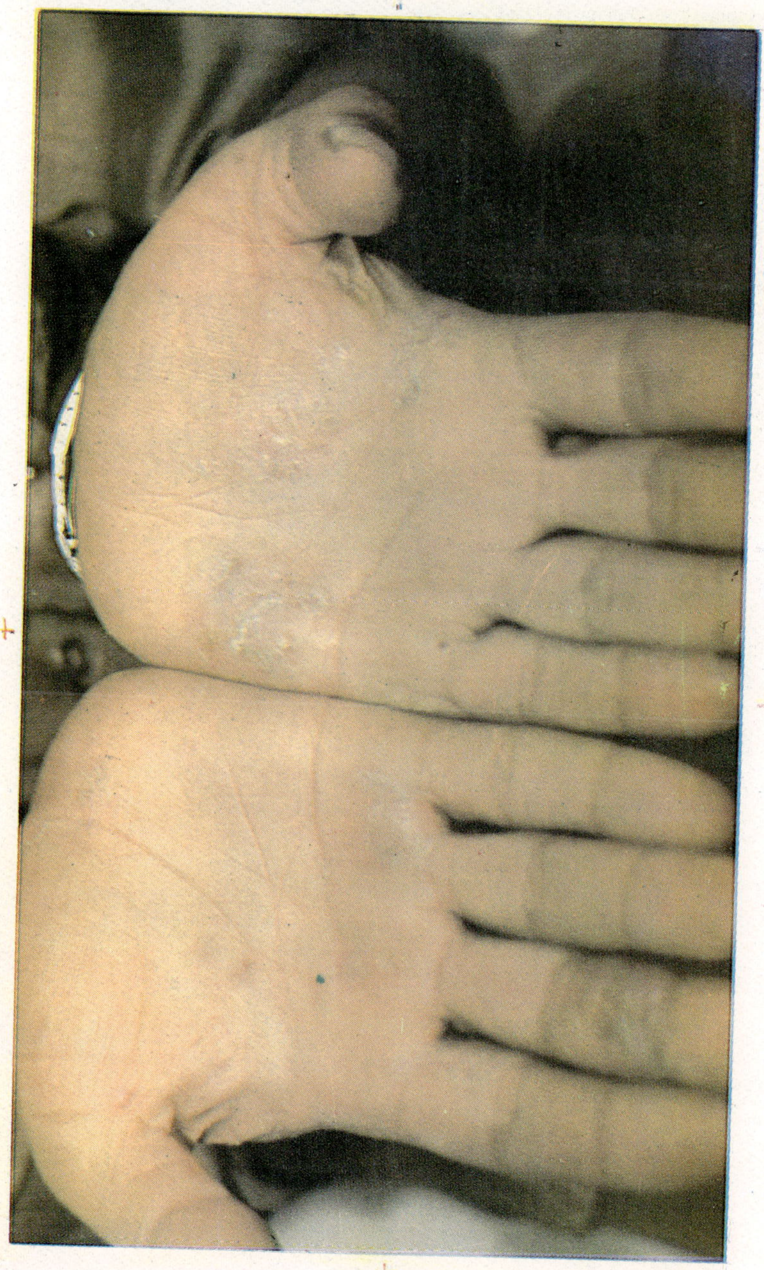

BEFORE

ECZEMA TREATED WITH ANAGALLIS

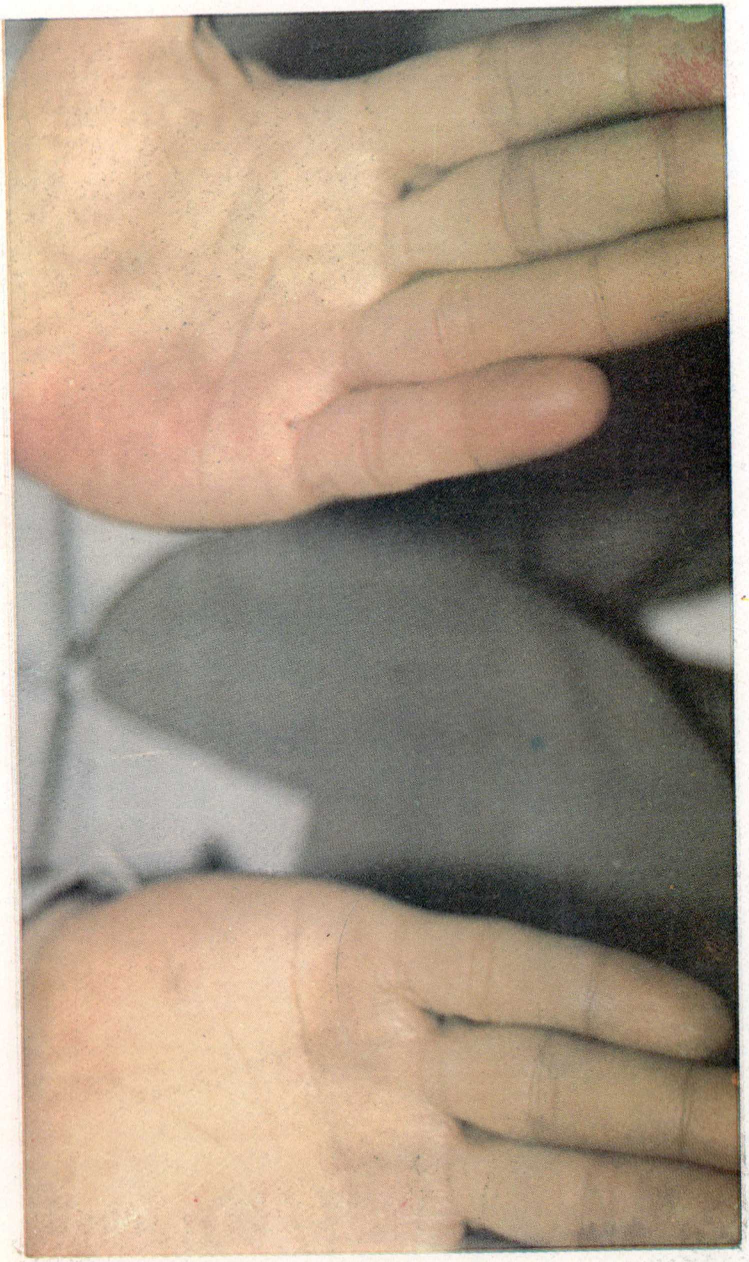

AFTER

of income because of his inability to work. Hence reassurance on all these accounts is very important in winning his confidence, and thus his co-operation in treatment. Tactful bedside psychotherapy pays dividends in all cases.

2. Elimination of predisposing, exciting and complicating causes. In one individual, more than a single cause may be at play. Where it is impossible to remove a known cause from a patient's environment, attempts should be made to desensitize or hyposensitize him. To prevent recurrence, advice should be given to the patient regarding exposure to causes. Anyone suffering from contact eczema, for instance, should be advised against exposure to the possible sources of the causative allergens and allergo-immunologically related substances. Patients with infective eczemas should be advised regarding the sources of infection the building up of resistance against infection with specific autogenous and stock vaccines, etc. Improving the general state of nutrition is also important.

3. Palliative treatment must be properly carried out to effect a complete cure. Half-hearted measures carried out in an inefficient manner, far from being helpful, are demoralizing. The principles of symptomatic treatment are :

Correction of Environment

(a) Moderate atmospheric temperature and humidity help recovery, whereas heat, sweating, high humidity (particularly in the monsoon), dust and unhygienic surroundings, have an untoward influence. Poverty and backwardness of the people are great obstacles especially when the climate is extreme. A change to a moderate climate should be recommended to a patient suffering from chronic eczemas.

(b) Rest to the affected part may be recommended; bed rest becomes necessary in generalized eczemas. With rest, healing is accelerated; that is why hospitalization is so beneficial for chronic, resistant cases.

(c) Diet should be simple; salt and fluids should be cut down. Sattvik (vegetarian food without spices and beverages like tea, coffee, alcohol) is helpful in bad cases. In acute disseminated eczemas, it is advisable to put the patient on light food for a few days to help the body to get rid of toxic substances. In allergic eczemas, eliminative diets may be tried.

(d) The protection of the affected part is desirable; more so, in exogenous eczemas where a cotton bandage or a glove or a mask ensures complete protection from offending agents. Cotton wool must never be employed in bandaging, it retains heat, thereby worsening the eczema.

(e) Patients should be asked to refrain from scratching as far as possible. In difficult cases, particularly in infantile and atopic cases, physical restraint with splints and bandages may be necessary.

Homoeopathic Approach to Contact Dermatitis

The role of Homoeopathic physician in the treatment of contact dermatitis is pivotal. He should be a good detective with powers of observation and detection, almost, like those of Sherlock Holmes.

It is very essential to hear the history of the patient carefully. Patch test should be done to confirm the diagnosis, as many a times dermatitis and eczema are confused in routine practice.

The important point that one must remember is, that the eruptions develop briskly, spreading far beyond the original point of contact. It has an ill-defined margin, fading at the periphery, associated with brisk oedema and uniform vesiculation. Hence it is essential to have what we call homoeopathically "an unprejudiced history".

Once the history is noted, the next step would be to locate the causative factor responsible for the development of contact dermatitis; e.g., plants, cosmetics, clothings, medicaments, industrial and occupational agents, etc.

(1) Careful description of the lesion present, e.g., vesical erythema.

(2) Abnormal sensation like burning itching.

(3) Thermal modalities.

(4) Various aggravating and ameliorating modalities.

One should then evolve the complete conceptual image of the patient, the relation to the general mental and emotional state and concomitants if any.

(5) Elimination of exciting causes, mentioned above is a must for permanent cure. Dermatitis, as a rule is a curable condition, hence every effort must be made to cure the lesions.

Occasionally, contact dermatitis is superadded with secondary bacterial infection, focal sepsis, or emotional stress. Hence care should be taken to treat them as their presence may retard cure.

Sometimes, with the best of homoeopathic treatment, the patient may not improve or the cure is retarded, because of the following conditions :

(1) India, being a tropical country with heat and humidity.
(2) Prevailing unhygienic conditions.

CONTACT DERMATITIS

Aethiops : The appearance of *Aethiops* in characterized by eczematous lesion, the lesions are painful to touch with severe itching sensation. It is usually indicated in person with syphilitic or scrofulous diathesis. The lesions very rapidly suppurates. and form thick scabs.

Anacardium : The appearance of the skin of Anacardium patient is bright red with excessive itching and burning sensation < in bed, > evening to midnight. To start with, there is a presence of scarlet red rashes with tiny blisters and unbearable itching, gradually they turned into thick yellow crust. The more the patient scratches, worse the itching beomes locally person feels > by heat, hot bath and in the sun occasionally itching is better by eating. Also it is indicated when the skin symptoms are suppressed by the use of skin ointment.

Apis : The appearance of the rash is fiery red; child rubs the affected part with the fingers quite vigorously. This is due to stinging burning, sticking, smarting sensation experienced by the child. This is worse evening and night and warm application. Better by cold application. The affected parts is swollen and has a bloated appearance. The part is very hot to touch. If the child is covered, it becomes very uncomfortable. Child feels better in open air.

Badiaga : The skin is extremely sore to touch with formation of reddish blue or reddish brown rashes. The patient is < touch, cold air. Better heat, warm room. It is frequently indicated in person with scrofulous diathesis.

Comocladia : Scarlet red eruptions or rashes is the characteristic appearance of comocladia. They are accompanied by severe itching and burning sensation. It is > night, > open air, scratching. The lesions have tendency to ulcerate easily.

Cantharis : Canth. is characterized by small ulcerations with exudations of watery discharge and small blisters. The child is very restless due to burning sensation and feels better when washed with cold water. Affected part is so sensitive that the child will not allow anyone to touch.

Euphorbia Lathyris : The lesion usually begins on the uncovered parts and then spreads over whole body. They are rough, scaly and accompanied by burning when scratched. They form deep rhagades < in the cold air, > closed room, sweet oil application.

Graphites : It affects folds of the skin throughout the body characterized by great itching, worse at night. There is a burning sensation. There is a characteristic thin, sticky, acrid, offensive, gluey discharge which oozes from the skin. The affected part burns after scratching and there is tendency to form cracks and fissures. When skin is cleaned with warm water it agg. Better in open air.

Hepar-Sulph : Skin is extremely sensitive to any contact, especially, plants, animals, etc. The skin is unhealthy with tendency to suppuration and uceration. There is burning and itching < cold air, cold application winter. Dermatitis is frequently encountered in Hep Sulph patient after exposure of mercury or its compounds. The odour from the skin is either offensive or sour.

Juglans-Regia : The skin lesions chiefly affect face, neck, back, and axilla. They are accompanied by itching < night, washing. The tendency for eruptions to suppurates with formation of thick crust.

Merc-Sol : Itching becomes pleasant on scratching more at night in bed on getting warm. After scratching there is burning and skin becomes rough and secretes a thin acrid fluid with small vesicle formation. Surrounding lymph nodes are enlarged and tender. Affected part may bleed when scratched. Part is dirty and odour is offensive. Part affected is prone to suppuration and ulceration. Burning is worse from scratching and warmth.

Mancinella : The lesions are characterised by formation of vesicles and large blisters as from scalds. The vesicles when broken discharge yellow serum. Patient in general is > by heat.

Rhus-Tox : The erythematous rash of *Rhus-Tox* is characterized by tiny vesicles which tends to become crusty with itching and burning which is better by warm fomentation. Here the child likes affected part to be covered as the skin is sensitive to cold air. Slightest exposure to damp and cold makes the child uncomfortable by worsening the rash. Rash is prone to suppuration and crust and then one gets vesicles with small abscesses.

Rhus-Venenata : The lesions typically affect hand, face, genitals, thighs, characterized by erythematous rash with vesicles, with excessive itching < night, hot water.

Xerophyllum : The skin is characterised by erythema with vesication. Stinging, burning and itching < cold application > hot application. The area around knee is the typical side affinity for the drug to develop dermatitis. The surrounding area is inflammed. The skin is rough and feels like leather.

In acute cases, apply a mixture of *Calendula* Q with water in a ratio of 1:3.

Some Examples of Occupational Dermatitis

Occupation	*Causative Agent*	*Homoeopathic Drugs*
Agriculture	Plants Insecticides.	Anacardium, Rhus-tox Petroleum
Automobiles	Oil Petrol, Paints	Petroleum

Occupation	*Causative Agent*	*Homoeopathic Drugs*
Buildings Workers	Cement	Calc-sulph
	Lime	Calc-carb
Pharmaceutical	Dyes	Sulph
	Chemicals	Psor
	Solvents	Graph, Carbo-Veg
House wife	Soaps	Calc-s
	Vegetables	Graph
	Artificial flavour	Nat-m
Doctors	Iodine	Iodium
	Streptomycin	Streptomycin
	Sulphonamide	
Painters	Turpentine	Terbinthinum
Painters	Printer's ink	Plb-met Carb-v
		Sulph
Rubber workers	Dyes, Glues	Sulph
Tar workers	Tar	Carb-an.

Homoeopathic Approach to Eczema

Treat the patient and respect the skin, — should be the golden rule of thumb whilst treating an eczema, that is to say, there is no eczema, but an eczematous patient.

It is such a common dermatological condition that practically one in every ten individuals has or has had eczema in the past. Since we do not know the exact aetiology of eczema, many factors, endogenous as well as exogenous are blamed for its causation. From the homoeopathic point of view, one has to give importance to the fundamental or the predisposing cause and that is familial predisposition.

Not only should history of eczema be enquired in the past of family, but also its duration, site, signs and symptoms present at that time with modalities and concomitants, along with treatment taken at that time should be carefully and meticulously recorded.

I would like to go one step ahead, and declare that the way we have tubercular, scrofulous diathesis, we also have an eczematous diathesis. It is those patients with eczematous diathesis who have a strong predisposing or fundamental cause to develop the said eczema. Therefore, during their span of life whenever patients with such diathesis come in contact either with any of the following :

(1) Sensitizers
(2) Irritants
(3) Infections
(4) Drugs
(5) Emotional stress
(6) Focal septis
(7) Climatic change
(8) Dietetic factors etc.

Then they exhibit various patterns of eczema namely, infective, atopic, infantile, seborrhoeic, etc.

Miasmatically I would put eczema as a multiple miasmatic condition.

To start with every eczema has psoric phase characterized by erythema, vesicle associated with pruritus, and a serous discharge. This is followed by tubercular phase characterised by pustular discharge which is due to secondary infection so common amongst eczematous individual. There is formation of lots of crust, following this stage comes the sycotic phase characterised by pigmentation and lichnification and finally we come to the syphilitic phase characterised by scar formation also occasionally we come across an eczematous patient, wherefrom vesicular stage, ulceration develops. This also indicates a syphilitic phase.

A homoeopath should always be on guard not to permit an acute eczema into a chronic phase either by giving suppressive therapy or not selecting the correct similimum, further if factors like (1) Scratching, (2)Chemical trauma, (3) Climatic strains, and (4) psychogenic stress are not checked than the eczema progresses quickly to a chronic phase.

Homoeopathic Treatment of Acute Eczema

It is not true that always one should prescribe an acute durg in acute phase of eczema; many times one gets a picture of deep acting drugs like Sulphur or rare occasional nosodes like Tuberculinum.

We build the acute totality with the help of the following :

(1) Ailments from, if any.
(2) The look of eczema.
(3) The discharge.
(4) Itching with modalities.
(5) Concomitants, if any, associated with it.
(6) Any other P.Q.R. symptoms available.

If the selected remedy is a short acting drug, then one should start with giving it 3-4 times a day and a following remedy every 3rd day.

Further repetition should be considered only after enquiring in detail about the symptoms just mentioned in the totality. Never start with a deep acting drug in acute eczemas as far as possible until you are too sure.

Once the acute eczema gets completely cured, do not forget to evolve the constitutional drug and interpose either a constitutional remedy or a nosode, depending on the dominant miasm present at that time. this is chiefly to prevent recurrence or suppression of the eczema if at all by the acute remedy.

Homoeopathic Treatment of Chronic Eczema

The main reasons for the eczema to become chronic are :

(1) Non-elimination of exciting, predisposing and complicating causes.

(2) Treatment of acute eczema with suppressive measures like faulty selection of similimum using strong topical ointments, local application of strong acids to burn the skin.

Two things should always be kept in mind while treating a case of chronic eczema :

(i) In cases of infective eczema resistance of the patient should be built up against the infection by repeated administration of intercurrent remedies like nosodes and constitutional remedy wherever applicable.

(ii) In cases of allergic eczema one should try to desensitize the individual by giving the allergies in potentized form on the principle of Isopathy, e.g. in cases of congress grass eczema. Congress grass in 30 potency to be given repeatedly over a prolonged period.

It should always be remembered that half-hearted measures, carried out in an inefficient manner far from being helpful, are almost always demoralising to the patient.

Aethiops : *Aethiops* typically affects persons with scrofulous and syphilitic diathesis who are prone to easy suppuration. The lesions are characterized by formation of thick crust with pus beneath the discharge which is extremely acrid.

Eczema in individuals after abuse of mercury.

Alnus : Eczema associated with gastric disturbances situated specially on the fingers, characterised by crust and pustules.

Eczema that tends to ulcerate easily, angry looking eczema associated with glandular enlargement.

Aethusa Cynapium : Eczema in children, especially during dentition; it typically affects the area around the joints with itching and burning sensation > local application of heat.

Skin is cold and covered with cold, clammy sweat, Lymphatic glands swell like strings of beads. Eruption itches when exposed to heat.

Alumina : Eczema of the scalp, nails are the typical sites. Eruptions are humid, scabby, scurfy with gnawing itching sensation. They bleed easily when scratched. < evenings; < alternate days, from heat of bed, at full and new moon; from eating potatoes > open air (*Baryta carb*). Dry skin even in hot weather. Eczema that appear periodically, especially in winter. Skin feels as if white of egg had dried on its surface.

Ammonium Carb: Eczema on bends of extremities; excoriation between the thighs and above genitals, < wet application. Violent itching, after scratching burning blisters appear. Eczema in individuals with scrofulous diathesis who dislike washing.

Ammonium Mur : Eczema especially on hands, wrist, shoulders, tips of fingers. Eczemas which are associated with desquamation of the skin, with a fine brown exfoliation.

Itching is > applying cold water in the evening. Eczema is worse during menses. They bleed very easily on touch and friction.

Eczema in individuals who are fat, bloated, with lax muscles, who are indolent and sluggish and who are prone to frequent gastric upset like vomiting and diarrhoea.

Anacardium Oriental : Eczema that chiefly affects, fingers, eyelids, face, scrotum, chest and around neck, vesicles that become pustules very early.

Multiple vesicles which later confluent and discharge a yellow transparent fluid, hardening to a crust. The discharge is acrid and excoriating. The eruption tends to spread from left and right.

Itching < scratching, eczema in individual with neurotic personality of nervous, hysterical women.

Anthrokokali : Eruption typically affect the hands, tibia, shoulder and dorsum of feet, where it produces vesicles and pustules. There is considerable itching appearing during the night and disappearing in the day time. Eruptions decrease with appearances of the full moon. The skin has got tendency to develop cracks and ulceration. Eczema in individuals with bilious affection.

Antim Crud : Eczema especially on face, genital organs and extremities, neck, chest and back.

Suppurating, yellow crusted eruption, painful to touch and easily detached; a green serous pus oozes out from beneath. The thick hard, yellow crust, irritating the surrounding parts, itching violently; < from application of poultices, bathing, working in water, alcohol and in the sun.

Eczema in individuals who are gluttons in their eating habits and frequently suffer from gastric troubles.

Antim Tart : Impetigenous eczema; vesicles surrounded by a red areola, with itching, chiefly above nose, neck and shoulder and back of the ears; the eruptions leave a bluish red mark. It is indicated in individual who has ailments from ill effects of vaccination.

Apis-Mellifica : Eruptions sting and burn like bee stings, sensitive to touch, chiefly in circumscribed spots all over body, causing itching and restlessness, < by heat and > exposure to air. The skin is dry and hot alternating with gushes of sweat. Eczema developing in individual after suppressed eruptions.

Ars Alb : Eruptions typically affect, scalp, face, extremities genitals, margins of hair. They are dry and scaly or with vesicles, having fetid and acrid discharge. Sensation of itching and burning < at night, in cold air, scratching > application of warmth in general.

Eruptions bleed on scratching. Skin symptoms alternate with internal affection like asthma.

Ars-Iod : Small vesicles which burst and discharge an acrid fluid with severe itching and burning < night, application of cold. Itching is so violent that patient scratches till it bleeds. Eczema of beard < washing. Eczema in individual tuberculous, scrofulous or syphilitic diathesis.

Asterias-Rubens : Eczema on thighs, legs, ankles and in steps itching vesicles break and forms small ulcers which spread superficially; it typically affects individual with cancerous, scrofulous and sycotic diathesis. Eczema are typically left sided.

Baryta-Carb : Moist vesicular eruption, with formation of thick crust, itching, burning, causes the hair fall out; skin is humid and sore. Eczemas of fat dwarfish children with swollen lymphatics, enlarged tonsils who take cold easily.

Berberis-Vulgaris : Eczema of anus and hands with severe itching, burning, and smarting < scratching, > cold application circumscribed pigmentation following eczematous eruptions. Eruptions that leave a brown stain. Eczemas in individual with arthritic, nephrotic and urinary complaints.

Berberis-Aquifolium : Eczemas typically affection affects scalp and extends to face and neck. Dry eczema in individual with chronic catarrhal affections. Itching of the scalp is followed by severe scaling.

Borax : Eczema affects fingers, toes and nails. There is a sensation of itching and stinging.

The appearance of skin is dry, wrinkled and wilted. Eczemas tend to ulcerate with slightest friction.

Bovista : Eczemas affection back of hands (baker's and grocer's itch) mouth, nostrils and bends of elbows and knees, eczemas especially when the skin is irritated by repeated washing. Eruptions are moist and vesicular with formation of thick crust or scabs, with pus beneath. There is no relief in itching from scratching. Itching < by warmth. The skin is flabby to feel, blunt instruments leaves a deep impression in it.

Bromium : Eczema covers entire scalp like scab, dirty looking, offensive discharge. The scalp is tender to touch. Profuse moist eruptions in armpit and perineum.

Caladium : Burning vesicular eczema on chest, forearm and vulva; alternating with attacks of asthma; the sweat is so sweet that it attracts flies.

Calc-Carb : Eczemas appear on the occiput and then spread to the face. Eczema on neck, around navel and flexures of extremities, on scalp there is thick large, yellow scab with thick bland pus under the crust; itching not very intense but on awakening from sleep person is apt to scratch his head till it bleeds. Eruptions < by water. Eruptions are assoicated with cold feet as if damp stockings on them; chalky stool; skin inclined to ulcerate.

Calc-Sulph : Eczemas affecting the scalp and extremities with formation of greenish, brownish or yellowish scab. There is severe itching followed by scratching and bleeding,< warm application, > cold application. Skin is unhealthy and is prone to abscesses and carbuncles. The discharge is yellow, thick and lumpy.

Cantharis : Eczema affects scalp, genital's extremities. Eruptions begin in a small spot and spreads so as to involve a large surface, with a watery discharge underneath the scalp. There is intense burning with itching < warmth, > cold application. Eczema typically affects right side. Eczema usually associated with urinary complaints.

Causticum : Eczema chiefly affects nape of the neck, around the nipple, around the mouth. There is presence of itching worse at night, evening, open air, with formation of thick crust which tends to ulcerate. It is better from heat, warmth of bed. Indicated in person where eruptions are suppressed by local application of mercury or sulphur.

Chelidonium : It has got especial affinity to affect the ankle and foot, where it tends to develop chronic eczema, characterized by formation of vesicles, pustules and scabs with excessive itching. Better by eating; also lips and above nose are also affected, where it develops painful vesicles and pustules which later turn into crust.

It usually affects the right side is suited for those individuals who suffer from bilious and pulmonary disturbance.

Chrysarobinum : It typically affects the ears, eyes, legs and thighs. There is presence of dry scaly eruptions with scabs and pus from the vesicles, a foul smelling discharge with crust formation, tending to become confluent and to give the appearance of a single crust covering the entire area. Violent itching which leads to burning which is worse in warmth.

Cicuta-V : It has an affinity to develop eczema on scalp, chin, upper lip. There is presence of whitish scurf with oozing from purulent eruptions, which later become confluent and starts drying down to hard lemon crust, like dried honey. There is no itching whatsoever with eczema. Suppression of eczema leads to disease of the brain.

Clematis : Eruptions appear on occiput, nape of the neck, face and lower legs. They itch violently with profuse desquamation vesicles and pustules. Easily colloid the skin and ultimately develops flat eating ulcer with thick crust. Eruption moist during increasing moon. Dry during waning moon. They are worse when washed in cold water. Eczema develops after suppressed gonorrhoea with glandular enlargement.

Comocladia : Eczema appears on extremities around the eyes. There is presence of redness all over the skin with formation of multiple pustules. There is presence of itching which is worse by warmth and at night. Better by scratching and in open air. It is indicated in those eczemas which recur periodically.

Conium : Eczema affecting face, arms and mons veneris. Moist vesicle with bluish sticky discharge forming hard crust. Itching is worse by scratching. Eczema developing in old person after being over heated.

Copaiva : Eczema consisting of small vesicles, itching and pricking with severe inflammation in parts. Denuded epithelium.

Croton-Tig : Almost all parts of the body are affected; face, genitals, eyelids, soles of feet, temples and vertex. There is a presence of small vesicles, pustules, blisters, which get clustered, or may burst too. There is violent itching and burning after eating; worse at night, better gentle scratching, better after sleep.

Curare : Moist eczema of face and behind ears, scrofulous children; presence of small vesicles on scrotum with serous exudation forming squamous scab, with intense itching, worse in the evening and night.

Dulcamara : Affects the scalp, cheeks, forehead, chin, extremities. Itching vesicles that pass into suppuration and become covered with a thick brown or yellowish crust. The discharge coarsens the skin causing loss of hair. There is itching followed by scratching and bleeding. Itching of the skin diminishes after formation of crust, but remains sensitive to contact and bleeds after scratching; the eczema tends to become worse before menses.

Euphorbia Lath : The eruption starts on the face and spreads all over the body, they are characterized by itching, burning and smarting sensation. Worse by touch, worse in cold air; better by sweet oil applicaton. When eczema is scratched, it forms deep ragged ulcers.

Graphites : Folds of the skin, vertex, scalp, ears, extremities, around anus, are some of the common places where *Graphites* develop eczema. Eczema is humid and scurfy with formation of dirty crust which ooze foul acrid gluey discharge; it mats the hair together and leads to formation of deep rhagades with ulceration. Eruptions bleed easily on scratchng. They are worse from heat and they are better by cold. Eczema of fat, blonde women with scanty menses. Extreme dryness of skin with inability to perspire.

Hepar Sulph : It affects scalp, genitals, folds of scrotum and thighs. There is presence of foul moist eruption which tend to ulcerate. they are very sore and sensitive to touch. They itch violently on rising in the morning; there is presence of thin, acrid, offensive discharge from the eczema. Eczema in individual with coldness of palms and soles.

Hydrastis : Eczema on margin of hair, in front of head, worse coming from cold into warm room, oozes after washing; itching when warm; scalp and face with thick crust which upon removal, expose red, raw patches. Eczema in individual with tendency to profuse perspiration and unhealthy skin.

Juglans Cin : Eczemas especially on lower extremities, sacrum and hands. There is presence of itching and pricking when heated. Worse when heated. Itching is associated with burning and redness. Eczema associated with dyspepsia and bronchial irritation and scrofulous swelling.

Kali Ars : It produces dry, scaly eczema especially affecting bends of arms and knees.

There is presence of severe itching, worse in warmth. from walking and undressing. Eczema developing in individual with malignant disease.

Kali Bi : Eruption starts on ears and spreads over the ear, with formation of greenish crust which oozes whitish thick matter. Eruptions tend to ulcerate. There is sensation of itching which is worse from heat and hot weather. Eczema, gastric complaints and rheumatism alternates with each other. Eczema developing in individual with suppressed catarrh.

Kali Brom : Eczema that affects chest, shoulder and legs. Moist eruption which at a later stage turns into pustules and finally leads to scaling.

Kali Carb : Eczema especially on abdomen and around nipples. Eruption dry at first, but when scratched exude moisture. Sensation of burning as from a mustard plaster in the eczema.

Kali-Mur : Eczema develops after vaccination with oozing from inflammed skin whitish opaque muco-purulent discharge. Eczema from suppress stomach and menstrual disorder.

Kali Sulph : Eczema of *Kali-sulph* is characterised by abundant desquamation. There is scaling of epithelium leaving the base, moist and sticky, the discharge is yellow, slimy and sticky. There is presence of violent itching and burning sensation which is better by application of very hot water.

Lappa Major : Eczema affecting head and face, moist eruption oozing foul discharges. Formation of greyish, white crust with destruction of the hair in the surrounding part. Eczema in individual with tendency to form boils.

Ledum Pal : Eczema of individuals who are chronic alcoholics. The eczema is dry without any discharge with sensation as if lice were crawling over the surface. There is a sensation of itching worse from heat, motion and at night. Eruption only on covered parts.

Lycopodium : Eczema that are associated with urinary, hepatic and gastric disorders. Eruptions start on back of head; also on hands, thick crust which easily bleed, oozing of fetid moisture. There is presence of violent itching; worse from 4 to 8 pm; from getting heated, from poultices, better from cold air or uncovering the parts. Eczema in individual who have tendency to develop blood boils and abscess.

Manganum Acetium : It is indicated in chronic eczema with amenorrhoea < menses or menopause, perspiration. Itching better by scratching. itching on palms, with red spots, lips sore. Rhagades in bends of joints, with soreness. Deep cracks in bends of elbows, etc. Burning in small red spots, on chest, arms, hands and feet accompanying rheumatism.

Mercurius : One of the important remedy for moist eczema. Eruptions are humid, foetid, thick yellow discharge or yellow crusts form on scalp; vesicular and pustular eruption. These eruptions are surrounded by irregular margins. Itching is worse by warmth of bed, with pain from scratching and tendency to bleed. Excessive odours viscid perspiration, worse at night. Complaints increase with sweat and rest: all associated with a great deal of weariness and prostration.

Mercurius Dulcis : Eczema over whole body — the eruptions are of round copper coloured spots; in centre are dry papules. Inflammation with plastic exudate. Skin is flabby and ill-nourished with swollen glands.

Mezerium : Eczema affects especially those parts of the skin that are normally deficient in fat. There is intolerable itching, compelling the patient to scratch and has to change position. Vesicles are full of serous exudation, especially on nose and back.

Itching is better in bed, from touch, burning and change of position after scratching. Scurf like fish scales on back, chest, thighs and scalp. Scabs thick, lamellated, like rupia, blood secretion beneath, they look like chalk and spread to brows, nape and throat. Honey like crust above mouth and cheeks, worse from undressing. Eruptions ulcerate and form thick scabs under which purulent matter exudes. There is marked thirst and scrofulous tendency.

Muriatic Acid : Eczema on back of hands and face. Papular and vesicular eruptions with violent itching. Blood boils, pricking when touched. Ulcers; painful, deep, putrid, covered with scruf, on lower legs, with burning at their circumference. Worse in damp weather, before midnight. There is marked restlessness, frequently changes the position, but soon grows weak and very debilitated.

Nat-Ars : Squamous eruption, scales thin, white and when removed leaves the skin slightly reddened if scales remain; they cause itching; worse when warm and from exercise.

Nat-Carb : Eczema solaris. Inclination to perspire easily. The skin dry, rough, cracked. Itching like fleas over whole body. Eruption on finger-tips, knuckles and toes. Vesicular eruption in patches and circles. Eczema on dorsum of hands. Soles of feet raw and sore. Worse from summer heat. Mental exertion; changes of weather, sun, least draught. There is great debility caused by summer heat.

Nat-Mur : Affects the margins of the hairy scalp; flexures of skin, knuckles skin behind the ears and covers mouth and eyelids. Persons with oily, dry, harsh, unhealthy skin who are always worse when at seashore. Eczema in person with a habit of eating too much salt, raw, red inflamed eczema. Eczema oozing a corrosive fluid more so at 10 am; in warmth and during exercise. Discharge decreases when lying down.

Nitric Acid : Affects anus, vertex, temples, genitals, auditory meatus. The eruptions bleed easily when scratched and there is splinter-like pain. Eczema of the anus with long lasting pain in rectum after stool. Adapted to person with gouty diathesis and person who craves sweets.

Nat-Sulph : *Nat sulph* is indicated in very moist eruptions with much oozing of fluids. The secretions are more watery than sticky. Vesicular eczema, the thin watery discharge exuding from stiff, swollen fingers. The palms of the hands are raw and sore with fine blisters. The itching is worse when undressing.

Oleander : Adapted to person with a very sensitive skin. There is violent itching eruption, bleeding and oozing. There is absence of sweating. Vesicular eruption on scalp in children. Humid scaly eruption on back part of head and behind ears with itching. Itching as from lice. The symptoms are first better but later become worse from scratching.

Petroleum : Affects occiput, scrotum perineum, thighs, back of hands, webs of toes. Yellowish-green, thick crusts on face and neck, discharges profuse, excoriating. Pain as of slight burn in denuded area. Itching, moist sore places or cracks in skin. Inflamed skin heals with difficulty. Skin symptoms are always worse in winter.

Nux-Juglans : Vesicular eruption with itching associated with burning vesicles tend to be on cracked surface. There is greenish discharge which stiffens the linen, large blood boils on shoulders and in hepatic region which are very painful.

Phytolacca : The skin becomes dry, shrunken, pale. Papular and pustular lesions. There is itching, but too sore to allow any scratching, or made worse by scratching. The skin is hot and dry. Erythematous blotches, irregular, slightly raised, pale red ending in dark red or purple spots. Worse in damp, cold weather, night. Better in warmth, dry weather Aching, soreness, restlessness, prostration are market associated symptoms with glandular affections.

Pilocarpus Microphyllus : It is one of the well indicated remedy for dry eczema. Persistent dryness of skin. There is excessive perspiration from all parts of the body. Unilateral sweat. It is a powerful glandular stimulant.

Plumbum Met : The skin is rough, dry, scaly, feels dry and cool yellow or pale bluish. Serous infiltration and puffy appearance of skin. The patient is sensitive to open air, to touch, especially on arms and eyelids. Skin is wrinkled, shrivelled and drawn over the bones.

Primula Obconica : It is one of the important remedy for moist eczema of face. Papular eruption on chin. Burns at night. Eczema on arms, wrists, forearms, hands, papular and excoriated. Cracking over joints and fingers. Eruption between fingers, purple blotches on back of hands.

Great itching, worse at night, red and swollen like erysipelas. Small papules on a raised base. Skin symptoms accompanied by febrile symptoms.

Psorinum : Eczematous eruption after severe exertion, accompanied by sensation of tension and swelling.

Eczema behind ears, on scalp and in bends of elbows and armpits, accompanied by abscesses affecting bones; humid eruption on face. Raw red oozing, scabs around ears. Offensive discharge from eczema around ears. Intolerable itching. Offensive discharge from eczema around ears. Intolerable itching. Skin has a dirty, dingy look. Crusty eruption all over. Eruption of small vesicles, quickly filling with a yellow lymph, painful, sore to touch. Worse change of weather in hot sunshine, from cold; dread of least cold air or draft. Better by heat, warm clothing. Evening summer. Eruptions disappearing during summer, but reappearing when the cold weather comes on. Psoric constitutions, subject to glandular and skin affection, with tendency to diarrhoea.

Ranunculus Bulb : Vesicular and pustular eruptions. There is thickening of skin and formation of hard, honey scabs. Vesicular eruption on face appears as from a burn, smarts as if scalded, vesiculation followed by scabbing and this by a renewal of vesicles, attended by burning and itching. Coarse itching in hollow of hand. Crawling in skin of fingers. worse in open air, atmospheric changes, wet stormy weather, cold air brings on all sort of ailments.

Rhus-Tox : Fine, vesicular, crusty eczematous eruptions. More around the genitals. Eruptions alternate with dysentery. The skin is sensitive to cold air. Itching is worse in the hairy parts. Burning eczematous eruptions with tendency to scale formation. Moist eruptions on head beginning with small yellow vesicles with red areolae, forming thick horny crusts and scabs which eat off the hair. Eczema worse on change of weather, during wet weather and in winter.

Rhus Venenata : Vesicular eruptions with intense itching which is relieved by application of hot water; and is worse at night. Dry eruption on back of hands during winter which disappears in spring.

Ruta Graveoleus: Eczema of the palms, hands and feet with unbearable itching. Itching is worse after eating meat.

Sarsaparilla : Affects persons emaciated shrivelled skin which lies in folds. Eruptions which come in summer and spring; also after abuse of mercury. The base of the eruption is inflamed, crusts get separated in open air and the adjoining skin gets chapped.

Sepia : Acts on face, vertex, occiput, bends of joints. Eruptions during pregnancy and lactation. Itching vesicles and pustules with soreness of skin. Eruption is dry or moist and discharges, copious offensive pus like fluid, which when dry, cracks and exfoliates. Itching is worse in the open air and better in a warm room. Itching changes to burning when scratched.

Silicea : Acts on skin behind ears; skin of scrotum, hand, scalp and neck. Itching, burning, offensive, eruption ending in scabs discharging pus. Skin is sensitive to cold, patient wants to wrap up warmly. Unhealthy skin, every little injury suppurates.

REPERTORY OF ECZEMA

Skin eruption : ECZEMA — *Acon, Aeth, Aethiops, Alnus, Alum, Am-c, Am-m, Anac, Anthrok, Ant-c, Arbut, Arg-n, Ars, Ars-i, Astac, Aur, Aur-m, Bar-m, Bell, Berb-aq, Berb-v, Bor, Bov, Brom, Bry, Calad, Calc, Calc-s, Canth, Caps, Carb-ac, Carb-s, Carb-v, Castor-eq, Caust, Chrysar, Cic, Clem, Comod, Con, Cop, Crot-t,*

Cycl, Dulc, Euphorb, Flu -ac, Frax-am, Fuligo, Graph, Hep, Hippoz, Hydras, Iris, Jug-c, Jug-r, Kali-ar, Kali-bi, Kali-c, Kali-chl, Kali-m, Kali-s, Kreos, Lach, Lap-m, Led, Lith, Lyc, Mang-ac, Merc, Merc-c, Merc-d, merc-pr-rub, Mez, Mur-ac, Nat-a, Nat-m, Nat-p, Nat-s, Nit-ac, Nux-v, Olnd, Oxal-ac, Persicaria, Petr, Piloc, Phos, Phyt, Plb, Podo, Prim-v, Psor, Rad-br, Ran-b, Rhus-t, *Rhus-v, Sars, Sep, Solid, Sil,* Skook-ch, *Staph, Sulph, Sul-i, Syph, Terb, Thuj, Ustil, Vinca, Viol-t, Xerophyl, X-ray.*

Acidity with — *Nat-p, Vinca, Zinc.*
Acute — *Acon, Anac, Bell, Canth, Chin-s, Crot-s, Mez, Rhus-t, Sep.*
Alternating with internal affections — *Graph*
Anaemia with — *Calc-p*
Atrophy of infants — *Petr*
Bleeds easily and is covered with thick crusts, with fetid secretion beneath — *Lyc*
Blondes inclined to obseity in — *Graph*
Rodent — *Ars, Calc, Cic, Graph, Hep, Merc, Nat-m, Nit-ac, Rhus-t, Sep, Sil, Staph, Sulph.*
Scabida — *Anthrok, Dulc, Lyc, Sulph.*
Scrofulosa inveterata — *Iod*
Thick mild secretion — *Calc*
Of strumous persons — *Aethiops, Ars-i, Calc, Calc-i, Calc-p, Caust, Cistus, Crot-t, Hep, Merc-c, Merc, Rumx, Sep, Sil, Tub.*
Pustular (Impetigo) — *Ang, Arg-nit, Calc,* Calc-p, *Carbol-ac, Carb-s, Caust, Cic, Con, Crot-t, Jug, Kali-bi, Kali-i, Merc, Mez, Nat-m, Rhus-t, Rhus-v, Sil, Sulph, Terent.*
— *Chronic* — *Cinnab*
Figurata — *Ars, Calc, Clem, Con, Dulc, Graph, Lyc, Merc,* Thuja, *Sulph.*
Figurata tendency to spread — *Merc*
— with gastric complaints — *Iris*
— after abuse of mercury, in psoric constitutions — *Clem*
Pimples form scabs — *Carb-s*
Pustular — *Ant-t*
Recent case in adults — *Viol-tri*
Pigmentation in circumscribed areas following — *Berb-v*
Pregnancy and nursing during on face — *Sep*
Raw fluid destroying hair — *Nat-m*

Redness, small blisters, intense, itching — *Anac*
Recurrent — *Como*
Right side on, moist — *Canth*
Rubrum — *Acon, Alum, Am-m, Anac, Apis, Bell, Bov, Calc, Canth, Carb-v, Crot-t, Dulc, Lyc, Mez, Rhus-t, Sulph.*
Sea-shore, ocean, voyage, excess of salt - worse — *Nat-m*
Exudation dries into hard, lemon coloured scab — *Cic*
Scabs, thick and honey combed — *Hep*
Scabs, thick hard from which pus exudes on pressure — *Mez*
Scurfy — *Kreos*
Scurfy, discharging corrosive fluid, which eats hair, worse in edges of hair — *Nat. m*
Smarts as if scalded — *Ran-b*
Scratch the more they, greater the urgency to scratch — *Rhus-t*
Scratching one place itching ceases but appears at another — *Staph*
Scrofulous — *Dulc, Tell.*
Small thin white scurfs on surface — *Merc*
Sun exposure from — *Mur-ac*
Smarting burning when touched — *Canth*
Solaris — *Acon, Arum-m, Bell, Camph, Canth, Clem, Hyos, Nat-c, Mur-ac.*
Squamosum in conjunctivitis scrofulous — *Kali-bi*
Squamosum fifteen years — *Graph*
Stinging — *Merc*
Suppressed — *Cap-ac, Kali-s.*
Suppressed in epilepsy — *Kali-m*
Suppressed following vaccination — *Ammoniac*
Suppressed or deranged uterine functions — *Kali-m*
Suppressed, head of agg — *Mez*
Severe and stubborn of sweating parts of body, exposed to fumes of poison — *Merc-cor*
Thickening of skin and hard horny scabs — *Ran-b*
Tingling — *Rhus-t*
Tingling when she gets warm — *Kali-ars*
Urinary, gastric, hepatic, disorders with — *Lyc*
Suppressed urine agg — *Solid*
Ulcer large surrounded by smaller ones, some healing, some healed — *Phos*
Umbical — *Sulph*

Uterine functions suppressed or deranged from — *Kali-m*
Vaccination after with itching — *Rhus-t*
Vaccination after worse — *Mez*
cured by vaccination in two children — *Variol*
from vaccination with bad vaccine lymph — *Kali-m*
Vesicles small in neighbourhood of joints, itched, dried up rapidly and frequently recurred — *Phos*
Small vesicles, Smaller and flatter than mercurial eczema — *Cop*
Washing agg — *Ars-iod*
Watery vesicles — *Canth*
Weeping after taking cold, worse in warmth of room after having been in cold air, itching when warm, worse washing — *Hydras*
White secretions — *Kali-m*
Winter every for a number of years — *Merc*
Of twelve years standing — *Phos*
Head — *Agar, Ant-t, Arct-l, Ars, Astac, Aur, Bad, Bar-c, Bar-m, Berb-aq, Brom, Calc, Calc-s, Carb-s, Caust, Cocc, Cic, Clem, Dulc, Fl-ac, Graph, Hep, Hydr, Iris, Kali-ar, Kali-bit, Kal-m, Kali-s, Kreos, Lyc, Mez, Nat-m, Nat-p, Oleand, Petr, Phyt, Psor, Rhus-t, Sars, Sep, Selen, Staph, Sil, Sulph, Tellur, Tub, Ust, Viol-t, Vinc, Viol-od.*
Eyes around — *Bry, Sep.*
Eyelids on — *Bry, Clem, Graph, Hep, Mez, Rhus-t, Sep, Tell Thuja.*
Ear — *Ars, Arundo, Bov, Calc, Chrysarob, Graph, Hep, Jug-r, Kali-m, Mez, Lyc, Olnd, Petr, Psor, Rhus-t, Sanic, Scrophul, Sep, Staph, Sulph, Tell, Tub.*
Meatus in — *Bor, Graph, Kreos, Nit-ac, Petr, Psor,*
Face — *Alum, Ambr, Anac, Ant-c, Ars, Bac, Bar-c, Bor, Bell, Bry, Calc, Calc-s, Carb-a, Carb-v, Caust, Chel, Cic, Clem, Col, Con, Cornus, Crot-t, Cur, Cycl, Dulc, Ferr-i, Fl-ac, Graph, Hep, Hyper, Iris. Kali-ar, Kreos, Lach, Led, Lyc, Merc, Merc-i-r, Merc-pr-rub, Mez, Mur-ac, Nat-m, Petr, Phos, Ph-ac, Psor, Ran-b, Rhus-t, Sars, Sep, Sil, Staph, Sulph, Sul-ac, Sulph-i, Syph, Vinc, Viol-t.*
With serous exudate — *Petrol*
Spreading from back of head — *Lyc, Sil.*
— **like dried honey** — *Ant-c, Cic.*
Honey like crusts about mouth — *Mez*
Beard of — *Ars Iod*

Chin on — *Bor, Cic, Graph, Rhus-t, Sep.*
Mouth corner of — *Arund, Graph, Hep, Lyc, Rhus, Sil.*
Mouth around — *Mur-ac, Nat-m.*
Nose — *Ant-c, Caust, Cost, Rhus-t, Sep, Sulph.*
Temples about — *Alumin*
Epigastrium — *Ars*
Anus and rectum — *Nat-m, Nit-ac.*
Genitalia, female — *Caust, Dulc, Petr.*
— **male** — *Arg-n, Ars, Chel, Crot-t, Graph, Hep, Lyc, Nat-m, Nit-ac, Petr, Rhus-t, Sep, Sulph, Thuj.*
On Scrotum — *Calc, Crot-t, Graph, Nat-m, Petr.*
Pudendum — *Am-c, Ant-c, Ars, Canth, Crot-t, Hep, Plb, Rhus-t, Sanic, Sep.*
Perineum — *Petr*
Vulva, labia — *Rhus-t*
Neck and throat — *Caust, Lyc, Petr, Sep Sulph.*
Chest — *Anac, Ars, Calc, Calc-s, Carb-v, Cycl, Graph, Hep, Kali-s, Petr, Psor, Staph, Sulph.*
Axilla — *Carb-a, Hep, Jug-r, Lyc, Merc, Nat-m, Petr, Psor, Sep.*
Mammae — *Anac, Caust, Dulc.*
Nipples — *Graph, Sars, Sulph.*
Back — *Arn, Merc, Sil.*
Finger — *Lyc, Sil, Staph.*
Painful — *Arn*
Fingers, toes of with loss of nails — *Bor*
Lower limbs — *Anil, Apis, Ars, Bov, Chel, Jug-ar, Kali-br, Merc, Petr, Psor, Rhus-t.*
Thigh — *Petr, Rhus-t.*
Thighs between — *Nat-m, Petr.*
Knee — *Anil, Arn, Rhus-t.*
Knee hollow of — *Graph*
Legs — *Apis, Ars, Carb-v, Graph, Kali-br, Lach, Led, Lyc, Merc, Nat-m, Petr, Rhus-t, Sars, Sulph.*
Calf — *Graph*
Ankle — *Chel, Nat-p, Psor.*
Back of foot — *Merc, Psor.*
Extremities — *Anil, Arn, Ars, Kali-br, Merc, Pros.*
Joints — *Led, Phos.*
Flexures of joints — *Aeth, Am-c, Caust, Graph, Hep, Kali-ar, Man-ac, Nat-m, Psor, Sep, Sulph.*
Upper limbs — *Canth, Graph, Merc, Mez, Phos, Psor, Sil.*
Shoulder — *Petr*

Elbow — *Brom*
Bend of elbow — *Cupr, Graph, Mez, Psor.*
Forearm — *Graph, Merc, Mez, Sil, Thuj.*
Wrists — *Jug-c, Mez, Psor.*
Hand — *Anag, Ars, Bar-c, Berb-v, Bov, Calc, Canth, Clem, Graph, Hep, Hyper, Jug-c, Kreos, Lyc, Malandr, Merc, Mez, Nit-ac, Petr, Pix-l, Plb, Phos, Sanic, Selen, Sep, Sil, Still, Rhus-v.*
Back of hand — *Graph, Jug-c, Merc, Mez, Nat-c, Phos, Sep.*
Swelling hand with — *Psor*

A Case of Asthma and Eczema Alternating with Each Other

Patient of 25 years of age, suffers from eczema and asthma, both alternating with each other.

Started with eczema when he was about 7 years of age. Was treated with various ointments and lotions which "cured" the eczema. He was alright for some years; then he got a chill and was down with fever and severe cough; was hospitalised and was told he had pneumonia. After coming out of the hospital he was well for some time. One night, about midnight. he was woken from sleep with breathelessness and cough. Family doctor was called and he said, the patient had asthma. Treatment for asthma was continued for some months but the patient did not improve. Then all of a sudden the asthma went away and on came the attack of eczema. Treatment for eczema was started; but this time the eczema was not improved; and then come the attack of asthma. Patient was fed up with this see-saw affair and come to me to ask if Homoeopathy could help. I said, "Homoeopathy will certainly help, provided you have patience to continue. Homoeopathic treatment for a long time". I also said, "There are every chances that your eczema would aggravate to a great extent during the treatment and at that time if you get panicky all our efforts would be wasted."

On taking the case the following symptoms were recorded :

Asthma	Agg night, especially around midnight. Attacks generally start in the evening lasting till morning. Spasmodic attacks with rattling in chest. During the attack he can't sleep and has to be near an open window. If he goes out in the open air, he feels very much relieved.
Eczema	With tremendous itching amel by scratching; scratching followed by burning; agg heat.
Constitutional symptoms	Hot patient with desire for open air. Wears thin clothes in winter. Light sleep, waking up at slightest noise. Does not cover during sleep. Eats little in comparision to intake of water, drinks, a lot of water. Desires sweets.
Family History	Of eczema in mother; asthma in sister, gout in father.

The case was repertorised by using *Kent's* and *Knerr's repertories.*

Asthma after suppressed itch - p. 1017
Asthma evening - p. 1017
Asthma night - p. 1018
Asthma spasmodic - p. 1019
Asthma humid - p. 1018
Asthma after suppressed eruption in general - p. 1017.

The above was from *Knerr's Repertory.*

The following from *Kent's Repertory* :

Asthma Alternating with eruptions - p. 764
Asthma evening - p. 764
Asthma night - p. 764
Respiration difficult, wants doors and windows open - p. 770.

Respiration difficult, air in open amm. — p. 768
Eruption alternating with asthma — p. 1308
Desires sweets — p. 486
Air, open desire for, — p. 1344
Remedies agg. by heat — p. 1366.

Treatment was started with *Sulphur* 30, and was continued for two months. The patient improved slowly, but after two months there was a slight set back, when *Sulph.* 200 was given for three months. Patient improved still further, attacks of eczema and asthma are far apart and of less severity. After three months the patient was at a stand still, and so *Sulph.* 1M was given for two months, t.d.s. No attack of either of diseases for two months. The patient stopped coming. After a month of stopping the medicine, attack of asthma came on. Patient came back and *Sulph.* 1M was repeated and treatment continued for four months more; and the patient stopped coming again.

The treatment with *Sulph.* was started on 15-1-81; and continued till Dec. 81, when he stopped coming.

He remained well for one year and seven months; but on 27-7-83 came back again with no actual eczematous eruption anywhere on the body but itching of various parts of body which was not there till a month ago. Also he gets breathlessness in the middle of the night since last seven days. He suffered so much with these diseases that he did not want to take any risk of going without medicine.

Now the symptoms were :

Still the patient wants open air, doors and windows open, but that is in summer. When he came back to me it was rainy season. In rains he is not comfortable in open air and if it is very windy he has to close the windows. Last time when he came, sweating was of no characteristic importance; but this time he perspires profusely on head, especially at night.

Sulph. 10M t.d.s. was given for a week.
No change. In the meantime case was studied again and it was found that now *Calcarea carb* was indicated.

On consulting Allen's "Keynotes" :

"Longing for fresh air, which inspires, benefits, strengthens."
"Aversion to cold air; sensitive to cold, damp air".
"Head sweats profusely while sleeping."

On consulting Harvey Farringtons "Homoeopathy and Homoeopathic Prescribing" p. 104, Para, 31 :

"The action of C. C. on skin is less profound than that of Sulph. Nevertheless, it is indispensable when the latter remedy has failed to clear the skin and the patient's general symptomatology merges into that of *Calcarea* type."

So. C. C. 1m was given on 30.7.83 for 15 days. Not much change. C. C. 10m was given for 15 days on 15.8.83. Patient felt better. He does not get any itching of the skin, nor does he get any breathlessness at night, feels better in every way.

On 3.9.83, repeat for a month.

On 4-10-83 C.C. 10m was again given for two months. Patient remains in good health as seen in Nov. 85.

HOMOEOPATHY
Vol. IV — No. 9
Page No. 283

The following case was definitely provoking and is illuminating as showing how we are in the hands of patients and their guardians.

A little girl, aged 9 years, was brought. She was suffering from eczema behind both knees. This condition had come on when she was one year old, and in spite of a" previous treatment had not become improved, far less cured. On enquiry found, amongst other treatments, exposure to X-rays had been tried. This put away the eczema from the knees and brought it out on the child's abdomen. This case was tackled with great happiness and with corresponding depression, as for three months treatment failed to do other than to change the character of the eruption. One day, on calling to see the child, the mother said, would I not think of giving the child *Iodine.* I asked why should this be done, and was told that every time the child went to the seaside, the skin went bad again. Let me say here that this had never been hinted to me, in spite of my request that I should be told everything, and despite a very lengthy questionnnaire.

Immediately, the child got *Med.* The present state of affairs is that two months after her dose, the skin is perfectly healthy and the eczema gone. It cleared up in a week after her powders of *Med.* If you refer to the repertory, you will find only one drug given there for amelioration at the seaside.

THE HOMOEOPATHIC HERITAGE
No. 8 — August 1983
Page No. 372 — Case No. 1056

Parotidinum

A little Nosode case has been sent to us. Weeping eczema, between fingers and all over body, intensely itching, which had persisted for ten years in spite of much treatment, was cured by *Parotidinum* 200 — a few doses, repeated at need, six weeks later. The indication being, 'Past history'.

One becomes more and more convinced, as one gains in experience, that to CURE it is imperative to give, or to interpose a dose or two of the most perfect antidote to the ancient malady, viz., its own self, potentized and given in the nonlethal manner of Homoeopathy, only as required, and by the mouth. Burnett in regard to his special one, *Tuberculinum* or *Bacillinum*, said emphatically, to those who desired to use them otherwise, 'Hands off!'

THE HOMOEOPATHIC HERITAGE
No. 13 — December 1983
Page No. 568 — Case No. 1109

Case of eczema behind the ears, on the scalp, and in the bends of the elbows and armpits, accompanied by abscesses afecting the bones. Nothing relieved, but the affecting eruption disappeared to reappear again, years after, on the wrists. There was then a patch on each wrist as large as a half dollar with intense itching, preventing sleep, with constant desire to scratch. *Psorinum* mm; in two days the patches had doubled in size and in a week more they had extended to the dorsi of the hands between the metacarpal bones, but in another two weeks they disappeared entierely.

THE HOMOEOPATHIC OUTLOOK
Vol. XV — No. 2 (1955)
Page No. 63
Eczema of 25 years cured (S.R. Wadia)

Patient's Name : Mrs A.A. Choksey; *Age* : 73 years.

The patient has eczema since the last 25 years. Location bends of the elbows and knees, thighs, hands (Knuckles) and feet also between the webs of the toes. The skin has become hard with fissures oozing a sticky fluid. She is worse in winter, better by hot or very hot application, specially the itching. The skin that is affected has changed and looks pigmented dark though the patient is fair. She always takes a hot bath. Her thirst is normal.

Temperament : She is sad and very worried about her prolonged illness. She has no peace of mind due to intense itching. Her memory has become dull recently.

Past Illness : Operated for hernia, cataract and fracture right wrist seven years back. Had Herpes Opthalmicus three years back. For her skin condition she has consulted practically each and every specialist. She was treated for seven long years at K.E.M. Hospital, Parel. Light therapy was given by a famous doctor and various injections to no avail.

15-11-52 — A single powder of *Sepia* 200 was given.

25-11-52 — Report after one week patient was much better, the dark colour of the skin has started fading. The skin is slightly softer but itching still persists. *Placebo* was prescribed and externally oil coconut.

29-11-52 — Patient better, itching less. The patient wanted to go to Broach and asked my permission which was granted. Placebo.

15-12-52 — I saw her today after her return from Broach. The itch is much better in the flexors but the hands specially the knuckles and feet are still itching and there is slight oozing. *Sepia* 200 a single dose was given.

After the second dose the patient kept on improving not only the skin was better but her mental condition improved too. She is happy now. The patient comes to me every week and placebo is given as usual with best results.

25-3-53 — Slight itching on legs again. *Sepia* 200 one dose.

These three dose of Sepia was all that the patient required to cure her skin condition perfectly. The skin which was rough pigmented and dirty looking is now pearl white. The patient came to wish me a Bon-Voyage on 26-3-54 before I left for England with a present for me when she was perfectly well. This is the magic of the minimum dose.

THE HOMOEOPATHIC OUTLOOK
Vol. II — No. 11 (1941)
Page No. 355 — Case No. 11

Eczema

A baby 12 months old, has had eczema pretty much all over her body since 10 days old. She had had all the ointments, lotions and external applications that several physicians could think of, but no internal treatment. If ointment was put on her face, the eczema went to the arm; if suppressed on the arm, it went somewhere else, and had been doing so for a year.

We had a typical *Calcarea* baby fat, sweaty head, no teeth, constipated, catches cold all the time, does not walk or creep.

Calcarea 1m, 10m, and 40m, and no external applications practically cured the eczema in less than four months. The usual number of teeth had come; she stopped catching cold, and was a well baby.

THE HOMOEOPATHIC HERITAGE
Eczema Capitalis
August 1987 — Page No. 448

Was called to see Miss Edna S. aged 4½ months. Mother stated that she had been under the care of different Allopathic physicians both in this city and in Toronto for 3 months, but was constantly getting worse; one physician had told her that nothing could cure the baby until it got its teeth, at which time it would cure itself. So, in her prejudice, to try Homoeopathy.

While under Allopathic treatment it had all kinds of ointments applied, both patent and prescribed ones, and had also taken from the Toronto physician quantities of 'Cod Liver Oil' and 'Syrup of Hypophosphites.' The following is the history of the case while under treatment as it occurs from time in my case book :

3-1-1884 — Patient had an eruption on face and scalp since she was six weeks old. Cheeks covered with moist eczema discharging watery pus, forehead and scalp covered with a dry, scalpy eczema,. Large, yellow scabs formed on face, secreting a thick yellow pus underneath discharge quite profuse, itching sometimes almost intolerable; baby very fair, exceedingly fat; fed on cow's milk appetite ravenous, vomits thick curds; alternate constipation and diarrhoea; stools very hard, pale and chalky at first then loose, containing indigested material. Before eczema appeared its head used to sweat profusely. *Calc. carb* 200 followed by placebos for one week.

10-1-1884 — Eczema on cheeks drying up dry scabs on forehead and front of scalp. General health better; bowels regular and natural; does not vomit at all. No discharge from eczema; dry brown scabs. Continue placebos.

14-1-1884 — Scabs on forehead scaling off, are of a greenish yellow colour and as large as a silver dollar, skin under scabs seems to be healing, general health much improved, not fleshy. *Calc.c.* 200, 2 doses in one day and placebos.

18-1-1884 — Face presents a much healthier appearance, only a scab here and there on cheeks, has cut two teeth without causing any apparent inconvenience. Placebos.

25-1-1884 — Baby still keeping in excellent general health. Not nearly so fat. Eczema improving. The mother says if was better two days ago than now. *Calc.c.* 200 as before.

31-1-1884 — Slowly improving. *Calc.c.* 20M. 2 doses.

9-2-1884 — Very marked improvement, face all healed up; only two or three scabs on scalp now. Placebos.

14-2-1884 — Almost well; skin still slightly rough. Child much stronger and healthier in every way, though not so fleshy. *Calc.c.* 40M one dose.

24-4-1884 — Since last record, child has enjoyed perfect health, has cut several teeth with no symptoms of any return of the trouble. The only topical application which was allowed was pure rain water, and that used sparingly and with great care.

In this case the special indications for the remedy were found elsewhere than in the eczema although that also corresponded to the remedy.

THE HOMOEOPATHIC OUTLOOK
Vol. II No. 4 (1940)
Page No. 97

Homoeopathic Treatment of Eczema

From ancient times all schools of medicine considered *Sulphur* a remedy par excellence for eczema. The picture of the *Sulphur* patient as dirty and Water-shy is often correct, but from experience, I can say *Sulphur* has never disappointed me in clean patients. A typical symptom is that the *Sulphur* eczema is dry and scaly, itching especially evenings, in the warmth of bed and is worse from washing. The *Sulphur* eczema is found especially on the forehead at the hairline, genitals and flexor surfaces of joints.

I also like to give *Sulphur* to produce reaction. Often we find that a well chosen homoeopathic remedy is apparently not able to affect the eczema, and it is not always possible to explain this. Possibly there is a weakened physical reaction, or other obscure factors play a role. In many cases I have experienced that *Sulphur* caused an extraordinary reaction in the sense of a primary aggravation, and that then the eczema disappeared suddenly after a while, or that now the suitable homoeopathic remedy could better develop its action. I have seen patients who suffered from eczema (usually as so — called seborrhoeic eczema) and asthma. If now the asthma was treated successfully, then often the eczema was aggravated and vice versa. Such patients often react to *Sulphur*. However, in such cases it is difficult to solve the question of dose. I have seen improvement from low as well as from high potencies. In combination with *Arsenicum* one can often relieve such patient of their distressing condition.

Arsenicum with *Sulphur* in large doses is used today extensively by the dermatogical school; how much of the often outstanding results belong to the credit of homoeopathic medicine action, I do not wish to decide.

The *Arsenic* skin eruption is usually dry, seldom moist, combined with severe burning of skin. Itching is not so prominent. There is aggravation from scratching and cold. The skin bleeds easily and is covered with crusts. Open air and radiated heat are unpleasant to the patient. *Arsenicum* seems to be especially valuable in degenerative processes, so often caused by eczemas of the aged and in suitable forms of diabetic eczemas.

Graphites has often been found to be an excellent eczema remedy. Its domain is the chronic form, but often one must have much patience till its action becomes evident. Its type is the slow, thickset, indolent and gluttonous patient, women have delayed and weak menses. It is strange that these people do not perspire; but the women have much 'flying heat'. Eczemas behind the ears and on occciput, often very moist with tough, yellow crusts, and that is characteristic. Callosities on hands and feet remind one of *Graphites*. Aggravations of all symptoms in evenings is often marked.

Antimonium crudum is the opposite of *Graphites* in many ways, perspiration is one of its characteristics. Its eczema is usually moist, begins with purulent pustules in face. Impetigo in children is one of its great fields of action. The tongue is usually coated with bad,, flat taste mornings. Chronic digestive disturbances. the patient is very tired and lazy, may have severe horny calluses, especially on the feet; deformed nails.

Calcium has lately played a prominent role in dermatology. In itching eczemas it has often acted splendidly but again in other cases which seemed to be the same, it failed. Perhaps in these cases there was no *Calcium* type as in the others. I have found that *Calcium* type : fat, phlegmatic, easily perspiring patient, women who menstruate too early and profusely, respond often very well to *Calcarea carbonica*. Important is, that though skin getting wet is not tolerated, there is a craving for water. Cold, moist feet fit well into the picture. Warmth relieves. In children's eczema *Calcarea* often acts well. I generally try to learn whether or not patients have had eczema or milk crust in younger years, which indicate circumscribed eczema on the hands of young girls which resists all other therapy respond well to *Calcarea carbonica*. *Natrum muriaticum* must not be forgotten here, as it often exactly suits these cases.

Baryta carbonica for children as well as for the aged is well indicated in many instances, and especially in backward children.

Petroleum has the chronic eczemas in the fall and winter with cracked skin, which does not heal well.

Sepia is pre-eminent in eczemas in the climacteric or at its end, if they also have small, very itchy vesicles on the fingers worse from water. Of course, there should be other *Sepia* symptoms too. During summer one must be sure that it is not a case of mycosis from athlete's feet. In such cases anti-parastic treatment must be instituted and a constitutional remedy should be given, like *Calcarea* or *Silicea*.

Lycopodium is a valuable remedy in eczema : itching severely, bleeding from scratching; disturbed digestion. Bulimia satisfied by a few bites; flatulency not relieved by passing of gases. I mention these symptoms because they are the opposite of *Carbo vegetablis*, which is also efficient in the treatment of chronic leg ulcers of older people. Often it is advisable to alternate with *Calcarea fluorica*.

Thuja occidentale can be used in facial seborrhoeic eczema, especially if there exists also an oily condition of the hair. There are women who distinctly show the *Thuja* type.

Croton is especially for eczema of scrotum with terrible itching.

Silicea is a constitutional remedy which should be tried repeatedly in many cases.

Berberis vulgaris in eczema with much uric acid, often accompanied by troubles of joints and bladder.

Acidum nitricum is for itching and eczema, rhagades and moist conditions.

All these remedies have this in common. They are especially valuable in chronic cases from disturbed metabolism, or when they are constitutionally indicated. For acute eczema with redness and swelling of skin, vesicle formation, the following briefly mentioned remedies must be compared :

Belladonna when skin is tightly drawn and hot; during infectious diseases and intestinal disturbances.

Apis is similar : oedema of skin, stitching pains; no thirst.

Rhus toxicodendron : acute blisters on skin, intensely itching and burning. Often after colds and change of weather.

Cantharis : when acute eczema is preceded or soon followed by bladder troubles.

Not to be forgotten : Formic acid therapy (internally, or preferably hypodermically or intravenously in medium aqueous potencies).

HOMOEOPATHY AND COMPARATIVE MEDICINE
Page No. 108 — Case No. III(i)

A Case of Eczema

Patient, Ashok Dey, aged 19, was suffering from Eczema. He was under the treatment of the local allopathic doctor but without any beneficial result, although he has spent nearly about Rs. 20 for the medicine. I examined the patient and noticed that the muco-cutaneous outlets of the body were red. There was an offensive odour emanating from his body, and he told me that there was severe itching of the eruptions which was worse at night, especially while he lay himself on the bed to sleep at night. I gave him *Sulphur* 200, one does on that very morning and repeated the same after a fortnight. These two doses cured him completely and there was no need for any external application.

THE HOMOEOPATHIC HERITAGE
Case Reports :
Case No. 2 - Page No. 395

Male : 39 years.

12-3-76 — Eczema dry, 20 years old on left leg with whitish eruptions near genitalia, nates and finger joints. Antibiotics gave temporary relief. Had been operated for appendicitis. His father and one of his children a daughter too have similar eruptions on the same leg, affected parts burn with severe itching. Patient's salt intake abnormally high.

On the totality of symptoms he was put on *Nat-mur* 200 T.D.S. Very much improved by 13-9-76, when he stopped the treatment.

2-12-80 — Reported again, but the eruptions were confined to a small area above the ankle. *Nat-mur* 200, one dose caused severe agg. SL for 10 days. Thereafter *Nat-mur*, 6 brought about complete recovery by 12-5-81.

There has been no return of symptoms till date.

INDIAN JOURNAL OF HOMOEOPATHIC MEDICINE
Page No. 59 — Case No. 2

Infantile Eczema with Secondary Infection — Arum Triphyllum 30.

Master P. aged 6 years suffering from Eczema for two years came to me from Bhopal. Eczema was spread all over the body but particularly more around the mouth. There were pustular eruptions with reddish erythema around them at many places. It was ulcerated and was discharging thin watery fluid. Itching was so violent that the child would go on scratching even if the surface bled. Itching was aggravated at night, aggravated by exposure to heat and during rainy season.

He had been on homoeopathic treatment earlier and has been given *Graphites*, *Hepar sulphur*, *Silicea* and Biochemic drugs. Earlier he had been treated with local ointments also. The first prescription of *Bacillinum* 200, based on family history of pleurisy with effusion made no effect on the skin but the dry cough he was having,disappeared. *Antim. crud.* later made no improvement. I prescribed Arum *triphyllum* 30 next on the basis of the violent itching which drove the patient to scratching even if the surface was raw and bleeding. Improvement was noticed from next day onwards. *Arum triphyllum* was given four times a day.

INDIAN JOURNAL OF HOMOEOPATHIC MEDICINE
Vol. 9 - No. 1 (1975)
Page No. 15

My wife suffered from very severe eczema. In spite of careful prescribing — *Graph.* was her remedy — she had recurrent attacks with violent itching. I had a cousin who was suffering for five years from TB. His remedy was *Phos.* He had bleeding P.R. during cloudy weather. I continued to give him *Phos.* At a stage he developed eczema with burning, oozing, bleeding, etc. He used to run like a made man due to the itching. But finally we gave him *Ac. fl.* and he was cured. For the last 5-6 years he has no illness at all and enjoys the best of health. He had a h/o having been given paraffin for many years for constipation. In these cases I think paraffin was being eliminated as in my wife's case, she had taken some petroleum product in her early years.

HOMOEOPATHY AND COMPARATIVE MEDICINE
June 1957
Page No. 102 — Case No. III

Eczema and Goitre Cured :
(Dr. Truman Coates)

A graduate of 'Old School' in 1888, although willing, yet anxious, to accept the good wherever found and knowing our limitations, a few years ago I strayed into neighbouring pastures led by a case of very stubborn eczema in a woman of middle life. The trouble at times, especially after becoming heated from undue work in sunshine, covered her face, hands, exposed parts of her arms, the skin being very red and exasperatingly itchy and thick.

After repeated failures in my efforts and of those to whom I applied for assistance, I sought for help in the domain of Hahnemann, when I was recommended to give *Skookum*

Chuck 3x, four tablets a day and to my surprise and our thankfulness the case was cured in two weeks, the lady never had an itchy skin again and the skin cleared up entirely. If we have anything in our school that will do this, it was my misfortune to never find it.

A year ago a lady of fifty-seven years came to me for relief from a pain in her right brow, toward the temple, attacking her at frequent periods nearly all her life. Three years previously I corrected her eyestrain with lenses, which dissipated at least half of her suffering. I gave *Magnesia phos.* somewhat irregularly for a few weeks, with but partial relief from pain, but to our surprise and real joy a goitre on right side, in size very noticeable even through an ordinary collar was gone; not a vestige was left. I at once began research for such and found in Dr. Vondergoltz's Biochemical Manual, *Magnesia phos.* is the second remedy he recommends for goitre. To this day the goitre is not to be seen.

I might continue relating further results, especially in nasal catarrh and adenoids in cases of children from eight to seventeen years, but the foregoing is likely enough for my maiden effort in new company.

INDIAN JOURNAL OF HOMOEOPATHIC MEDICINE
Vol. 10 - No. 2 (1976)
Page No. 82 - Method 3

A woman, twenty-seven years of age, for four weeks suffered from a dry, papulous, violently itching eczema of neck, upper part of chest and wrist, during six weeks prior to the outbreak of the eczema, the patient became sleepless, lying awake for hours. Upon one dose of *Coffea* 200, which covered both disorders the eczema disappeared within a week, the sleeplessness the next night. The patient was told that the remedy was administered for the eczema; the disturbance of sleep was purposely not mentioned.

In this method remedies which cover several disorders are given to the patient and the patient is told that they are given for one of them. The influence on the other disturbances can thus critically be observed and any suggestive influence is avoided.

INDIAN JOURNAL OF HOMOEOPATHIC MEDICINE
Vol. II - No. 2 (1977)
Page No. 59 - Case No. 1

Infantile Dermatitis — Arum triphyllum 200

Master N. Aged 1 year 8 months. In June 1965 developed eczema relieved by local application of Hydrocortisone. In September 1965 eczema relapsed again on the left cheek and was treated similarly. In November 1965 spread to both the cheeks, abdomen, back, legs and arms with violent itching day and night. Face was swollen, moisture on scratching, and the patient did not want to cover. The child craved for indigestible substances like Pencil, chalk, earth. Stools were hard, at times streaked with blood. Fissure in Ano.

Family History : Sister — Psoriasis; Mother — Alopecia Areata. Mother's sister — Asthma; Father — Urticaria and — Grandfather — Diabetes. There was a strong history of Allergy in the family.

The following drugs were given : *Graph* 30, *Acid nitricum* 200, *Kali-sulph*, *Lachesis*, *Sepia*, *Rhus-tox*, *Ratanhia*, *Pulsatilla*, but ultimately it was *Arum triphyllum* 200 to which he responded and the eczema started clearing up.

THE HOMOEOPATHIC HERITAGE
No. 5 - May 1983
Page No. 196 - Case No. 973

Eczema

Mr. G.B 72 years old, told me he suffered, when he was about 40 years, from an obstinate eczema which had extended from the feet to the sexual parts, then onto the trunk, and at last to the eyelids and scalp. But for the eczema, he thought at that time, that he was very strong and in perfect health. It required years of various treatment and the use of numerous ointments to suppress little by little this eruption, traces of which are still to be seen on the scalp and eyelids. During more than twenty years since the time he had at last succeeded in ridding himself of his eczema, he suffered from frequent influenza, then from bronchitis, which little by little turned into asthma. He attributes all these phenomena, from which he never suffered before to chills and these grew worse in spite of every care. Little by little rheumatism set in (a question of time perhaps) which made him suffer cruelly, in the shoulders, hands and lower limbs. Every winter he had one or two attacks of lumbago and sciatica, without mentioning attacks of bronchitis and asthma.

Now he has a pityriasic erythema on the scalp, dry eczema of the eyelids and conjunctivitis. The skin all over the body is extremely dry and covered with little white scales, especially abundant on the limbs. When auscultating the globulous thorax, one hears a loud ronchi and numerous sibilances spread about. The cough is noisy, paroxysmal, turns loose and dry. Solar plexus painful when pressed, when the patient is standing (signal pain according to Leven), which denotes a gastric ptosis. The liver very sensitive to touch, continues beyond the ribs a little. The patient complains of lack of appetite and constipation. Dry arthrities of the shoulders and knees. Heart normal, Pulse 75. Tendon reflexes not very much marked. Numerous nodosities around the articulations of both hands. The nails of the big toes are very much thickened. The patient is frequently disturbed in his sleep by his cough and after 5 in the morning he cannot sleep at all.

The story and the complex of the present symptoms clearly indicate *Sulphur*. On January 27, I gave *Sulphur* 30 every morning in the plus method. On February 3 the patient returned saying : "I feel better, I sleep better till 6.30. The cough disappeared two days ago, the breathing is deeper, the stairs much less difficult to ascend. I have an appetite again, my bowels. evacuate two or three times a day." The only shadow in the picture is the increase of rheumatism nearly everywhere. I gave Placebo.

On February 27, the above mentioned improvements are maintained. The head is lighter, the mind more active, the ideas clearer. The itching and the erythema of the scalp have disappeared. The eyes are getting better. On the contrary, the rheumatic pains are stronger in the hands and feet. "An extraordinary thing, doctor, my previous perspirations and my eczema of 20 years ago, on the genitals, hands and feet have returned. I don't want to recommence this remedy of yours." I warn my patient and tell him to abstain from any external medicinal application and I speak to him of the law of cure explaining to him that his symptoms are following exactly the desired direction less

From the above downward (the head is better, the lower parts of the body worse).

From within outward (the cough, asthma, breathing, digestive functions are very much improved, whilst the extremities show serious aggravation).

And in the reverse order of the coming of the symptoms (reappearance of the previous eczema and perspiration). Of course, I give Placebo.

On April 2, I see my patient again. He declares that his state has rapidly improved, until a recent journey during which he indulged in an indiscretion of diet, which brought a strong aggravation of all skin symptoms. The rheumatism is better but has not completely disappeared. I order a dose of *Sulphur* 200 and Placebo. (The duration of *Sulphur* 30 was 10 weeks).

On July 6, the patient returns to thank me. He is cured and wishes to make me endorse his opinion.

CHAPTER 10

Erythematous Rashes

Erythema is one of the commonest primary lesions of the skin. It is produced by the dilatution of the cutaneous blood vessels. If the dilatation is accompanied by increased permeability, redness and oedema of the skin are produced, features of urticarial eruption, quite familiar to everyone, as commonly seen in nettle rash. At times the cutaneous blood vessels are so irritated and damaged, that they permit the whole blood to pass through, as in purpuras (haemorrhagic rashes). Thus, it will be seen that these three lesions, erythema, urticaria and purpura, depend upon the degree of stimulation of damage to the cutaneous vascular system. In every case, an erythematous lesion must be felt for induration or infiltration, either by palpation with gloved fingers, or with pointed dissecting forceps. Simple erythema has no resistance or infiltration of underlying tissues. Granulomas, however, like tuberculosis and leprosy have erythema plus filtration. Generalized erythema and infiltration of the whole integument is termed erythroderma.

Erythematous Rashes

The causes of erythematous rashes are as follows :

Localized erythema due to local external causes.

1. Traumatic — injury, pressure, bedsores, intertrigo, napkin rash.

2. Chemical — Dermatitis and eczema.

3. Heat, cold, light — Burn, frost-bite, sunburn.

4. Infective — Erythema in the early stages of impetigo, insect bite.

Generalized erythema, usually bilateral and symmetrical, due to a systemic internal cause.

1. Specific causes :

   (a) Syphilis.
   (b) Exanthemata.
   (c) Drug — eruptions.
   (d) Toxic erythema — focal sepsis, intestinal — food and its products.

2. Non-specific causes, described on morphological basis. They are definite disease entities, though the causes are indefinite.

   (a) E. Nodosum.
   (b) Induratum.
   (c) Lupus erythematosus.
   (d) E. Pernio.
   (e) E. Multiforme.
   (f) Other rare erythemas.

Erythema may take the form of localized or generalized — macules or sheets. Asymmetrical, localized redness is usually due to a local, external cause. Injury produces redness; pressure may result in bedsores. Chemical and thermal burns, insect-bites, bacterial infections, dermatitis and eczemas produce erythemas, at least, in the early stages. Bilateral and symmetrical widespread eruptions are usually due to an internal cause.

Erythema Multiforme

It is an affection uncommon in tropical countries, being a disease found mostly in the temperate climate. It occurs most often in young adults, and in the spring and autumn.

Etiology : It is considered to result from sensitization to products of infection and drugs. The infective group includes haemolytic streptococcus infection of the nose and the throat. The common offending drugs are barbiturates, sulphonamides, phenolphthalein and salicylates. So a search for a septic focus, and an enquiry into the drugs taken, should always be made. Quite often the patient himself volunteers of history of sore throat preceding the attack of erythema multiforme. Sometimes the disease is related to visceral disorders like allergic purpura or rheumatism or lymphogranuloma venereum or herpes simplex infection.

Clinical features : The onset is acute with mild fever, malaise and perhaps other constitutional symptoms. The lesions are multiple and polymorphic; they are distributed symmetrically on the dorsum of hands and feet, the forearms, the legs, the face and neck. Predominantly, the lesions are oedematous erythematous macules and flattened papules. Nodules, vesicles and bullae are uncommon. Bullous lesions can occur as such, generally starting on erythematous bases. Mucous membranes are usually spared, but a few lesions may be found in the mouth. The colour of the macular and papular cutaneous lesions changes from crimson-red to a purplish and even bluish colour. At times, concentric rings of various colours may be found in the lesions (erythema iris is a common annular lesion with a red centre). The cutaneous lesions are asymptomatic except for mild burning and smarting. Erythema multiforme is rarely associated with a gastro-intestinal disturbance, arthritis and haemorrhages. Severe erythema multiforme with predominantly extensive bullous eruption of the skin and mucous membranes, sudden onset, high fever and prostration, is often termed as Stevens Johnson disease, or Syndrome. The eyes urethra and respiratory tract may also be involved.

Pathology : The histopathological picture varies with the clinical picture. In all cases, the dermis shows dilated capillaries and infiltrate consisting mainly of lymphocytes. There may also be polymorphs and eosinophils. In bullous lesions, there is a typical sub-epidermal bulla while in maculopapular, epidermis shows spongiosis and intra-epidermal oedema.

Prognosis : The individual lesions last from several days to weeks. The whole attack lasts from two to four weeks. There is a tendency to recurrence, unless the causative factors are completely eliminated. Sometimes, there is a likelihood erythema multiforme bullosa being clinically mixed up with dermatitis herpetiformis and pemphigus (Percival). One can follow the other.

Differential diagnosis : It is made from other erythematous and vesiculobullous lesions and occasionally from urticaria. In the later, the diagnostic features are : asymmetrically distributed weals with whitish centres, marked itching, the short duration of the disease, and the absence of constitutional symptoms.

Main differentiation is from lupus erythematosus, dermatitis herpetiformis and pemphigus.

Lupus erythematosus shows typical butterfly lesions on the face, chronic infiltrated erythematous patches, follicular plugging and scarring. Dermatitis herpetiformis is seen as grouped polymorphic rash on forearms, scapular region and lower back, accompanied by marked itching and typical histopathology. Pemphigus bullae develop on normal skin. (bullae in erythema multiforme which develop on erythematous areas) and there are lesions in the mouth. Nikolsky's sign and Tzanck test and positive for acantholysis.

Toxic Erythemata

It is a wide but useful term for a group of erythematous conditions, apart from exanthemata, syphilis and drug eruptions, which one comes across in practice. These erythemas are, on their own, specific, though morphologically, they present varying pictures, and have no strict association with cause. Occasionally the term, Toxo-Allergic Rash is employed. The morphological names do not convey anything to the clinician. On the contrary, they are responsible for a great deal of confusion and misunderstanding.

As the name suggests, toxins reaching the skin produce such an erythema. These toxins include products of focal sepsis in the ear, nose, throat, teeth, intestines, urinary tract,etc., products of digestion and metabolism, acute illnesses, fevers rheumatism, drugs, injections and so forth. Clinically, lesions occur symmetrically and are usually widespread. The trunk, the upper parts of the extermities and the face are generally affected. Erythema may be morbiliform, scarlatiniform, roseolar or chronic, migratory variety. Erythema fades on pressure. The condition lasts from days to weeks, depending upon the cause. The eruption may be accompanied by mild constitutional disturbances like low-grade fever, headache and joint pains. Besides, there are local subjective symptoms of the causative toxic focus.

Toxic erythemas are very common. Selectively affected are children and young adults. Before the label of toxic erythema is given, pityriasis rosea, drug eruptions, secondary syphilis and infectious fevers, must all be definitely ruled out.

The treatment is usually simple. All obvious causes must be removed.

ERYTHEMA NODOSUM

Diagnostic Hallmarks:

1. Distribution : anterior lower legs.
2. Pain and tenderness.
3. Lack of response to antibiotic therapy.

Clinical Presentation:

Erythema nodosum is characterized by the pressence of large (4 to 10 cm) non-scaling, red, painful, lesions on the anterior surface of the lower legs. The smaller lesions appear as slope shouldered nodules whereas the larger lesions appear as flat topped plaques. Ulceration is never seen. On palpation the lesions are slightly warm and very tender. The distribution may be unilateral at first but later in the course of the disease both legs become involved. Generally no more than 6 lesions are present at any one time. Almost all of the lesions occur on the anterior shins or around the ankles. Occasional lesions develop above the knee, on the thigh or posteriorly on the calf. Ankle and knee swelling with redness and tenderness is rather commonly found. Erythema nodosum occurs considerably more often in women than in men.

The rapidity of onset together with tenderness and warmth on palpation often suggests the presence of cellulitis. However, the presence of more than a single lesion, a duration of more than several days usually allow for differentiation. Superficial thrombophlebitis also occasionally mimics erythema nodosum but it is rarely if ever bilateral.

Course and Prognosis:

Individual lesions resolve over a period of 10 to 20 days but even as the first lesions disappear one or more new ones begin to develop. Because of this sequential development, the entire course of the disease may last for months. Recurrent episodes occur in occasional patients but they are not commonly seen. Healing occurs with post inflammatory hyperpigmentation but not permanent scarring develops.

Pathogenesis:

A definitive etiology is not often found. However, the following causes should be considered : (1) **Medications** — Erythema nodosum is seen quite commonly with birth control pills containing large amounts of estrogen; it has been occasionally reported with use of sulfonamides, iodides and bromides. (2) **Infection** — Erythema nodosum occurs in association with blastomycosis coccidioidomycosis, histoplasmosis, Yersinia infection and streptococcal infection. Tuberculosis was important historically.
(3) **Autoimmune disease** – Erythema nodosum rather frequently accompanies chronic inflammatory bowel disease. Erythema nodosum rarely occurs with dysproteinemia, malignancies or the ingestion of foods, food dyes or food preservatives but is commonly found in early pregnancy and in association with sarcoidosis.

The reason for the female preponderance in erythema nodosum is unknown but perhaps estrogens play a facultative role allowing other, often undetermined, causes to act as true etiologic agents.

The skin lesions themselves may develop as a type of vasculitis. Circulating immune complexes together with the deposition of complement and immunoglobulin within the lesion have occasionally been demonstrated but the histologic picture is that of a lymphocytic, rather than neutrophilic, process.

Therapy:

The discomfort of erythema nodosum is due to tissue distention which is in turn caused by the presence of inflammation. Treatment revolves around the use of leg elevation and bed rest. For patients who wish to avoid bed rest, the use of elastic wraps or support stockings may be very helpful.

PALPABLE PURPURA (VASCULITIS OF THE NEUTROPHILIC TYPE)

Diagnostic Hallmarks.:

1. Distribution especially marked on the lower legs.
2. Non-blanchable petechiae.
3. The petechiae are slightly palpable.

Clinical Presentation :

Purpura is the general name for the escape of red blood cells into the skin. Purpura occurs in two forms . Petechiae and ecchymoses. Petechiae are small lesions, that is, macules and papules. Ecchymoses are large lesions, that is patches and plaques. The purpuric lesions of neutrophilic vasculitis consists entirely of petechiae; ecchymoses are not found. Moreover, since the petechiae form in association with the presence of a perivasular inflammatory infiltrate, the petechiae are usually palpable. This accounts for the term palpable purpura.

The smallest lesions of neutrophilic vasculitis occur as pinpoint dots which, early in the course of the disease, are bright red in colour. At the lesions age they become increasingly violaceous or even blue-black in colour. The smallest lesions may not be palpable but they are usually accompanied by at least a few larger, palpable papules. These larger lesions are sharply marginated violaceous papules 2 to 10 mm in diameter. They are characterized by the presence of a minute centrally located blue-black infarct or tiny haemorrhagic vesicle. Both the small and the large lesions of neutrophilic vasulitis fail to blanch when they are compressed by a glass microscope slide. The lesions are asymptomatic.

The lesions of vasculitic purpura first develop on the lower legs but in the more severe cases there may be spread to the rest of the body. Clustering of lesions, particularly over joints, is often notable.

These vasculitic lesions occur in a variety of closely related syndromes such as allergic vasculitis, hypersensitivity angitis, leukocytoclastic angitis, necrotizing angitis and Henoch-Schoenlein purpura. The skin lesions in these syndromes are identical both clinically and histologically. Moreover, the condition themselves overlap to the point where they are often indistinguishable. For these two reasons there is an increasing trend to consider all of these terms as synonymous and to "lump" them under a single title of neutrophilic vasculitis or palpable purpura.

The lesions of vasculitic purpura are easily recognizable on a clinical basis. A coagulation survey is usually carried out to eliminate non-vasculitic diseases such as thromobocytopenic purpura.

Course and Prognosis :

The prognosis of vasculitic purpura depends largely on whether or not internal organs are involved. When internal involvement is not present there is little morbidity and the disease runs an uneventful course over 10 to 20 days. On the other hands involvement of the nervous system, kidneys or lungs result in considerable morbidity and the possibility of death from the disease. Intermediate syndromes with only skin, joint and gastro-intestinal involvement are less troublesome.

Pathogenesis:

A definitive cause for the presence of vasculitic purpura is not often found. However one or more of the following possibilities should be considered : (1) **Medications**. Vasculitic reactions are particularly likely with allopurinol, iodides and sulfa type drugs to include the chlorthazides, frusemide and the sulfa antibiotics. (2) **Infection**. Sterptococcal infections and hepatitis B viral infection are the most common of the infectious causes. (3) **Autoimmune disease**. Vasculitic purpura is seen frequently with lupus erythematosus. It has also been associated with rheumatoid arthritis, chronic inflammatory bowel disease and Sjogren's syndrome. (4) **Dysproteinemias**. Cryoglobulinemia and polyclonal gammopathies are frequently associated with vascultic purpura. (5) **Malignancies**. Vasculitic purpura occasionally occurs in the presence of leukemia, lymphoma and myeloma.

Biopsy of the purpuric skin lesions reveals endothelial swelling and disruption of small blood vessles located in the upper dermis. Extravasation of red blood cells is notable around the disrupted vessels. Polymorphonuclear leukocytes are found surrounding the vessels and in most instances are also present within the vessel walls. Nuclear fragments from disrupted neutrophils (Leukocytoclasis) are also present. Fibrinoid deposits may or may not be found within the vessels.

Immunofluorescent studies of biopsies from purpuric vasculitis usually reveal the presence of immunoglobulin and complement. These findings, together with the demonstration of circulating immune complexes suggest that the blood vessel disruption is due to immune complex deposition.

MISCELLANEOUS PETECHIAL AND ECCHYMOTIC DISEASES

Purpura which occurs without inflammatory change (i.e. non-vasculitic purpura) can be divided into two groups : (1) an intravascular type characterized by disorders of coagulation and (2) an extravascular type characterized by faulty mechanical support for blood vessel walls.

The former includes conditions such as thrombocytopenia, hemophilia and platelet aggregation disorders. Clinically these intravascular disorders are accompanied by the presence of non-palpable petechiae, cutaneous ecchymoses and evidence of internal bleeding in the form of nosebleeds and gingival oozing.

The latter includes conditions such as steroid induced purpura and actinic (senile) purpura. Clinically these extravascular disorders are accompanied by the presence of non-palpable petechiae and cutaneous ecchymoses but they lack evidence of systemic bleeding. That is, nose-bleeds and gingival oozing do not occur. Actinic purpura occurs only on sun damaged skin whereas steroid purpura occurs anywhere on the body.

Erythema Multiforme — Homoeopathic Apporach

The above condition demonstrates typical multimiasmatic evolution. The illness starts with constitutional symptoms like fever, malaise, etc., and then gradually develops odematous erythematous macule of various shades of red, especially red, crimson-red, purplish-red, bluish-red, etc., very rarely one develops bullous eruption. The lesion usually disappear in few weeks with a strong tendency to recurrence.

This clearly exhibits psoric miasm (Erythema) gradually progressing to sycotic (bullous).

IMPORTANT POINTS TO BE NOTED DURING HISTORY

1. H/O indigestion of drugs like :
   = barbiturates = phenolputhalne :
   = sulphonamide = salicylates :

2. Every case to be taken to locate septic focus in the body especially nose, throat.

3. Since erythema multiforme is the result from sensitization of products of infection and drugs; it indicates disruption of the immune system one should rule out any other associated condition like allergic purpura, herpes simplex infection, rheumatism, etc.

4. The most important point to consider is that it is a selflimiting condition which usually disappears in few days to weeks, hence homoeopathic treatment is aimed at reccurrence of lesion and treating the septic focus if any.

The approach to the problem should be carefully observing :

(i) The lesion (site, character, colour, duration, onset).
(ii) The associate, constitution symptom.
(iii) The deriving miasmatic background from past and family history.

In my view erythema multi-forme falls under tubercular miasm chiefly because :

(1) Abboerant immune reaction.
(2) Tendency to recurrence.

I would like to caution the treating physician that the bullous variety can, in a few occasions be fatal, hence utmost precautions should be taken whilst treating the patient homoeopathically.

Drugs

Antipyrine : Intense pruritus, acting on vasomotor centre it causes dilation of capillaries of skin and circumscribed patches of hyperaemia and swelling. Antipyrine causes leucocytosis. Excessive perspiration.

Boracic Acid : Erythema multiforme more on trunk and upper extremities. Oedema around eyes. *Boracic acid* arrests fermentation and putrefaction.

Copaiva : (Bullous eruption. Dark coloured or bright red, elevated, intolerable itching).

Uneasiness during two days, followed by a very hard chill, which is succeeded by heat and an eruption which gives rise to intense itching and pricking of skin, but without any catarrhal symptoms; on third day fever subsides and eruption grows pale; on seventh day has a mottled appearance; the eruption does not wholly disappear for 5 days. No desqumation. Erysipelatous inflammation, especially around abdomen.

Vespa : Erythema multiforma. Intense itching, wheals macules and swellings with burning, stinging and soreness. Better by bathing with vinegar. Erythematous blush on left half of body from head downwards lasting, 8 - 10 days and desquamating followed by rheumatic pain in left instep.

REPERTORY OF ERYTHEMA MULTIFORME

Antpyr, Ars, Bell, Bor-ac, Dry, Chlol, Chlor, Coca, Cop, Crot-t, Gels, Jug-ac, Kali-br, Kali-i, Merc, Nat-c, Petr, Phos, Phyt, Rhus-t, Sil, Stram, Ter, Thuj, Vespa.

Cervical region — *Chlol, Gels, Hyos.*

Chest discoloration red — *Apis*

Eruptions : Penis — *Petr, Samb.*

Stevens Johnson Syndrome
Dr. Mirza Arwar Baig, M.B.B.S., Ph.D.

It was an evening of first August 1986. I was busy seeing patients at my clinic. A young gentleman entered my chamber with a request to see his ailing mother who was in a critical condition lying in a hospital with no hopes of recover. At first, I refused to go since I had a painful experience about the Hospital Staff who never co-operate with a homoeopath; moreover the people contact a homoeopath only in such dying moments. But on his insistently requesting me, I ultimately agreed.

Next day, while accompanying him to hospital, he told me that his mother was a diabetic and had developed some skin problem which appeared in the form of eruptions over her chest. Those eruptions were very painful. The family doctor diagnosed it was Herpes zoster and had treated her but without improvement. Other specialists were consulted too, but nothing helped. A leading skin specialist was called in, but his medicine had severe reaction over her whole body. At this stage she was hospitalized. Days passed without even relief, rather she became worse. All sorts of medicines (some of them imported) were tried but in vain.

When I reached the hospital, the Staff nurse and a Houseman accompanied me. They thought me to be a dermatologist, since every other day some new doctor was visiting her. She was lying quietly as if in Coma, looking like a burns case. Her whole body was painted with gentian violet. There were lots of blisters, small and large, some of them broken with peeling of skin and serous discharge.

Her eyes were half open and filled with exudates from the necrosed margins of her eyes which looked as if bitten by a rat. Her face was swollen with signs of inflammatory changes inside her mouth and nasal tract as well; her lips were necrosed and swollen. On the whole, it was looking as if she had been thrown into a boiler. It was a horrible sight to look at.

She was in toxic condition an advanced stage of shock. The drip was on, she was breathing with difficulty since there was some pleural effusion as well. The urine output was scanty since there were inflammatory changes in the kidneys and bladder also. She was last seen by a very famous dermatologist who had diagnosed this group of symptoms — as Stevens-Johnson Syndrome.

Stevens-Johnson Syndrome is a condition where mucosa and skin are involved. It gives rise to various group of symptoms. Mucosal involvement may be oral, ocural or genital. The bullae which for lead to extensive ulceration and pseudo-membrane formation haemorrhagic crusts, purulent or Catarrhal Conjunctivitis. Corneal ulceration, severe balanitis, vulvovaginitis and urethritis. Whereas skin involvements give rise to variable size of large and small bullae which contain clear or haemorrhagic fluid with severe constitutional symptoms. Allopathic treatment is with antibiotics and steroids of adrenocorticotropic hormones (ACTH). The prognosis is grave, spontaneous recovery rare and severe cases are always fatal.

For Homoeopathy it was a simple case. Though she was in a stage of shock she responded well to every question. She told that she felt as if she is lying on burning sand. She was thirsty but could not drink. Every attempt was very painful. She could not eat nor see because of constant oozing of stuff in to her eyes. She could hardly eat, pass stools. She could hardly pass a few drops of urine which caused severe cutting and burning pains.

She was disgusted with everything,i.e., to eat, to drink, to see and to urinate. Guided by those symptoms, a few doses of *Cantharis* 30 t.d.s. was given for 3 days — with great relief in 24 hours. The same day her mental condition improved. The next day she could drink and urinate. Third day she could eat and pass stool. The recovery was very rapid. On fourth day she wanted to go home. A patient who a couple of days ago was in dying condition was asking to go home. The hospital authority did not believe that this remarkable improvement was the result of homoeopathic medicine.

By the time she went home within a week the bullae had dried completely and she was discharged from the hospital against medical advice.

After going home the burning pains while passing urine recurred again and she was given a few more doses of *Cantharis*. Skin was not falling off in the same way as when one removes his socks or hand-gloves. Natural healthy skin was forming. She could see, eat, drink, pass stool and urinate without any difficulty. All this happened in a week's time and she resumed her routine work. She was later treated for diabetes according to her constitution.

13 Imamwada Road,
Bombay — 400009

PURPURA

Purpura implies a haemorrhagic eruption. If it is punctuate, it is called a petechial haemorrhage; if it is large in size, it is called ecchymoses. To begin with, eruption is bright-red; however, it differs from erythema in that the redness does not disappear on pressure. It changes colour like a bruise, becomes dark-red, bluish, and then disappears in a couple of weeks. Localized purpura is due to localized injuries, sprains, blows, insect bites, needle punctures etc. Generalized or widespread purpura signifies severe damage to the blood vessels by internal toxins, allergens or disturbance of the platelet or coagulatory mechanism. It should be viewed with concern, and the opinion of a medical expert should at once be sought.

Causes of Purpuric and Haemorrhagic Conditions

1.	Hereditary	:	Haemophilia. Hereditary haemorrhagic thrombo-asthenia. Hereditary haemorrhagic telangiectasia.
2.	Fevers	:	Typhus Smallpox Scarlet fever Rheumatic Meningitis.
3.	Toxic	:	Nephritis Septic focus Snake venom.
4.	Drugs	:	Phosphorus, arsenic and anaesthetics (liver damage), Benzol, N.A.B. sulphones (bone marrow depression). Salicylates, Penicilllin, Irgapyrin, (P), Sedormid, sulphonamides, serac vascular damage).
5.	Allergic and anaphy-lactoid	:	Henoch-schoenlein purpura (drugs and toxic).
6.	Liver disease (Jaundice)	:	Acute yellow atrophy (including drugs, circirrhosis of the liver).
7.	Splenic disease	:	Felti's, Banti's, Gaucher's syndromes.
8.	Bone marrow	:	Thrombocytopenia — essential and idiopathic and symptomatic. Aplastic — anaemia Carcinomatosis Pernicious — anaemia Drugs.
9.	Nutrition	:	Scurvy Cachexia Vit. K. and deficiency.

10. Mechanical : Hypertension, polycythemia vera, venous thrombosis and convulsions.

Only occasionally do people with purpuric and haemorrhagic conditions seek the help of a dermatologist, because these diseases come under the department of internal medicine. Hence, they are only mentioned here, with the exception of allergic and anaphylactoid purpura. A case of purpura calls for detailed history and examination. Laboratory aids are usually resorted to do for the following : the tourniquet test (Hess's), platelet count, coagulation time, bleeding time, clot retraction, prothrombin time, fibrinogen content of the blood, and a complete blood and bone marrow examination. These tests are ordered according to the provisional diagnosis.

Purpuric haemorrhages are common in thrombocytopenia (both idiopathic and symptomatic), allergy and anaphylaxis, hereditary haemorrhagic thrombo-asthenia and telangiectasia, liver diseases and scurvy. In others, there is only a tendency to increased bleeding.

Allergic and Anaphylactoid Purpura

Synonym: Henoch-Schoenlein Purpura

The common symptoms are : purpuric spots usually on the lower limbs and buttocks, less so on the other parts of the body, urticaria, joint pains, visceral haemorrhage causing intestinal colic and malaena, and constitutional symptoms like malaise, fever headaches etc. The onset is sudden, and relapses are common. Occasionally, nephritis occurs. The blood count shows eosinophilia

Causes

1. Streptococcal infection — tonsillitis, pharyngitis etc.
2. Drugs like penicillin, sera, salicylates; Irgapyrin (P), Sulphonamides etc.
3. Rarely food allergy.

Prognosis : It is good in an average case. In the severe, fulminating variety with kidney involvement, the prognosis is bad, and death may occur. In cases with recurrent causes, relapses occur.

Treatment : 1. Rest in bed, light food and reassurance. 2. Treat the cause, eradicating streptococcal infection with anti miasmatic constitutional remedy and by withdrawing drugs that have produced toxic effects.

Homoeopathic Approach to Purpura

I have purposely discussed this topic of purpura with skin therapeutics, as frequently patients visit a homoeopath for the purpuric spots.

Since there are multiple aetiologies for the purpura, it is wise to wait till the exact cause of purpura is detected.

On first consultation, patient should be advised tests e.g. platelet count, coagulation time, bleeding time, clot retraction time. prothrombin time. If the result of the above list is not confirmatory then one should advise more invasive methods like bone marrow investigation.

I would like to mention in a table various homoeopathic drugs indicated for specific aetiology.

	Aetiology	*Homoeopathic Drugs*
1.	Hereditary factor	Deep acting constitutional remedies.
2.	Fevers	*Arnica, Carb -veg, Baptisia*
3.	Toxic	*Carb-veg, Lachesis, Crot-hor*
4.	Drugs	*Ars, Carb-veg, Sulph*
5.	Liver Disease	*Lyco, China, Phos*
6.	Spleen Disease	*Phos*
7.	Bone Marrow	*Thyrodinum, Phos*
8.	Injury	*Arnica, Led-p*

Whilst treating a case of purpura, the homoeopathic improvement should be in liason with the various parameters described above. Constant watch should also be kept for anaemia, which is so common in this condition.

Occasionally, other than constitutional medicines, sometimes we may have to prescribe drugs chiefly for the haemorrhagic cases if the purpura is very severe.

I shall now discuss various important drugs for purpura.

Arnica : It helps in absorbing after violent contusion bruises and tearing of the fibres and capillaries. Skin black and blue. Purpura miliaris. Dusky Mottled Skin :

Tendency to develop crops of small painful boils. Symmetrical eruptions. Itching sensation shifts from place to place.

Ars. : Paroxysmal appearance of petechiae. Purple petechiae on chest, neck, abdomen, genitals and thighs. Reddish or bluish spots on the skin.

Burning and itching sensation with purpura. Skin rough dry. Shrivelled and wrinkled.

Petechiae with eruptive fevers. Alternates with internal complaints.

Baptisia : Used for septic conditions of blood; livid spots all over body.

Purpuric spots associated with typhus, typhoid and variola. Burning all over the skin.

Carb-V. : Blood seems to stagnate in the capillaries, causing blueness, coldness and ecchymosis. Plexus of the veins, formed by a dilatation of the capillary vessles with violent haemorrhage after the slightest injury. Burning in various places agg. night and in bed. Purpuric spots associated with jaundice and typhus. Ptalengesecia in children coldness and purpuric fever with great soreness.

China-S : Purpura associated with smallpox, plague, gangreneous and cancerous affections. Great exhaustion with purpura. Skin flacid and sensitive to touch.

Crot-Hor : Extravasation of blood from skin. Blood fluid, dark, non-coagulable, leaking through vascular wall everywhere. Skin very sensitive, especially right half of body. Sore sensation ameliorated with pressure.

Purpura associated with jaundice, diphtheria, grave situation. Purpuric spots develop purple colour. Patient has tendency to develop septic condition, gangrene, carbuncle, furuncle.

Ham : Passive Haemorrhage, ecchymosis. Sore bruised sensation. Acting on the coats of veins. It causes relaxation with consequent engagement. Varicose diathesis; constant oozing from small wounds.

Lachesis : Haemorrhages and extravasation, red and black streaks on skin. Purpura with intense prostration. Purpura associated with diphtheria, jaundice, typhoid, scarlatina, spotted fever, septic fever. Bluish black discoloration of skin. Purple spots and ecchymosis on back, chest, extremities.

Phos. : Purpura haemorrhagica, ecchymosis, phosphorus disorganizes the blood, causing fatty degeneration of blood vessels in every tissue and organ of the body, giving rise to haemorrhage. Purpura associated with jaundice, variolla, sepsis.

Burning, itching, stinging, sensation compelling the patient to change the position.

Distended veins. Black blood oozes from the skin.

Rhus-Ven. : Small ecchymosis great weakness and soreness, sleeplessness and restlessness.

Sec-Cor. : Multiple haemorrhages, petechiae.
Vesicles filled with black blood. Enormous prostration even to fainting.

Sulph-Acid : Ecchymosis especially in old people.
Extreme weakness, exhaustion and trembling all over the body.
Bluish spots on forearm.
Reddish blue discoloration.
Tendency to develop carbuncles, boils, gangrenes, cicatrices.

Terebinthena : Purpura haemorrhagic. Skin warm and moist, skin sensitive. Fresh ecchymosis. Dropsy.
This is associated with typhus, typhoid, nephritis, jaundice and dropsy.

SOME IMPORTANT ANTI-HAEMORRHAGIC REMEDIES

Achillea : This remedy affects the capillaries and produces profuse, painless, bright red fluid haemorrhages chiefly from nose, lungs, wounds, uterus, etc. There is a bruised sore sensation with congestion. There is presence of spasms at convulsions, especially after suppression of haemorrhages. The other characteristic symptoms are as follows : Ill-effects of operations for stones billious renal etc. (continuous high fever).

Adrenalin : *Adrenalin* in potency is a powerful vasoconstrictor. It typically affects the sympathetic ending, notably the splanchnic area, it helps in checking capillary, haemorrhages from all parts of the body, especially nose, ear, mouth, throat, larynx, rectum, uterus and bladder.

Arnica : Bleeding caused by injuries, falls, blows, concussions and contusions. Patient feels a soreness as from a bruise in the part where the blood issues. The blood vessels are relaxed, causing ecchymosis with blue-black spots. Any kind of exertion causes haemorrhage. It typically produces haemorrhages from various parts; e.g. retina, nose, uterus, lungs. An important concomitant is that (1) muscles feel very sore all over, (2) bed feels hard or full or rocks, (3) foul breath and taste.

Bothrop : Haemorrhage from every orifice of the body. It helps in dissolving thrombosis. Broken down constitutions. Great lassitude and sluggishness. The venom of the snake is most coagulating, hence on potentisation, it is expected to be useful in thrombosis and thromboembolic, phenomena. It typically affects the intracranial blood vessels and blood vessles of lower limbs and retina. There is great lassitude and sluggishness with profuse perspiration and nervous trembling.

Bovista : Relaxation of the entire capillary system, favouring haemorrhagic diathesis. Puffy condition of the surface of body from sluggish passage of blood through the veins. There is presence of bleeding early in the morning during sleep at night. Bleeding from gums on sucking them. Especially adapted to persons of scrofulous diathesis. There is marked languor and lassitude.

Cactus-Grandiflorus : Cactus has marked action on the circular muscles of the blood vessles; it favours the formation of clots speedily. Pulselessness, panting and prostration with sensation of constriction and the periodicity concomitants. There is profuse epistaxis with haematuria, haemoptysis. Patient is extremely chilly with tendency for the patient to maintain persistent sub-normal temperature.

China Officinalis : *China* affects the blood, making it thinner and improverished. It weakens the heart and impairs circulation, producing congestion and haemorrhages. The main cause of ailments in *China* is profuse loss of fluids. Profuse, exhausting haemorrhages, nearly exsanguinating the patient; haemorrhages with loss of sight, faintness, tinnitus and great nervous prostration. Blood often dark and clotted. Haemorrhage from orifices of the body. Coldness of face and body. Patient gasps for air and desires to be fanned. Adapted to persons of thin, dry, bilious constitution with gastric troubles.

Cinnamonum : *Cinnamonum* acts best when there are repeated small haemorrhages which are caused by lifting, straining, overstretching or taking a false step. Profuse flow of bright red blood; haemorrhages from bowels; haemoptysis, epistaxis. Post-partum haemorrhage, uterine haemorrhages. Haemorrhages in persons prone to hysterical attacks, especially when following the haemorrhage.

Crotalus Horridus : The venom of the rattle snake has a marked haemorrhagic action. Haemorrhages of dark fluid, non-coagulating blood from all orifices of the body. Patient even has bloody sweat and bloody pus. Suited to broken down, debilitated or old persons. Haemophilia.

Erigeron : Profuse haemorrhages of bright-red blood. Persistent gushing haemorrhages. Vomitus or stools of pure blood. Haemorrhage from bladder. Uterine haemorrhage with painful micturition. Bleeding haemorrhoids. Patient gets epistaxis instead of menses.

Ferrum : *Ferrum* relaxes the blood vessels causing bright red haemorrhages with small clots. Haemorrhages associated with flushing. Patient becomes pale, bloated oedematous with cold skin pitting on pressure, particularly about the joints. Adapted to anaemic young persons with false plethora and a strong concomitant is the gastric symptom. Patient who look strong but are easily fatigued.

Geranium : Profuse haemorrhages from lungs, stomach, uterus (postpartum) in persons with a tendency to habitual sick headache. Haematemesis in gastric ulcer.

Hamamelis : *Hamamelis* acts principally on the coats of the veins of rectum, genitals, limbs and throat; causing relaxation and engorgement. Parts from which haemorrhages occur, feel sore and bruised. The patient exhibits no alarm and anxiety concerning the bleeding. Very useful in open painful wounds, with weakness from loss of blood. Passive non-coagulable haemorrhages. Haematemesis of black blood.

Ipecac : Profuse, bright-red steady flow of blood usually accompanied by nausea. Haemoptysis caused by slightest exertion. Whooping cough with bleeding from the nose and mouth. Patient suffers from haematuria which is accompanied by nausea and cutting in abdomen and urethra. Profuse, bright-red, steady or gushing uterine haemorrhages.

Nitric Acid : The haemorrhages of *Nitric acid* consist of bright blood or bloody water. There is easy haemorrhage. Haemorrhage from the uterus with pain in back and pressure as if the uterus would be forced down and out of the vagina. Uterine haemorrhage after curettage. Especially suited to dark haired persons with rigid skin and muscle with bleeding from the bowels. Haemorrhage from rectum after removal of piles. Painful piles which bleed easily. Epistaxis of dark clotted blood.

Phosphorus : The haemorrhages of *Phosphorus* come from any part of the body, particularly from lungs and stomach, when associated with Bright's disease. Small wounds bleed much; they heal and break out again and bleed. *Phosphorus* causes fatty degeneration of blood vessels and also disorganises the blood itself.

Sabina : The bleeding of *Sabina* consists of bright red blood with clots in it. The bleeding may at times be dark or pale. Especially adapted to uterine haemorrhages in hot blood women with a gouty diathesis. Pain from sacrum to pubis or reverse with haemorrhages from uterus. Important concomitant symptoms are : (1) Violent pulsations, (2) Heaviness and indolence of body. The patient always feels worse in a warm closed room.

REPERTORY OF PURPURA ECCHYMOSIS

Acon, Aeth, Anth, Arg-n, Arn, Ars, Ars-i, Aur-m, Bad, Bar-c, Bar-m, Bapt, Bell, Bellis-p, Berb, Bothrops, Bov, Burs-p, Bry, Calc, Camph, Canth, Carb-v, Cham, Chin, Chin-a, Chlol, Cic, Coca, Cor-r, Cop, Cor, Crot-h, Cub, Cupr, Cur, Dulc, Euphr, Ferr, Ham, Hep, Hyos, Hyp, Iod, Iodf, Jug-r, Kali-chl, Kali-i, Kreos, Lach, Laur, Led, Merc-s, Mur-ac, Nux-v, Par, Petr, Phel, Ph-ac, Phos, Plb, Puls, Pyro, Rhus-t, Rhus-v, Ruta, Sal-ac, Sec, Sil, Sinap, Solid, Stram,

Sulph, Sul-ac, Sulphon, Supraren-ex, Tab, Tarent, Tarn, Ter, Ver-v.

Advancing — *Terb*
Blow slight from — *Agar, Arn.*
Blue with muco-purulent diarrhoea — *Kali-br*
Bruise from slight — *Sulph*
Chorea in — *Lach, Nux-v.*
Livid — *Carb-v*
Extensive — *Sec*
Fevers in — *Apis*
Miliaris — *Acon, Am-c, Am-m, Arn, Bell, Coff, Dulc, Sulph, Sul-ac.*
Metritis — *Sec*
Old age — *Con, Sars*
Organs internal in — *Hippoz*
Senilis — *Ars, Bar-c, Dry, Con, Lach, Op, Rhus-t, Sec, Sul-ac.*
From least touch or pressure — *Lach*
Typhus or Typhoid in — *Ars, Bapt, Bry, Crotal, Cup-m, Ham, Nit-ac, Ph-ac, Phos, Rhus, Sinap, Sul-ac.*
Urticaria with — *Lob*
Red spot over whole body, on parts covered with clothing — *Phos*
Returning yearly — *Crot-h*
Scorbutic — *Lach.*
Spots full of bluish dark blood, all over body except face and hands — *Rhus*
With fever and soreness — *Carb-v*
With haemorrhages from all mucous membranes and vomiting of blood and mucus — *Sal-ac*
Spine on — *Ver-v*
Caused by excessive use of salt, bloody diarrhoea after — *Nitr-sp-d*
Viper bite — *Camph*
Eye — *Acon, Aeth, Am-c, Arg-n, Ars, Bell, Cact, Cham, Chicr, Con, Crot-h, Cupr-ac, Erig, Glon-v, Ham, Kali-bi, Kali-chl, Kreos, Lach, Led, Lyc, Lyss, Nux-v, Phos, Plb, Ruta, Sul-ac, Ter.*
Right — *Con*
Coughing from — *Arn, Bell.*
Lids — *Arn, Led.*
Mouth — *Crot-h, Lach, Phos, Psor, Ter.*
Mouth dark red blood — *Antr, Ter.*
Tongue — *Phos, Plb.*

Abdomen — *Phos*
Chest — *Ars, Cop, Kali-i, Lach, Phos, Sul-ac, Stram.*
Back Cervical region — *Ars*
Lumber region — *Merc-c, Vip.*
Upper limbs — *Berb, Cop, Cupr, Lach, Phos, Phys, Sec, Sul-ac, Ter, Vip.*
Hand back of — *Berb, Lach, Phos.*
Fingers — *Coca*
— **lower limbs** — *Lach, Phos, Sec, Sul-ac, Tereb.*
Leg — *Crot-h, Kali-i, Lach,* ***Phos****, Sec*
Extremities eruptions — *Ars, Aur-m, Berb.*
— **lower limbs** — *Am-m, Ars, Kali-i, Phos.*

CHAPTER 11

Psoriasis

It is a common, chronic and non-infectious skin disease characterized by well-defined slightly raised, dry erythematous macules with silvery scales and typical extensor distribution.

Etiology : It is world-wide in distribution. Contrary to earlier belief, it is fairly common in the tropics; though undoubtedly, it is more prevalent in the temperate climate. Psoriasis is a chronic disease; its course is punctuated by intermissions and remissions. Attacks are more common in winter than summer; the eruption has a natural tendency to clear up with a warm weather. In the tropics, a fair number of attacks develop in the monsoon (rainy season).

The exact etiology is still unknown. According to most workers, it is a heredo-familial disease brought on by stress, viz., anxiety, mental trauma, fever, physical injury, digestive upsets,etc.,on a genetic constitution. Transmission is by a single, irregularly dominant gene. Recent histochemical studies and also studies of vasculature, neural population and family tree have provided double proof of genetic transmission. Streptococcal infection, presence of diabetes and purines in the diet are the other precipitating factors. Pressure and trauma seem to determine the localization of psoriasis.

Pathology : Psoriasis appears to be largely a disorder of keratinization. The basic defect is rapid replacement of epidermis in psoriatic lesion (3 to 4 days instead of 28 days in normal skin). In addition, there are marked vascular changes in upper dermis in the form of tortuosity and dilatation.

Histochemical studies have revealed an increase in both oxidative and anaerobic metabolism with increased pentose, glycogen, purines, sulphydral groups and soluble proteins and a decrease in activity of dipeptidases.

Histology is characteristic and consists of (i) Parakeratosis. (ii) Thinning of supra-papillary portion of the stratum Malpighii. (iii) Elongation of rete pegs. (iv) Oedema and clubbing of papillae. (v) Micro-abscesses of Munro. (vi) Dilated and tortuous capillaries in upper dermis. (vii) Oedema and round-cell infiltration in the papillae and upper dermis.

Clinical features : Typical distribution is extensor. The areas commonly affected are the scalp, back of elbows, front of knees and legs and the lower part of the back of the trunk. The nails, the palms and the soles may also be affected in the average case; but the mucous membranes may be rarely involved.

Clinically, psoriasis exhibits itself as dry, well-defined macules, papules and plaques of erythema with layer-upon-layer of silvery scales. The typical lesions are coin-shaped; by confluence, big plaques of the size of the palm of a hand (or even bigger) or figurate areas may be formed. When a psoriatic lesion is scratched with the point of a dissecting forceps, a candle-grease-like scale can be repeatedly produced even from the non-scaling lesions. This is called the Candle-grease sign (Tache de bouge). The complete removal of a scale produces pin-point bleeding (Auspitz sign). The lesions are slightly raised above the surface of the skin, but there is no induration Psoriasis is normally characterized by the absence of itching, but in tropical countries, patients complain of slight or moderate pruritus which, if accompanied by secondary psychogenic stress and lichenification, is more marked. Psoriatic lesions may develop along the scratch lines in the active phase; this is called Koebner's phenomenon (other common disease in which Koebner's phenomenon occurs are : warts and lichen planus).

The central clearing of the circular lesions produces ringed lesions-Annular Psoriasis.

The scalp is involved in almost all cases. It shows thick, scaly papules discretely distributed all over, with intervening areas of normal skin. The lesions are dry, and there is no matting of hair, the latter comes out straight through the scales. Psoriasis of the scalp never causes loss of hair and baldness.

Nails show three types of lessions : (a) pitting, (b) separation of the distal portion of the nail from the nail-bed and walls, and (c) thickening of the nail, accompanied by the collection of hyperkeratotic debris under the nail. The face is relatively spared but lesions may occur along the scalp border (Corona psoriatica). The palms of the hands are involved more commonly than the soles of the feet. Lesions consist of well-defined patches of hyperkeratosis and fissures, on erythematous bases. Lesions are bilaterally symmetrical. Occasionally psoriasis starts on the palms and soles; it may be confined to these areas (Psoriasis inversus).

Pustular Psoriasis : Sometimes though rarely, there is the complication of pustule formation and crusting on an erythematoscaly base. These pustules are sterile. Lesions commence on the prominences or on the soles as pin-head pustules appearing in crops and in time a patch is produced which is red and exfoliating and is studded with pustules. Pustular psoriasis must be distinguished from ringworm, acrodermatitis perstans and bacterides.

Flexural Psoriasis : As stated above, the typical distribution of psoriasis is extensor. Occasionally, flexural psoriasis may occur when flexures like the groins, axillae and infra-mammary regions are involved. The lesions lose their dryness in these areas; hence scaling is reduced. Some degree of itching is present in this variety.

Psoriasis Arthropathica : In a small percentage of psoriatic patients, there is involvement of the joints resembling rheumatoid arthritis. This combination is termed psoriasis arthropathica. The joints of the fingers, feet, ankles, knees and sacroiliac are selectively affected; these joints are swollen and painful. The psoriatic eruption and the involvement of the joints may increase or decrease simultaneously. Nail changes are usually present. Radiological changes are characteristic and consist of osteoporosis followed by increased density, diminished joint space, erosion of joint surfaces followed by eventual destruction of the ends of bones. Ultimately, the joints become deformed.

Guttate Psoriasis : Though the normal course of psoriasis is chronic, there occurs occasionally an acute attack in the form of guttate psoriasis. In this variety small discrete papules develop rapidly all over the body, particularly the trunk, the arms and the thighs. Acute guttate psoriasis is usually precipitated either by an acute illness like tonsillitis or a sharp mental stress or physical injury. It is more common in children than adults.

When a rapid spreading and joining together of individual lesions takes place in psoriasis, it becomes generalized and may produce an erythroderma-like picture viz. generalized erythema and scaling of the whole of the integument. Some typical individual lesions can always be detected in this variety, the history also helps to differentiate it from the other causes of erythroderma.

Diagnosis : It is based upon :

1. The family history of psoriasis.
2. The typical distribution of the lesions of the scalp, elbows, knees, the front of the legs, back and nails.
3. Well-defined, non-indurated, dry, erythematous areas with silvery, layer-upon-layer scaling.
4. The Candle-grease sign, Koebner's phenomenon, and pinpoint bleeding upon removal of the scale (Auspitz sign).
5. Little or no itching.
6. History of previous attacks, and seasonal variations of the disease.
7. Typical histopathology.

Differential diagnosis : In the majority of cases, the diagnosis of psoriasis is usually easy if the above mentioned features are borne in mind. A typical case may create diagnostic problems. The following conditions must be particularly considered in differential diagnosis :

Syphilitic psoriasis : The history reveals an illicit exposure and the development of chancre; the rash is less scaly, and shows some degree of induration, mucous patches and lymphadenopathy. The V.D.R.L. is positive.

Seborrhoeic dermatitis : The scalp patches are diffuse, ill-defined and moist, the hair is matted and tangled in the crust, the crusts are greasy. Body lesions affect the flexures, the sternal and inter-scapular regions; they do not have either sharply defined borders or silvery, dry scales.

Pityriasis rosea : A short history, centripetal distribution, a herald patch and typical oval lesions with cigarette-paper like centrifugal scaling.

The flexural lesions must be distinguished from those in tinea cruris, intertrigo, seborrhoeic dermatitis; the nail lesions, from the lesions in tinea unguium, eczema, paronychia and syphilis; the palmar lesions, from the other causes of hyperkeratosis; the guttate variety, from lichen planus, and the erythroderma type from the other cuses of erythroderma.

Prognosis : A permanent cure is not yet known, though individual attacks can, almost always, be controlled satisfactorily. Disease is non-infectious. General health and longetivity are unaffected though the majority of patients suffer from the disease on and off throughout their lives. The course is chronic with varying periods of intermission (from weeks to years). The outlook is never either sure or bright, but one should avoid an attitude of defeatism. The whole position must be explained to the patient, and then he should be encouraged to persist with the treatment till all the lesions have disappeared; this brings down the relapse rate. The disease does not leave scars. There is only faint staining which disappears slowly. The nails gradually assume their normal appearance after the attack has aborted.

Flexural, erythrodermic and pustular psoriasis take longer to heal than the typical variety. The palmar and nail lesions are rather resistant to treatment.

Complications in psoriasis are infrequent. The conditions which can complicate psoriasis are : joint involvement (psoriasis arthropathica) which can cause disability, even crippling; exfoliative dermatitis; eczematization caused by scratching and infection or the use of irritants; lichenification brought on by scratching in neurotic individuals.

Homoeopathic Approach

Since modern medicine has a very limited role to play in case of psoriasis, Homoeopathy comes as a rescue, not only as a palliative, but also as curative in a vast majority of cases. In certain obstinate cases, it is difficult to achieve the cure.

The homoeopathic treatment should lay stress on :

1. Impressing upon the patient that the treatment should be continued till the last lesion has disappeared.

2. The general health of the patient should be maintained, and the exciting causes should be studied and eliminated as far as possible.

3. The patient's life should be regulated, so that no undue stress affects either body or mind.

4. A moderate firm climate, frequent sun baths, before the onset of winter are very useful in bringing down the relapse rate.

As regards the treatment of individual attacks, the pattern of inquiry and analysis is as follows :

(i) Adequate information in relation to past and family history should be extracted from the patient, as psoriasis is a heredio-familial disease. Also, past and family history of streptococcal infection, diabetes, gout and injurious (physical and mental) should be inquired because psoriasis is frequently associated with the above conditions.

PSORIASIS TREATED WITH CALC. SULPH.

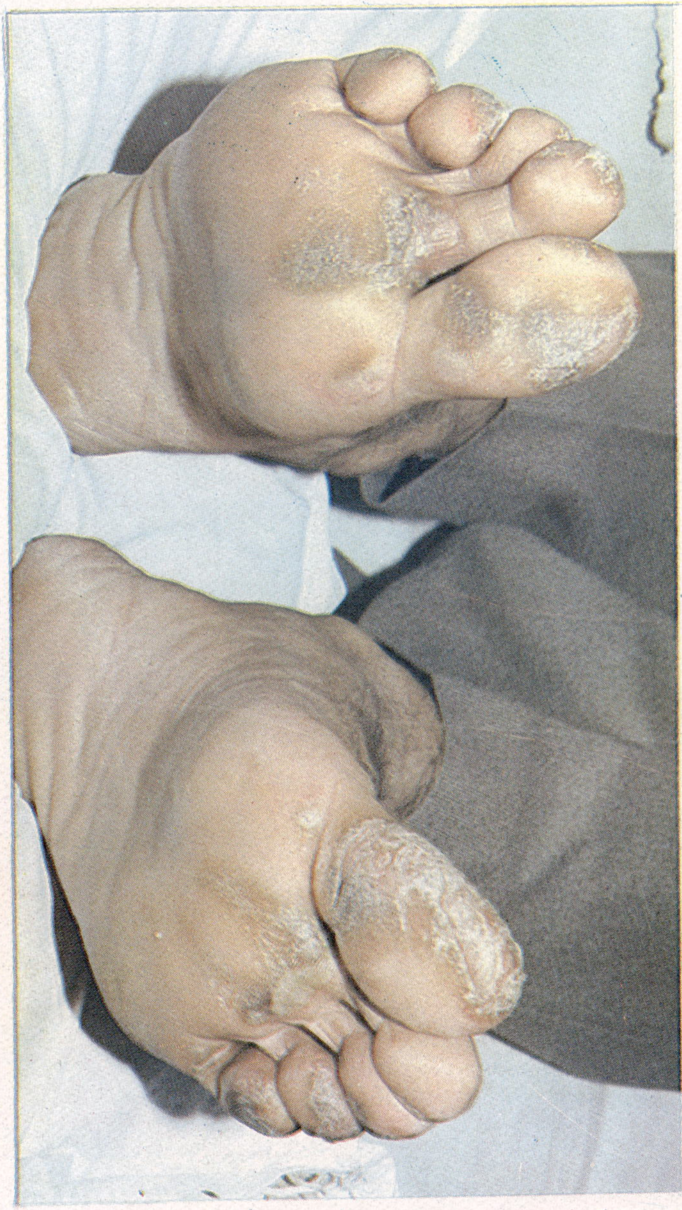

BEFORE

PSORIASIS TREATED WITH CALC. SULPH.

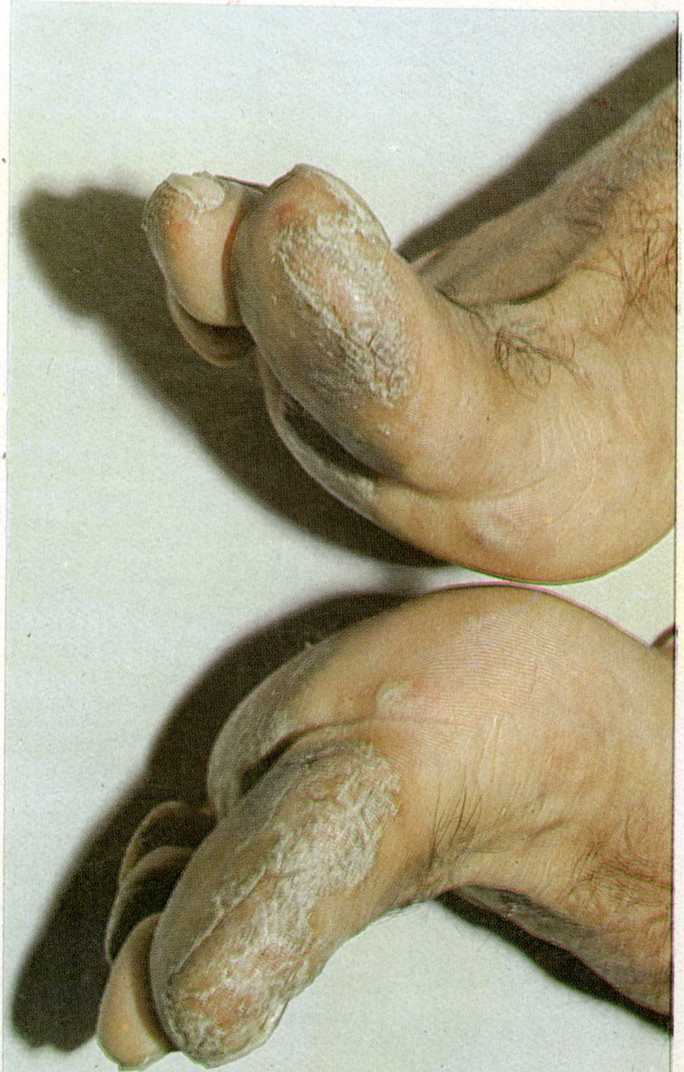

DURING

PSORIASIS TREATED WITH CALC. SULPH.

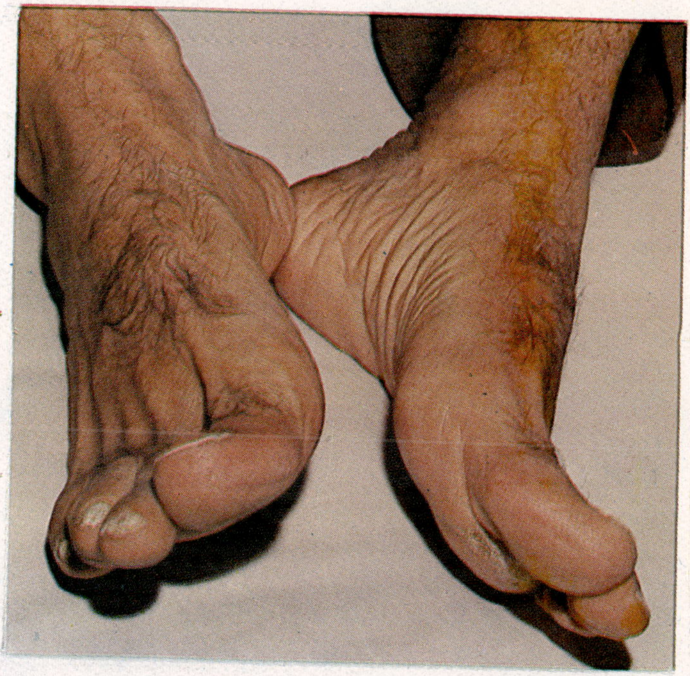

AFTER

(ii) Methodical recording of the remission and relapses chronologically is very useful. In every individual there are different exciting factors, aggravating and ameliorating factors, hence they should be recorded after thorough evaluation.

(iii) Individual lesion should be examined in detail for characteristic location, cracks and ulceration, general appearance of the skin, itching with its modalities and any other concomitant symptoms.

(iv) The life situation of the patient including the mental state should be evolved, as it is a known fact that relapses do occur during stressful situation.

Finally a homoeopath should always keep in mind that psoriasis is a chronic disease; its course is punctuated by intermissions and remissions. Attacks are more common in winter than in summer. The eruption has natural tendency to clear up in the warm weather.

Homoeopathic Remedies | Psoriasis |

Ars-Alb : The appearance of the skin is dry, rough, scaly, dirty and shrivelled. The eruptions are frequently accuminate with excessive scaling. There is severe burning sensation in the eruption which is worse in the evening, at night and by cold application, it is better by warm application. Psoriasis has a tendency to alternate with internal affections.

Ars-Iod : The psoriasis is characterised by marked exfoliation of skin in large scales leaving an exudating surface beneath it. There is intense burning with itching. The patient scratches violently till it bleeds. The psoriasis is worse in dry cold weather, even though *Ars-iod* is a hot patient, skin symptoms are better by local application of heat.

Borax : The skin of hands and face is covered with multiple psoriatic eruption. There is furfuraceous peeling off of epidermis. The psoriatic lesions ulcerate easily, especially from slightest injury. Here the psoriasis is worse in warm weather and better in cold weather. There is a sensation of cobweb on the skin. It typically affects individuals who are excessively nervous, frightened easily and sensitive to sudden noise.

Calc-Sulph : The psoriatic eruptions are chiefly located on the scalp, extremities, back. The appearance is scarlet red with lichenification of the surrounding skin. There is severe burning and itching which is worse in warm room, from warm bath and better by cold application and cold bath. Due to presence of secondary infection, the psoriatic eruptions suppurate, which heal with the formation of thick yellow scabs. There may be a greenish-yellow, acrid and offensive discharge.

Chrysarobinum : Psoriatic eruption especially around eyes and ears. There is presence of violent itching with tendency to formation of thick crust. The lesions may get infected and can form an eczematous patch which is associated with acrid, foul smelling, pustular discharge.

Clematis Erecta : The most unique feature is profuse desquamation, with severe itching, worse washing in cold water. Psoriatic eruption are present on face, hands and scalp, especially around occiput. The eruption has a characteristic modality that it gets worse during the ascending (waxing) moon and as the moon descends (waning), the eruption is better. Presence of psoriasis in individuals who are exposed to gonorrhoea or syphilis; also individuals who have consumed compound of mercury either locally or internally.

Cor-Rub : Psoriasis on palms and soles. The patient is too cold when uncovered and too hot when covered, feels better by artificial heat. Presence of psoriasis in individual with nervous temperament.

Graphites : Folds of the skin. e.g., ears, buttocks, groins, bends of joints are the important site for eruptions. The eruptions are absolutely dry with little desquamation and more cracking. The cracks bleed very easily and exude a gluey moisture. The eruptions are typically agg. with local application of heat. The presence of psoriasis in persons who are obese, chilly and constipated. Psoriatic eruption alternating with digestive complaints.

Iris-Ves : Presence of irregular psoriatic patches with shiny scales is the most important characteristic symptoms. Persons with oily nose, greasy taste in the mouth and fatty stool are characteristic. The eruptions are worse in spring, autumn and hot weather. Eruptions typically affect the right side. Psoriasis is associated with gastric derangement.

Kali-Ars : It is one of the most chilly patient to develop psoriasis. The patient is extremely chilly that he wants to warm himself enough even in summer. There is severe sensation of burning in the lesion accompanied by intolerable itching which is worse undressing, night, walking, warmth. The eruption tends to be better during monsoon season. It typically affects individuals who are restless, nervous, anaemic and they may have a family or past history of malignant disease.

With every change of weather, the psoriatic eruption, enter the phase of relapse.

Kali Bromatum : The eruptions are present on chest and back. The causative factor in the above case is ill-effects of worry, loss of business, loss of reputation and embarrassment, or illness of near and dear ones. As *Kali brom* also has an affinity for sexual sphere, ill-effects of lascivious fancies, satyriasis or nymphomania, could produce psoriatic eruption. The skin of the patient, is cold, and numb to feel. The patient, in general, feels well when he is busy mentally as well as physically.

Kali Sulph : This tissue salt of Dr. Schussler has mar-ked affinity on skin, where it causes des-quamation, also the Koebner Phenomenon can be observed in such patients, as a patient tends to develop eruptions after injury.

There is sensation of extreme burning and itching which is worse in evening, in a warm room, but definitely better in open air and by local application of very hot water. Scalp and other hairy parts of the body are chiefly affected.

Lycopodium : The appearance of the skin is dry, thick and indurated. The psoriatic eruptions are full of fissures with little itching and desquamation. The eruption tries to ulcerate early during the course of sickness.

It typically affects individuals who grow old prematurely, who are intellectually keen, and who have ill-effects of fear, fright, anxieties, loss of vital fluids. Patient gets a good sense of relief whenever cold applications are applied on the lesion. However one should remember that burning sensation of *Lycopodium* is always better by local application of heat (*Alumina, Ars, Caps, Carbo-veg., Sec. Cor*).

The psoriasis is associated with urinary, gastric and hepatic discorders.

Manganum Aceticum : The eruptions chiefly affect the flexures of the joints, extremities.

The eruptions are characterised by deep cracks, which do not bleed much (Petr). But they do have violent itching which is worse whenever the patient perspires. It is better by scratching. Psoriasis here is accompanied by menopausal symptoms. Also the eruption becomes worse during menses. Psoriasis present in individuals who also suffer from diabetes mellitus.

Merc-Sol : The skin has a general tendency to free perspiration, but the patient is not relieved thereby, the skin is always moist. The skin around psoriatic eruptions is excoriated like raw meat. The eruption are prone to early suppuration and ulcerations. There is a sense of itching which is worse at night in bed.

Presence of psoriasis in individuals who have history of suppressed gonorrhoea.

Mezereum : Scalp, extremities, are the parts that are covered with psoriatic eruptions. The eruptions are accompanied by excessive itching which is worse after a warm bath.

The itching changes location on scratching. The eruptions tend to suppurate early and ooze acrid, gluey, moisture with thick crust and pus underneath. also ulceration sets in the lesion quite early which are painful to touch and warmth.

Presence of psoriasis in individuals with suppressed eczema and bad effects of vaccination.

Nitricum Acidicum : The skin is dry, eroded and cracked in every angle. Multiple psoriatic eruptions are present with zig-zag and irregular margin. The appearance of the lesion is like raw flesh. The cracks within the lesions ulcerate easily and are extremely sensitive to pain and touch. There may be presence of burrowing pus within the lesion. The skin is extremely unhealthy and may have large jagged warts at various places. There may be itching in the lesions which is worse on undressing.

It is suitable for individuals who have yellow discoloration, who are of spare habits and who have a tendency to catch cold or diarrhoea. Bad effects of maltreated syphilis and gonorrhoea.

Petroleum : One of the chilly remedies with tendency to develop deep cracks, in angles, nipples, finger-tips.

Psoriatic eruptions develop in winter season and get aggravated periodically.

Early formation of thick, hard, yellowish green crust is the most characteristic symptom. The eruption itches violently and one must scratch until they bleed. The parts become cold after scratching. Psoriatic eruptions typically affect the occiput and the groins. The psoriasis is associated with long lasting and lingering gastric complaints.

Psoriasis usually follows after unusual mental strains, fright and grief. Also psoriasis develops after skin diseases are suppressed by local applications.

Sulphur : The skin is dry, rough, wrinkled and scaly. The eruptions break out on almost any part of the body having following characteristics.

There is voluptuous violent itching which is aggravated at night, in bed, < scratching and washing.

The skin burns whenever the patient scratches. The skin surrounding the eruption is excoriated. The psoriasis usually gets worse during spring time and in damp weather. Psoriasis develops after any other skin disease is suppressed by local measures. Psoriasis alternates with various other internal ailments e.g., asthma.

It typically affects individuals who are stoop shouldered, unwashed, tall and lean, untidy with offensive body odour.

It is to be thought of in chronic and obstinate cases of psoriasis or it should be given after an acute exacerbation of a psoriatic attack to prevent relapse.

Thyroidinum : The skin is extremely dry in appearance. Psoriasis is associated with obesity. It typically affects those cases of psoriasis which took a long time to evolve. The eruptions are symmetrical with serpigenous margin.

Psorinum : The psoriatic eruptions disappear in summer only to occur in winter. The skin is dirty, rough, scabby and greasy. Nape of the neck, scalp, folds of the skin and groins are typically affected. Eruptions itch intolerably which are worse by heat of bed.

The patient scratches till it becomes raw and bleeds. It is usually indicated when well related remedies fail to relieve or permanently cure or when Sulphur seems indicated but fails to relieve.

Psoriatic eruption developing after maltreated infectious diseases or long lasting grief reactions. The patient is extremely chilly and hungry with foul carrion-like odour.

THE HAHNEMANNIAN GLEANINGS
Vol XXX No. II (1963)
Page No. 499

A girl aged 20, had been suffering from psoriasis of two years' duration and had the typical eruptions on the folds of the elbows, knees and behind the ears. She gave us many symptoms of *Causticum* including the characteristic symptom that the whole skin condition almost completely cleared up without any treatment in the rainy season. We prescribed *Causticum* in various potencies. The response to every dose was very satisfactory but the condition always relapsed. Ultimately we put her on *Causticum* given in water, diluted and succussed every day. The response to this method of dosage was much better than to the single doses and the whole condition cleared up after about six weeks of such repetition. She has now been free for the last three months.

Of course, knowing the nature of the disorder, that it has long periods of remissions and exacerbations, we are most reluctant to conclude anything at this stage but this much can be stated that the response to the repeated doses of medicine given in water was superior to that of the single dose and also that such repeated dosing did not provoke any aggravation.

HOMOEOPATHY
Vol IV No. 4
Page No. 129 - Case No. 5.

Man of 37. Psoriasis since 1915 on elbows, knees and legs. Was given *Pulsatilla*. This helped very greatly and was followed by *Ars. iod.* which cleared up the condition.

A FEW CASES OF PSORIASIS TREATED WITH HOMOEOPATHIC APPROACH

Dr. R. P. Patel, Kottayam.

Psoriasis

It is a chronic, relapsing disease of unknown etiology characterized by sharply defined, dry, scaling, erythematous patches, covered with adherent silvery-white scales. The eruption is usually symmetrical and most commonly affects elbow, knee, scalp, nails, and the sacral region.

When etiology is unknown. Homoeopathy has good field to prove its efficacy by following the chronic miasmatic theory of Dr. Hahnemann.

Psoriasis according to chronic miasmatic theory, is a condition of three great miasms – Psora, Sycosis and Syphilis. It has more of Psora, a pinch of Sycosis and lot of Syphylis and hence needs anti-psoric, anti-sycotic, anti-syphilitic medicines. As it is of chronic nature and relapsing type it is stubborn to cure but it is amenable to Homoeopathy.

Dr. Kent has mentioned the following rubrics on page 1316 in the repertory.

Eruptions :

Psoriasis : *Alum, Ambra, Am-c, Ars, Ars-iod, Aur, Bor, Bry, Bufo, Calc, Cal-s, Canth, Carb-ac, China, Clem, Cor-r, Cupr, Dulc, Iod, Iris, Kali-ars, Kali bich, Kali-carb, Led, Lob, Lyco, Mag-carb, Mang, Mer, Merc-cor, Merc-i-r, Mez, Nit-ac, Nuph, Petr, Phos-ac, Phos, Phyto, Psor, Puls, Ran-b, Rhus-t, Sarr, Sars, Sepia, Sil, Sulph, Tell, Teucr, Thuja.*

Diffusa : *Ars, Ars-iod, Calc, Cic, Clem, Dulc, Graph, Lyco, Mer-i-r, Mez, Mur-ac, Rhus-t, Sulph, Thuja.*

Inverterata : *Calc, Carb-ac, Clem, Kali-ars, Mang, Merc, Petro, Puls, Rhus-t, Sepia, Sil, Sulph.*

Syphilitic : *Ars, Ars-iod, Aur-m, Cor-r, Kali-br, Merc, Nit-ac, Phyto, Sars, Thuja.*

Some additional medicines : *Ant-t, Aster, Aur-m-nit, Berb-aq, Chrysar, Flour-ac, Hydrocot, Merc-sol, Nat-ars, Nat-m, Tereb, Thyroid, Tuber, Syphilin.*

Bowel Nosodes : *Morg-p, Mutabile.*

Case No. 1

Master M. aged 3 years (now 12 years) only son of an M.D. was brought to me with the following complaints continuously crying from the age of 4 months onwards. Holds breath for a long time. Cold attack frequently after whooping cough (Triple vaccine was given). Cold attack at least once a month with temperature. Suspected Diphtheria and anti-diphtheritic serum was given. Afterwards sneezing, catarrh, followed. Tonsils enlarged. Agg. mostly night time, wants to cover, very obstinate - Cries for a long time had convulsions once after long cry. Eruptions rough, scaly on forehead and axilla. Both father and mother being Doctors they did not like to give more antibiotics and steroids. Rather antibiotics failed.

4-7-77 — *Pertussin* 200, one dose at bedtime. 5 days after *Merc sol* 30/45 doses 3 times per day.

26-7-77 — Feels better. *Merc sol* 30/30 — M/E.

9-9-77 — Slight cold. *Merc sol* 0/3/30 — 3 times per day.

22-9-77 — Was better, but now eruptions are worse in forehead and in axilla. *Sulphur* 0/3/30 — M/E.

3-10-78 — Small eruptions on face which are red and rough. Wants to cover the body. Feels chilly. *Psorinum* 0/3/30 — M/E.

20-10-78 — Feels better. *Psorinum* 0/3/30. M.E.

10-2-82 — Small eruptions on forehead. *Psorinum* 0/3/30. M.E.

6-9-83 — Was better, but eruptions on scalp after eating *Psorinum* 0/3/30 M.E.

2-1-86 — Feels better. Stye in right eye. Eruption in axilla, agg. during winter. Feels chilly. *Psorinum* 0/3/30 M.E.

18-11-86 — Feels better. *Psorinum* 0/3/30 M.E.

Father has adopted Homoeopathy and he is prescribing in 35% of his cases with good success, but he has obsession with *Psorinum* and *Psoriasis.*

Case No. 2

Mr. B, aged 35 came to consult for Psoriasis Universal is of 12 years standing. Scaly patches all over the body, but mostly in both extremities. Thick scab formation on scalp also. Itching with bloody oozing. At times pustular discharge, i.e. secondary infections. Itching agg. by dust, fertilizers, also in winter, at night time. Loss of sleep. Feels depressed due to itching and loss of sleep. Irritable. Cold attacks with sneezing since many years with blocking of nose, Agg. in the evening. These complaints are better after Psoriasis. Hardness of hearing — both ears. Saliva tastes bad. F.H. Nil P.H. Skin trouble — Scabies in childhood.

Heat agg, Rain better. Sleep agg.

30-12-81 — *Gunpowder* 0/1/60 M.E. due to secondary infection and bleeding.

29-1-82 — Feels better, thickness of the skin better. *Gunpowder* 0/1/60 M.E.

17-6-82 — Eruptions with itching, but better than before. Cough with blocking of nose and sneezing. *Ars-iod* 0/3/60 M.E.

27-6-83 — Was better, sneezing cough, suffocation, loss of sleep, difficulty in breathing agg. night time. *Ars. iod* 0/3/60 M.E.

3-10-83 — *Ars-iod* 0/3 was continued and was better for asthmatic breathing, sneezing and eruptions.

15-7-85 — Pain in the abdomen, loose motion and vomiting after taking some meat preparation. *Ars* also 0/3/45, 3 times.

15-8-86 — Feels better, eruptions better, *Ars-alb* 0/3/60 M.E. and it was continued upto 11-9-86 with remission of all skin complaints except in the legs which are smooth with occasional itching. Thickness is no more.

2-2-87 — Gastric complaints with distension. Slight itching in the legs. *Carbo-veg* 0/3/60 M.E.

Case No. 3

Master B. aged 11 years. Came with Psoriasis. First started at 3 years of age as small eruptions on the legs, gradually spread to all over the body. These small eruptions were with red bases and over that thick scales were present. At some places joined together with indurated edges. These eruptions started during the treatment for primary complex with Streptomycin. It was thought to be the reactions of Streptomycin but later it was confirmed as Psoriasis. Agg. winter, night. Had external applications — Bactale, Deresalic etc. Now eruptions started on the scalp which are suppurated and had to use strong external ointment which has relieved to some extent.

Had Primary complex at 10 months of age, and was given 60 injections of Streptomycin, followed by Isokin and Ethambutol tablets for 1 year and 6 months. Now occasional chest pain and cold attacks. F.H. Mother, a touch of T.B., Rheumatism. Father - Tinea.
Wants cold bath, sleep better, desires fish. Mentally forgetful, irritable, obstinate.

12-2-86 — *Ars-iod* 0/3/60 M.E.

6-3-86 — Cracks with bleeding in the lesions with itching. *Ars-iod* 0/3/60/M.E.

7-4-86 — Itching severe, agg. at night time. No oozing. Eruptions more on gluteal region. Fearful. *Ars-alb* 0/3/60/M.E.

14-5-86 — Feels better. Itching better. Eruptions have subsided. *Ars-alb* 0/3/60/M.E.

28-6-86	—	Eruptions are better. Scalp eruptions subsided. *Ars-alb* 0/3/60/M.E.
8-8-86	—	Occasional headache. Skin symptoms subsided from scalp, body and legs. Slight roughness in legs. *Ars-alb* 0/3/60/ M.E.
29-9-86	—	Feels better, occasional itching. *Ars-alb* 0/3/60/M.E.
6-12-86	—	Headache at times. Skin symptoms are cleared off. Uses Olive oil. *Ars-alb* 0/3/60 M.E.

My favourite remedies are as follows, which are having better action in 50 Millesimal Potencies :

Ars-Iod : Where history of Tuberculosis is present in the patient or in the family. Dry, scaly eruptions. Bleeding when scales are removed by force. Raw skin looks like beef steak, when washed or cleaned.

Itching agg. by cold, night, change of climate. Marked exfoliation of skin in large scales. Secondary infection with enlarged glands and evening rise of temperature. Patient is allergic to dust or pollens with respiratory complaints.

Sepia : Woman's remedy, but useful in men and children. Dry scaly eruptions mostly of scalp. Thick skin with scab formation. Sticky discharge oozing with great desire to scratch with comb. Feeling that the head is covered with caps Psoriasis of nails, face, and scalp. Intense itching in nail bases. Agg. by taking fish in almost all skin complaints is a main feature of this medicine. Eruptions are mostly seen in folds. Fishy smell of skin like in Ichthyosis. Fissures or cracks in the lesions which are painful with stiffness. Skin symptoms are worse by washing, itching and sweat. Patient feels depressed after knowing the disease which seems incurable. Careless.

Nat-Mur : Flaky, dry skin with cracks. Eruptions mostly in folds which are painful. Watery oozing after scratching, which is worse in the morning, after sun exposure, heat. Face looks shiny with reddish glow. Skin texture is loose and rough. Patient likes salt but salt agg. all skin complaints. When salt is reduced symptoms get better. Oily skin, dry eruptions on margin on hairy scalp is the characteristic of Psoriasis of scalp. At times rawness and redness of eruptions in the morning when scales have fallen at night with itching and serum-like sticky oozing. Agg. at seashore due to salty atmosphere or moisture.

Psorinum : Chilly patient, wants to cover even in warm room. Cannot tolerate air-conditioned rooms. Dirty look, of the face and skin symptoms. Psoriasis mostly in folds with fissures and dry skin with white flakes. Intolerable itching. Warm room also agg. Crusty eruptions worse in cold weather, winter, better by covering and in summer. Cranky person.

Ars-Alb : Clean fellow, but looks dirty. Dry, rough, scaly skin, a perfect picture of Psoriasis. Itching, scratching and burning in this order are guiding symptoms. Agg. at night time. Patient takes pleasure in itching and scratching. Patient is restless but full of energy and activities. At times offensiveness of body odour with secondary infection after scratching with enlargement of glands.

THE HOMOEOPATHIC OUTLOOK
Vol XII - Page No. 39
Case No. 2

Psoriasis

Mr. S. age 45 years, was suffering from chronic Psoriasis for over fifteen years. He had large patches with raised edges all over the body, which were itching very severely, and the itching was worse at nights after getting warm in bed, and after scratching caused intense burning, and scales were falling in large quantities. The whole body was disfigured, and so he had to keep himself always covered up to avoid public attention. As he was a public official with outside duties, he was obliged to apply vaseline liberally over the whole body daily in the morning before he started for work, in order to avoid the itching and exposure of his bodily ailment to others. This involved much strain and personal inconvenience. He tried various remedies both internal and external with no effect, and wanted to try Homoeopathy as a last resort. He was nervous by temperament with a melancholy mood on account of his long suffering.

As his symptoms clearly called for Sulphur, I started with *Sulphur* 10M, and gave two doses of this potency with an interval of six weeks, and as there was some improvement in the itching and general condition of the patient, I gave him *Sulphur* 50M, at intervals of two months, two doses, and as the patient continued to make steady progress, I gave him *Sulphur* CM every three months. For a complete cure, I had to give him six doses allowing longer intervals between doses. When I met the patient after two years, he looked a different person altogether and was in normal health. He was very grateful for the complete cure effected through homoeopathic treatment. In this case, *Sulphur* was clearly indicated and had to be given in the highest potencies to produce the desired effect as the case had become very chronic and of several years' standing.

INDIAN JOURNAL OF HOMOEOPATHIC MEDICINE
Vol 10 - No. 1 (1976)
Page No. 30 - Case No. 2.

I was able to promptly relieve an aged man, who was suffering from a skin eruption, which looked like a hybrid between Eczema and Psoriasis. His scales were white, thick and shining. Eruption was oozing watery discharge at some places. It was not a case of Psoriasis. It did not satisfy me as *Graphites* nor as *Mezereum* and other well-known medicines. Saliva gathering and peeping out at the corners of his mouth while talking, was noted as one symptom when he was talking about his symptoms. 'Salivation while talking' Kent gives *Graph, Iris, Lach., Nat-c., Sabina.* Referring Iris in Boericke I found a description of skin symptoms which matched the condition of my case. The remedy helped the patient.

REPERTORY OF PSORIASIS

Skin Eruption Psoriasis :

Alum, Ambr, Am-c, Ant-t, Ars, Ars-i, Aster, Aur, Aur-m-n, Berb-ag, Bor, Bry, Bufo, Calc, Calc-s, Canth, Carb-ac, Chin, Chrys-ac, Cic, Clem, Cor-r, Cupr, Dulc, Fl-ac, Graph, Hep, Hydrocot, Iod, Iris, Kali-ar, Kali-br, Kali-p, Kali-s, Led, Lyc, Mang, Merc-aur, Merc, Merc-c, Merc-i-r, Merc-sul, Mez, Mur-ac, Naph, Nat-ars, Nat-m, Nit-ac, Nuph, Petr, Ph-ac, Phos, Phyt, Platenus, Psor, Puls, Radm, Ran-b, Rhus-t, Sarr, Sars, Sep, Sil, Strych-ars, Strych-p, Stellar, Sulph, Tell, Tereb, Teucr, Thuj, Thyr, Tub, Ustil.

Alternates with asthma — *Sulph*
Chronic — Rhus-t
Diffusa — *Ars, Ars-i, Bor, Calc, Cic, Clem, Dulc, Graph, Lyc, Mer-i-r, Mez, Mur-ac, Rhus-t, Sulph, Thuj.*
Discoloration of skin after — *Kali-a*
Furfuraceous, sometimes fissured and bleeding — *Lyc*
Guttata — *Ars, Fl-ac.*
Inflamed in a child — *Ars-i*
Inveterate — *Calc, Carb-ac, Clem, Kali-br, Mang, Merc, Petr, Puls, Rhus-t, Sep, Sil, Sulph.*
Itching — *Nuph*

Itching without — *Cup-ac:*

Palmaris — *Crotal, Kali-s, Petr.*

Patches irregular with shining scales, edges slightly raised — *Iris:*

Scales shining, white adhesive, looking like stearine — *Sep.*

Syphilitic — *Ars, Ars-i, Aur, Cor-r, Kali-br, Merc, Nit-ac, Phyt, Psor, Sars, Thuj.*

Secondary syphilis — *Merc:*

With ulcers on legs — *Kali-a:*

Eye, eruption, eyebrows about, psoriasis — Phos*:*

Genitalia eruptions scrotum, psoriasis — *Nit-ac, Petr, Thuj..*

Back, eruptions, psoriasis, patches — *Calc, Kali-ar, Mez.*

Extremities : **Eruption upper limbs psoriasis** — *Iris, Kali-ar, Kali-s, Rhus-t, Sil.*

Elbow psoriasis patches — *Iris, Kali-ar, Kali-s, Phos.*

Forearm, psoriasis — *Rhus-t:*

Hand, psoriasis diffuse — *Ars, Calc, Clem, Graph, Kali-bi, Lyc, Mez, Petr, Rhus-t, Sulph.*

Hand back of psoriasis, chronic — *Ars, Aur, Bar-c, Graph, Hep, Lyc, Maland, Petr, Phos, Phyt, Rhus-t, Sars, Sulph.*

Palm-psoriasis — *Aur, Calc, Clem, Coral-r, Crot-h, Graph, Hep, Kali-s, Lyc, Med, Merc, Mur-ac, Nat-s, Petr, Phos, Psor, Sars, Sel, Sil, Sulph, Sul-ac.*

Fingers — *Lyc, Teucr.*

Fingers first, psoriasis — *Anag, Teucr.*

Second finger psoriasis — *Anag:*

Knee, psoriasis — *Iris, Phos.*

Leg, psoriasis — *Kali-ar, Phos.*

Sole of foot psoriasis — *Phos:*

Psoriasis of prepuce, nails — *Graph, Sep.*

Psoriasis of tongue — *Graph, Mur-ac, Sep.*

Tongue, psoriasis — *Cast-eq, Kali-bi, Mur-ac.*

CHAPTER 12

Napkin Rash

It affects infants in the areas covered by the napkin. Lesions consist mainly of simple erythema, though they may become vesicular or even ulcerative. They are situated, most frequently, on the prominences, and may occupy the inner parts of the thighs, perineum and genitalia. Usually, the flexures are not affected, contrary to what happens in intertrigo. The causes of napkin rash are : wet or soiled napkins, soap left in the napkins after washing, strong ammoniacal urine, poor general health.

Differential diagnosis : It is made from other erythematous eruptions in this area, namely, congenital syphilis (it is accompanied by other syphilitic manifestations, rash on the palms and the soles, involvement of the anal region, the lesions are erythematous or bullous); thrush (moist, red areas with peeling at the edges, also thrush lesions in the mouth); intertrigo (confined to the flexures only) and tinea (the lesions are characteristic, besides, tinea is rare in infancy).

The primary area that is affected in this condition, is the thigh, perineum, and genitalia.

The following signs and symptoms should be carefully noted :

I. Erythema — Its extent, its colour.

II. Sensations — like burning, pricking, stinging, itching.
III. Thermal and time modalities.

Since napkin rash occurs in infancy, it is difficult to get symptoms. Hence the prescription has to be based on signs and observations.

If the irritation persists, then apply gently to the affected part a mixture of Calendula and Olive oil in the ratio 1:4.

Prophylaxis : Avoid use of wet or soiled napkins. Look for any soap left in the napkin after washing. Immediately change the napkin, if soaked with urine. Improve the nutrition of the child with a balanced diet.

Treatment : The most essential part of treatment is keeping the parts dry and exposing the parts to fresh air as far as possible.

Rubber and nylon panties must be avoided. Use of talcum powder should be strictly avoided. If there is a distressing itching then one should apply plain Castor oil.

Drugs :

Apis : The appearance of the rash is fiery red; child rubs the affected part with the fingers quite vigorously. This is due to stinging, burning, sticking, smarting sensation experienced by the child. This is worse in evening and night and warm application. Better by cold application. The affected part is swollen and has a bloated appearance. The part is very hot to touch. If the child is covered it becomes very uncomfortable. Child feels better in open air.

Cantharis : The Nappy rash of *Canth.* is characterized by small ulcerations with exudation of watery discharge and small blisters. The child is very restless due to burning sensation and feels better when washed with cold water. Affected part is so sensitive and the child will not allow anyone to touch.

Rhus-T : The erythematous rash of *Rhus-t* is characterized by tiny vesicles which tends to become crusty with itching and burning which is better by warm formentation. Here the child likes affected part to be covered as the skin is sensitive to cold air. Slightest exposure to damp and cold makes the child uncomfortable by worsening the rash. Rash is prone to suppuration and crust and then one gets vesicles with small abscesses.

Sulphur : The appearance of the rash is bright red with fine scales in between. The child is most uncomfortable at night in bed and while washing. The burning sensation in the rash is sensitive to draft of air, wind and washing. There is voluptuous itching and the child scratches violently. The rash alternates with other complaints e.g., asthma.

Intertrigo

It is a very common and annoying cutaneous affection.

Etiology : Plethoric, debilitated and over-dressed individuals with hyperhidrosis and sedentary habits are most prone to intertrigo, but in tropical heat, anyone can develop this complaint. In my own experience, people in good health, of normal weight, who wear comfortable clothes in the day allowing the free passage of air, and loose garments at night, and who do some exercise in cool, fresh air, usually escape intertrigo. It is an uncommon condition amongst the poor who live in the open. Friction caused by opposing surfaces of ill-fitting underclothing, heat and retention of sweat, are the important local etiological factors. The disease is most prevalent in the summer in hot tropical countries. Diabetes and gout are two other predisposing causes.

Clinical features : The flexures are the sites of affection. In order of frequency, the groins, the axillae, the cubital and popliteal fossae, are the areas commonly involved. The symptoms are : an uncomfortable feeling, burning and sometimes tenderness. A clinical examination will reveal redness which leads to maceration and may be to a linear superficial abrasion or fissure. The latter is found right at the angle of two opposing surfaces. There is no frank oozing of serum or crusting unless flexural infective eczema complicates intertrigo owing to secondary infection and eczematization. Moniliasis may also secondarily complicate intertrigo.

Differential diagnosis : It is made from tinea cruris. Here, the characteristic clinical features are : marked itching, sparing of the deepset angle of opposing folds, and inflammatory border of vesicles and pustules. The microscopic evidence of fungus is conclusive.

The prognosis is good if the disease is treated by an expert and the patient is co-operative.

It is one of the most common problems encountered in our daily practice. Usually a plethoric overdressed individual with hyperhidirosis and sedentary habits walks into our clinic and complains of an uncomfortable feeling, with burning and itching, especially in the groins.

This condition is more prevalent in the young age groups. The following points should be carefully noted in history taking :

(i) Site — Inguinal region, axillary region, cubital fossa, popliteal fossa.

(ii) Symptoms like burning and itching should be completely analysed in relation to its thermal and time modalities.

(iii) Intensity of the itching with scratch marks or ulceration also should be carefully enquired into.

(iv) Pigmentation which follows intertrigo should be carefully observed, for its colour and extent.

(v) Sign of secondary infection should be noted.

Treatment : Since intertrigo develops complication like eczema and monilial infection very easily, treatment should be carried out very religiously otherwise the excessive itching in the private parts become very annoying and demoralising.

1. The general health of the patient must be improved, and he should be instructed to lead an outdoor life, exposing the affected part, particularly to fresh cool air for atleast a couple of hours each day. If possible, he should work and live in an Air-conditioned room.

2. The affected part should be kept dry, cool and free from friction. They must be frequently oiled. Underclothing should be of cotton and must fit properly.

3. Tight jeans, jockey types of underwears and synthetic materials should be avoided.

4. Exercise — Raise the legs and separate them as far as possible. Repeat it 20-30 times.

5. A mixture of Calendula and olive oil in the ration of 1:4 should be applied gently to the affected part.

Drugs :

Aethusa-Cyn : Excoriation of thighs < walking. Itching eruption around joints. Profuse perspiration. Surface of body cold and covered with clammy sweat. Lymphatic glands swollen. Eruptions itching when exposed to heat.

Agnus : Corrosive itching on different parts of the body. > by scratching, but it soon returns. Grawing or itching in various parts.

Ars-Alb : Skin papular dry, rough, dirty looking, scaly < cold and scratching. Hot, itching and violent burning in the skin — Itching increased by scratching followed by bleeding.

Icy coldness of body. Parts painful after scratching. Disease begins as red spot spread like ringworm covered with silvery scales.

Bell : Dry and hot skin. Burning swelling, spreading suddenly. Alternate redness and paleness of the skin. Redness of several parts. Tense skin — scarlet smooth and shiny with heat, itching, burning.

Borax : Intertrigo difficult to heal. Dirty unhealthy skin. Every injury tends to ulcerate. Inflammation of the skin with chilliness, followed by heaviness and pulsation in the head.

Calc-C : Burning and itching more in morning and in bed. Dry, rough, unhealthy skin; as if covered with a kind of miliary eruption. Skin excoriated in several places. Intertrigo of lenticular red and raised spots with great heat. Skin sensitive to rubbing, must wash gently. Eruptions moist and scurfy thick scales.

Causticum : Soreness and violent itching in folds of skin, back of ears, between thighs. Ulcerative vesicles. Skin prone to intertrigo during dentition.

Chamomilla : Eruptions with itching and nocturnal tickling. Unhealthy skin. Rash of infants during nursing and skin moist and burning hot with bruising and smarting pain.

Fagopyrum : General and excessive itching with or without eruption, most marked on pubis, pudenda, whiskers and hairy portions of body generally < afternoon, 5 p.m. to 7 p.m. skin hot, swollen.

Graphites : Rough, hard obstinate dryness and absence of perspiration, rawness in bends of limbs, groin, neck and behind ears, unhealthy skin, violent itching and burning. Eruptions oozing out a sticky exudation.

Juglans : Itching all over the body. Itching in folds, burning, soreness < after perspiring, severe redness with new vesicles with increased burning and itching. Greenish yellow secretion from eruptions. Glandular swellings and suppuration. Worse when heated, from over exertion.

Kali-Brom : Moist eruption. Itching at night in bed and in a high temperature.

Lycopodium : Great dryness of the skin. Intertrigo, raw places bleeding easily. Skin unhealthy, corrosive vesicles. Nocturnal itching. Intertrigo between thighs and labia forming flat hard ulcers with inflamed edges. Eruptions first vesicular then dry. Itching violently, raw places bleed, covered with thick crust with fetid secretion beneath.

Merc-Sol : Itching so intolerable almost makes him crazy. Better cold air and when bed is cold. Worse warmth of bed. Almost constantly moist, free perspiration which gives no relief.

Mezerium : Violent itching worse bed, from touch compelling to scratching until epidermis is removed and denuded part is covered with a scab or there is repeated exfoliation.

Oleander : Biting, itching worse on undressing compelling him to scratch. Intense itching and insupportable nocturnal burning after scratching. Slight friction causes soreness and chafing, especially above the neck or between scrotum and thigh — want of perspiration.

Ox-Ac : Exceedingly sensitive skin — agg. from sweat, with smarting and soreness, mottled, marked in circular patches.
Perspires easily.

Petroleum	:	Itching at night. Skin dry, constricted, very sensitive, rough and cracked, leathery. Itching sore, moist surfaces with redness and rawness. External hard pressure not painful but a soft touch is unbearable.
		Cracks bleed easily.
Psorinum	:	Dirty dingy look.
		Itching when body becomes warm. Agg. in bed and from warmth. Scratches until it bleeds.
		Scratching gives temporary relief.
Sulph-Ac	:	Livid skin, redness and itching blotches.
		Distressing itching and tingling of skin with eruptions.
Sulphur	:	Dry, scaly, unhealthy skin.
		Itching, spots painful red and hot after scratching. Bleeds after scratching, recurring every night in bed. Violent on thighs and legs. Skin painful for a long time after rubbing as if denuded and sore.
		Itching, burning worse scratching and washing.
		Excoriation on folds.
Tuberculinum	:	Eruptions itching, blotches all over body with exception of face and hand. Intense itching worse at night.

REPERTORY OF INTERTRIGO

Acon, Aeth, Agar, Ambr, Agn, Ambr, Am-c, Am-m, Ant-c, Ap, Arn, Ars, Ars-i, Ars-s-fl, Bap, Bar-c, Bell, Bor, Bov, Bry, Bufo, Calc, Calc-s, Canth, Carb-an, Carb-s, Carb-v, Caust, Cham, Chin, Clem, Coff, Colch, Dros, Echi, Euphr, Fl-ac, Fago, Graph, Hep, Hydr, Ign, Iod, Jugl-r, Kali-ar, Kali-br, Kali-c, Kali-chl, Kali-m, Kali-s, Kreos, Lach, Laur, Lyc, Mag-m, Mang, Merc, Merc-c, Merc-s, Mez. Nat-m, Nat-p, Nit-ac, Nux-v, Ol-an, Olnd, Ox-ac, Op, Petr, Ph-ac, Phos, Phyt, Plb, Podo, Puls, Psor, Pyrog, Rhus-t, Ruta, Sabin, Sars, Scil, Sele, Sep, Sil, Spig, Squil, Sulph, Sul-ac, Syph, Terb, Tub, Vinc-m, Zinc.

Bleeding — readily — *Lyc*
Boring into with fingers, children (scarlatina) — *Arum-t.*
Children in — *Ant-c, Bar-c, Bell, Calc, Carb-v, Cham, Chin, Ign, Kreos, Lyc, Merc, Puls, Rut, Scil, Sep, Sil, Sulph.*
Children with bilious symptoms — *Nat-s*
Children in especially — *Graph*
Dentition during — *Caust*
Discharges in every outlet of body, acrid, excoriating skin, wherever they come in contact — *Sulph*
Dries and mummifies, new blisters form around — *Anthrac*
Erosions — *Arum-m, Fl-ac.*
Humid — *Bar-c, Graph.*
Infants — *Calc, Carbo-v, Cham, Graph, Hep, Kali-m, Lyc, Merc, Psor, Sep, Sulph.*
Antrophy of infants — *Petr*
Obstinate — *Hydras*
Pain as if excoriated — *Paris, plat.*
Prurigo — *Graph*
Like raw decayed meat — *Como*
Inclined to scab — *Kali-m*
Scratching after (must scratch it raw) — *Agar, Alum, Am-c, Ant-c, Arn, Bar-c, Bov, Calc, Carb-s, Caust, Chin, Dros, Graph, Hep, Kali-c, Kreos, Lach, Lyc, Mang, Merc, Olnd, Petr, Phos, Plb, Puls, Rhus-t, Ruta, Sabin, Sep, Sil, Squil, Sul-ac.*
Sore feeling — *Sulph, Til.*
Tettery, oozing and bleeds easily when scratched — *Merc*
When walking or riding — *Sul-ac*

Easily chafed from walking or riding also in children — *Ruta*

Anus — *Agnus, Alu, Ant-c, Ap, Ars, Aur-m, Bell, Berb. Caps, Carb-v, Caust, Colo, Cham, Gamb, Gels, Graph, Kali-bi, Kali-c, Mag-c, Nat-p, Nit-ac, Nux-v, Phos, Podo, Rat, Rhus-t, Sep, Sulph, Thuj.*

With diarrhoea — *Nit-ac*

With serious discharge — *Caust*

Moist, soreness when walking — *Nit-ac*

Feeling — *Asc-h, Ign, Merc.*

In prolapsus ani — *Apis*

Agg. night from heat of bed, rubbing, scratching, amel. — *cold and pinching* — *Petr* **in scrofula** — *Ars*

As if skin were rubbed off — *Carbol-ac*

By stools — *Apis, Coloc, Merc, Mur-ac, Nit-ac, Nux-m, Nux-v, Rheum, Sulph.*

In Chronic intestinal catarrh — *Ars*

In dysentery — *Urt-ur*

Thighs — *Amyl, Arum-t, Calc-p.*

Anterior worse sitting while — *Bapt*

Between — in children — *Am-c*

Between — during menses — *All-sat, Graph, Kali-c, Nat-s, Sars, Sulph.*

Between — when walking — *Graph, Ruta, Sulph, Sul-ac.*

Between — with watery secretion — *Goss*

Burning from acrid, menstrual discharge — *Am-c*

Between thigh and genitals — *Merc-s*

In hamstrings — *Nat-p*

Humid in folds, between scrotum and thighs — *Hep*

Red sore after riding — *Sul-ac*

On inner surface — *Sulph*

Forming flat, handlike ulcers with inflamed edges — *Lyc*

From corrosive leucorrhoea — *Sabina*

Painful in right — *Ham*

Painful on touching — *Aspar*

Feeling as if rubbed sore in skin, after waking — *Lyc*

Sore near scrotum place moist — *Carbo-v*

Perineum — *Alu, Arum-t, Aur-mur, Calc, Carbo-an, Carb-v, Caust, Cham, Graph, Hep, Ign, Lyc, Merc, Petrol, Puls, Rho, Sep, Sulph, Thuja.*

Of children particularly in groins extending to scrotum — *Ars*

— caused by stool (dysentery) — *Sulph*

Viscid, inodorous humor oozes — *Carbo-ar*

Excoriation — bends of joints — *Bell, Caust, Graph, Lyc, Mang, Ol-an, Petr, Sep, Squil, Sulph.*

Nates between — *Arum-t, Arg-m, Bufo, Carb-s, Graph, Nat-m, Nit-ac, Puls, Sep, Sulph.*

Thighs between — *Aeth, Ambr, Am-c, Anan, Ars, Aur, Bar-c, Bufo, Calc, Carb-s, Carb-v, Caust, Chin, Chin-a, Coff, Goss, Graph, Hep, Iod, Kali-ar, Kali-c, Kreos, Lyc, Meph, Merc, Nat-c, Nat-m, Nit-ac, Petr, Phos, Rhod, Sep, Squil, Sul-ac, Sulph, Thuj, Zinc.*

Knee bend of — *Ambr, Sep.*

Leg — *Lach*

Toes between — *Aur-m, Berb, Carb-an, Clem, Fl-ac, Graph, Lach, Lyc, Mang, Merc-i-f, Mez, Nat-c, Nat-m, Nit-ac, Ph-ac, Ran-b, Sep, Sil, Syph, Zinc.*

CHAPTER 13

Acne Vulgaris

Diagnostic Hallmarks

1. Distribution; face and shoulders.
2. Polymorphous lesions : Pustules, papules and comedones.

Clinical Presentation

A wide variety of lesions are found in acne, only a portion of which are pustules. Open comedones (blackheads) consist of a keratinous plug firmly situated at the orifice of a sebaceous follicle. Open comedones are black in colour because of the deposition of melanin granules in the multiple layers of compacted keratinicytes which make up the plug.

Closed comedones are dome shaped 1 to 2 mm papules. They are skin coloured rather than black. These, too, occur because of keratinous plugs in the outlet of the sebaceous follicle but here the plug lies below the surface of the skin at a point too deep to pick up colour from the surface melanocytes.

Pustules situated on an inflammatory base occur when the plugged ducts of closed comedones rupture with extrusion of the keratin plug and retained sebaceous materials into the surrounding dermis. This extrusion causes a brisk local neutrophilic inflammatory response. Thus acne pustules contain both a solid white keratin core and surrounding pus cells.

Inflammatory papules without a surmounted pustule occur when the plug together with the follicule rupture and induce inflammatory responses. All occur at a level too deep to result in a visible pustule. Inflammatory cysts and pseudocysts 1 to 2 cm in diameter occur when the process described above occurs even deeper at the level of the sebaceous gland itself. Such cystic lesions are often fluctuant and painful. Moreover, as opposed to the other lesion of acne, they heal with scar formation.

For all practical purposes acne first begins at puberty. The initial lesions in the early teen years generally consist of comedones and small pustules and these are usually found on the forehead and upper cheeks. During the late teen years the mix of lesions shifts toward larger, more inflammatory pustules and papules. These lesions generally occur on the lower cheeks, chin and jawline. Inflammatory lesions may also develop over the shoulders and upper arms. The diagnosis of acne is made on the basis of history and clinical examination.

Atypical Presentations Acne conglobata is the name used for the presence of multiple, deep, cystic, scarring, lesions over the face and upper trunk. It occurs predominantly in individuals with genetically malformed sebaceous follicles. One indication of these structural abnormalities is the presence of multiple, double ended comedones in the skin adjacent to cysts. Some individuals with severe acne conglobates have associated fever, leukocytosis and arthralgia.

The adminstration of phenytoin (Dilantin) to individuals already prone to acne has an adverse effect on the severity and duration of the disease. Administration of corticosteroids causes an acne-like folliculitis in which small pustules develop in considerable profusion on the chest, back and shoulders. Comedones and cysts are not found. Ingestion of large amounts of iodine also leads to the presence of an acneform eruption.

Acneform lesions are sometimes induced in men though occupational exposure to tars, cutting oils and chlorinated hydrocarbons and in women through the use of petroleum pomades as hair dressings. Babies occasionally develop a few acne lesions during the first month or so of life presumably as a result of maternal hormonal stimulation.

Acne excoriee des jeunes filles occurs when individuals neurotically pick at acne lesions. Because of this chronic picking minor acne lesions are kept inflamed and active for weeks or even months at a time.

Course and Prognosis

Generally the peak activity of acne is in the mid or late teen years with steady improvement starting around age 20. However, occasionally disease activity continues into the fourth decade. Women seem particularly prone to this long lasting form of acne.

Hormonal factors play an important role in the course of acne. Acne in general seems to be more severe in men. Cystic lesions which are common in men are only rarely found in women. In women a monthly peak of acne activity often occurs during the week prior to their menses. Acne tends to improve during the third to ninth month of pregnancy but rebound worsening sometimes occurs following parturition and cessation of lactation.

It is difficult to predict the future severity of acne at the time a young patient is first seen. The presence of cysts and a family history of scarring acne are, however, bad prognostic signs.

When acne is untreated, individual small papules and pustules resolve spontaneously in 7 to 10 days. Resolution of these lesions does not result in scarring even when some degree of picking is carried out. Large papules and cysts require several weeks to resolve and even then post-inflammatory colour changes may persist for months. Scarring is occasionally found at the site of deep seated papules and is almost invariably present following resolution of fluctuant cysts.

Pathogenesis

Acne is a disease of complex genetic and hormonal factors. Identical twins tend to have acne of equal severity and similar types. Parents who have had troublesome acne tend to have children with a similar problem. However, differences in severity of acne among siblings from one generation to the next suggest that genetics simply provides a permissive setting for other, acquired factors. Some of these are discussed in the paragraphs below.

Hormonal stimulation of the sebaceous glands by way of androgenic substances is a necessary factor in both men and women, Acne does not occur until puberty when such hormonal stimulation first begins to develop. Castrated men and oophorectomized women do not develop acne. Serum testosterone levels are at the most only slightly elevated in men and women with acne but little is known about the levels of other — androgenic hormones or for that matter about end organ hormonal metabolism. The importance of androgenic factors in women is underscored by the regular presence of rather severe acne in patients with polycystic ovarian disease and in those with sterol hydroxylase deficiencies.

Hormonal stimulation as described above leads to increased sebaceous gland size and to increased sebum output. The presence and severity of acne correlate in a general sort of way with production levels of sebum but even high sebum flow rates in the absence of follicular plugs does not cause acne.

The presence of a follicular plug is the proximate and necessary factor for the development of an acne lesion in any given follicle. Such blockages are caused by the accumulation of compacted, dead, cornified cells within the duct of the sebaceous gland or at the outlet of the follicle itself. Several hypotheses exist to explain the formation of these plugs; genetic malformation of the follicle; stimulation of follicular keratinization by bacteria present in the follicle; or hormonal effects on the follicle wall.

ROSACEA
(Acne Rosacea)

Diagnostic Hallmarks

1. Distribution : Vertical, central third of the face.
2. Pustules and papules against a background of erythema and telangiectasia.

Clinical Presentation

Rosacea is characterized by the presence of dusky erythema and telangiectasia over the nose and cheeks. Often the glabella and chin are involved such that the eruption forms a vertical line down the central third of the face. In the more severe cases pustules and erythematous papules also are found. Comedones do not occur. Men with long-standing rosacea sometimes develop a connective tissue overgrowth of the nose known as rhinophyma. This condition is colloquially referred to as potato nose. Rosacea is seen primarily in middle aged or older individuals. Those of Celtic and northern European background seem particularly predisposed to the disease. The diagnosis of rosacea is made on a clinical basis.

Course and Prognosis

Rosacea is a chronic disease characterized by periodic exacerbations and remissions. Gradual worsening with more permanent redness and telangiectasia occurs in some patients whereas in others the disease gradually fades out over a period of many years. Men with rosacea may eventually develop rhinophyma. Conjunctivitis, blepharitis and keratitis accompany the disease in some instances. Treatment leads to considerable cosmetic improvement but probably changes the ultimate course of the disease very little.

Pathogenesis

The cause of rosacea is unknown. Familial predisposition for the disease and the remarkable tendency for those of Celtic background to develop the disease suggest that genetic factors are important. Ingestants such as spicy foods, alcohol and beverages drunk at hot temperatures are widely believed to worsen the disease. Certainly they do temporarily increase the redness and prominence of the telangiectasia but it is not clear that they permanently alter the eventual course of the disease. Contrary to folklore, rosacea is not a sign of excess alcoholic intake. The pustules of rosacea appear to be follicular abscesses; they lack the component of keratinous plugging found in the pustules of acne vulgaris.

ACNE

Homoeopathic Approach

Acne vulgaris can be considered as one of the common diagnosis brought forward by the patient to a homoeopath. The problem should never be tackled with superficial, local acting remedies. Instead, deep acting constitutional remedies should be bombarded judiciously as soon as the complete totality is available.

Whilst treating acne, inquires should be made in the directions given below :

(1) The exact type of acne should be diagnosed e.g. acne vulgaris, acne rosaceae.

(2) The site is extremely helpful to select the appropriate drug e.g. I am able to prescribe *Carbo-veg* on many occasions when no other symptoms are available only its characteristic site of affection that is back. (Refer — Kent Repertory : Back eruptions — acne carbo veg).

(3) As certain whether :

(a) Is patient asymptomatic and has come to take preventive measures for recurrence of acne.

(b) Pustular and cystic variety where pain is the presenting symptom.

(c) When patient presents with lots of scarring and disfigurement of skin due to acne.

The above differentiation is a must as the course progresses and the line of treatment is quite different.

(4) Acne from homoeopathic stand point are known to be caused by various causative factors, e.g.,

(i) Menstruation and pregnancy.
(ii) Masturbation.
(iii) Food habits and allergies.
(iv) Emotions.

A sincere attempt to find the cause pays rich dividends. The following additional causes have been frequently observed in my practice. They are : (i) during stressful situations, especially amongst teenagers, (ii) after abuse of various cosmetics (iii) occupational that is exposure to various organic and inorganic chemicals.

(5) The aggravating and ameliorating factors should be noted, e.g., acne aggravated during summer — Bovista.

(6) Concomitant symptoms that are usually associated with acne should be noted. We have frequently observed that amongst the concomitant symptoms, constipation and G.I. upsets are two of the commonest out of the lot.

(7) Patient should be strictly advised not to apply any local medicaments on acne as this does not help in overcoming the tendency to develop acne. Instead patients should be encouraged to clean the face, preferably with hot water atleast 6-8 times a day without using any soap. This helps to remove the dust particles and the minute organisms (bacterial).

(8) The patient should be advised to have proper timing for their diet and to omit from the diet :

(i) highly seasoned and pungent food;
(ii) foods that are rich in fats;
(iii) high carbohydrates — Mithais, sweets, chocolates. Patient should be encouraged to eat plenty of green leafy vegetables and fresh fruits.

Exercise in fresh open air adds a feather to the cap of treatment.

(9) The recent trend to be on long term antibiotics to subside the acne should be discouraged.

(10) When the patient is passing through a stressful situation psychotherapy is often of tremendous help to cope up with the situation.

Eugeina Jambosia : It is specially indicated for indurated and painful acne along with comedones. The pimples are painful for some distance around. It is also useful for acne rosaceae. Skin cracks about toes, fissures between toes and nightly cramps in soles of feet become important concomitant symptom.

Berberis Aquifolium : The acne eruptions come in blotches. The rest of the skin is dry and scaly. Pimples extend from face towards the neck. It is an age old remedy to clear the complexion of the face.

Antim Crud : Pimples that chiefly affect the cheek and chin. Simple acne that turn into pustules and then gradually develop into boils. Pimples that are associated with gastric derangement. Skin of the patient has a tendency to develop cracks and warts. There is burning and itching sensation in the acne, worse night.

Carbo Animalis : Acne rosacea having sensation of burning and rawness in it. The skin has a tendency to develop ulcers with indurated glands, especially neck, axilla and groins.

Chrysarobinum : Acne rosacea that leads to easy formation of crusts. Acne is associated with violent itching.

Calc-Phos : The face is pale, yellowish, earthy, full of pimples. They ulcerate very easily and form deep scars. Also they tend to suppurate easily. Acne vulgaris in individuals who are tall, lean, anaemic with glandular enlargement.

Calc-Sulph : Tendency to suppuration after the pus has found its vent, comes within the range of this remedy. The face is full of pimples and pustules. The discharge is thick, yellow, lumpy and bloody. Obstinate pimples that refuse to heal early. Even though a hot patient, calc-sulph patient feels better by local heat.

Carbo-Veg : Pimples with mottled cheeks and red nose. Pimples developing in individual who is fat, sluggish, old, lazy and lifeless. Pimples that suppurate and have an offensive odour.

Cimicifuga : Pimples with facial blemishes in young women. Pimples that are associated with ovarian and uterine complaints. Acne in individuals who are nervous, depressed and oversensitive.

Conium : Pimples, small, red burning appear with scanty menses and disappear when menses are over. Pustular acne on the face that itch violently. The skin is discoloured red. Pustules rupture and form thick crusts. Acne alternates with the internal symptom e.g. diarrhoea.

Graphites : Acne that exudes a gluey moisture, but bleeds easily and has a tendency to develop thick crusts. Acne vulgaris before the menses. The skin symptoms alternate with the digestive complaints.

Juglans Regia : Comedones and acne of the face that itch violently. When the acne bursts, it forms thick crusts — Acne that are associated with menstrual irregularities.

Kali Brom : The face has a blotchy red appearance with multiple acne and especially during puberty. The scar remains after the acne had disappeared. Acne developing in individuals after sexual excess.

Kali-Ars : Pustular acne worse during menses. The skin is dry, scaly and wilted. There is intolerable itching which is worse from warmth.

Led-Pal : Red pimples on forehead and cheeks, stinging when touched. Pimples developing in individual after suppressed discharges or after absence of alcohol.

Oophorinum : Acne rosacea associated with ovarian dysfunction.

Medorrhinum : Acne and pustules come out in blotches of reddish colour during menses; worse after menses. The discharge from the acne has a fishy odour. Appearance of acne in individuals with history of sycòses.

Nux-Vomica : Pimples and acne that develop after excessive use of liquors and cheese. Pimples associated with gastric derangements.

Acid-Phos : Acne from onanism. Acne with loss of hair from beard. Acne that gradually turns into small painful boils with stinking pustular discharge.

Psorinum : Acne rosacea with dirty, rough, scabby, greasy skin.

Sulphur : Pale sickly face with bright red lips with multiple, painful acne. Acne associated with dry, rough, wrinkled, scaly skin. There is burning and itching sensation in acne which is worse at night in bed. Acne alternates with other complaints like asthma.

Sulphuric Acid : Acne rosaceae with obstinate constipation.

THE HOMOEOPATHIC OUTLOOK
Vol II - No. 10 (1941)
Page No. 303

Acne (Dr. T.S. Hoyne)

Acne is a very disfiguring disease owing to the fact that it selects the face by preference as its location. It is often mistaken for syphilis by the non-professional man than any other skin affection.

Acne tends to be chronic, and is obstinately resistant to treatment. Moreover, it is subject to periods of amelioration and aggravation without treatment of any kind. With proper diet and attention to hygiene, together with the homoeopathic remedy it yields to treatment in course of a few weeks to a few months.

It is an inflammatory structural disorder of the Sebaceous glands or follicles of the skin. Dirt plugs the outlet of many of the follicles, forming 'black heads', or comedones. According to Unna, however, the uniform blackening of these outlets is due to a pigmentary staining. It may be both, but it certainly is chiefly the former. Retention of the natural secretion or sebum causes irritation of the follicles and congestion of the surrounding tissue. Pressure of the skin with the finger nails squeezes out the secretion in little cylinders, generally regarded by the laity as worms. Some points suppurate and some intermediate follicles inflame, and pimples, as well as hardened masses, appear. It is a complete spoiler of a fine complexion and hence dreaded by the fair sex.

The cases that suppurate are those that become infected with some variety of the staphylococcus pyogenes or pus germ. The variety described above is the acne simplex. A more formidable kind is the acne rosacea, characterised by hypertrophy, redness, dilatation of the blood vessels and even neoplastic tubercles.

Acne simplex is the form most frequently met with. It is more common about the time of puberty. The direct causes are said to be local irritants, cosmetics, uncleanliness, exposure to heat, cold and wind, and the entrance of pus germs into the gland. The general causes are inappropriate food, too rich or too nitrogenous, masturbation, sexual excesses, uterine derangements, and debilitating diseases generally. It is most intimately connected with derangements, overactivity, etc., of the sexual organs, which accounts for its frequent occurence at the time of puberty. At this age the hair follicles and the sebaceous glands are very active, and many changes are taking place in the developing individual.

Certain drugs produce an acne — like eruption of the face — namely, Tar. Potassium bromide (forehead) and Potassium iodide. The habitual use of alcohol, especially in excess, is responsible for a good number of cases.

The superiority of homoeopathic treatment over the local applications and alternative drugs of the allopaths may be shown by a few illustrative cases.

Case 1
Mary, employed in the hospital, came to the clinic affected with acne. The eruption came out since she had worked in the laundry, never troubled in this way before, Menses had been missed twice, her feet were cold and damp all the time; she complained of them without being asked about it. *Calcarea carbonica* worked about magically, in three weeks her face was perfectly smooth and well.

Case 2
A.S. 30 years old, acne for several years. Owing to chronic rheumatic pains, had drunk a great deal of whisky, which, he says always relieved his pains, but made his face a good deal worse. The pains were worse during quiet and relieved by motion. He is weak and complains that he can do little work because his strength gives out. All liquor stopped and *Rhus* 30 given. He was well in about ten weeks.

Case 3

J.B. 16 years old, acne simplex on both sides of the face. Glands on the sides of the neck somewhat enlarged; skin generally yellowish; an unusual condition was that the skin of the face was very sensitive to touch. Acne is not usually a painful or sensitive disease. The sensitiveness, enlarged glands and pustules led to the prescription of *Hepar sulph*. Report in three weeks showed much improvement, fell back during fourth week probably from the discontinuance of the remedy. It was then represcribed, with improvement.

Case 4

K.E. 22 years old, acne simplex. Yellowish and unhealthy skin; every little injury suppurates; always worse during and after menses; glands of neck enlarged. *Hepar sulph* was given for about six weeks, with disappearance of eruption and better health generally. The symptoms in these two cases in different sexes were about the same and called for the same remedy.

Neither of these cases : is fully reported, but *Hepar*, has sensitiveness to touch, glandular swellings, suppuration, unhealthy skin and yellow complexion.

Case 5

G.C. 22 years old, acne for several years; has taken Sulphur, salts and other home remedies for it; takes cold easily, takes wine often; has suffered from suppuration of the glands of the neck, *Baryta carb* — cured.

Case 6

Man aged 25 years. Had syphilis; has taken much Iodide of Potash. Some weeks ago an eruption came upon his face. He considered it a return of his old trouble, which so affected him that he had serious thoughts of throwing himself in the lake. On the mental condition he was given *Aurum*, which removed the eruption in about two months.

Other remedies have cured cases to their credit — namely Nux-vomica, Graphites, Lycopodium, Ledum and Pulsatilla. Many more are placed in the repertories under acne.

REPERTORY OF ACNE

Acne : *Ant-c, Ars, Ars-i, Ast-r, Aur, Bar-c, Bell, Calc, Calc-sil, Calc-s, Carb-an, Carb-s, Carb-v, Caust, Chel, Con, Cop, Crot-h, Cyc, Eug, Graph, Hep, Iod, Jamb, Kali-br, Kreos, Lach, Led, Med, Merc, Nat-m, Nit-ac, Nux-v, Ph-ac, Psor, Pub, Sabin, Sanic, Sel, Sep, Sil, Sulph, Sul-i, Thuj, Tub, Uran-n.*

Black — *Ars, Ast-r.*
Cheese agg. — *Nux-v*
Emaciation with — *Abro*
Face-disfiguring — *Cop*
Hard — *Ars-i.*
Masturbation from — *Crot-h, Ph-ac.*
Menses, after agg — *Med*
Menses before agg — *Graph, Mag-m, Psor, Sep.*
Menses delayed — *Crot-h*
Menses scanty with — *Sang*
Obstinated — *Lapp*
Pustular — *Berb-sul-i*
Pustular body all over — *Calc-hyp*
Pustular menses during — *Kali-ar*
Scars, remaining after — *Carb-an, Cop, Kali-br.*
Sore — *Arn*
Summer Agg — *Bov.*
Women-young — *Cyc*
Becoming heated agg. — *Caust*
Fire, near a — *Ant-c*
Rosacea — *Agar, Ars, Ars-br, Ars-i, Aur, Aur-m, Bell, Buf, Calc-p, Calc-sil, Canth, Caps, Carb-ac, Carb-an, Carb-s, Carb-v, Caust, Chel, Chrysar, Cic, Clem, Eug, Hydr-ac, Iris, Kali-br, Kali-i, Kali-bi, Kreos, Lach, Led, Mez, Nux-v, Oophor, Petr, Plb, Psor, Rad, Rhus-r, Rhus-t, Ruta, Sep, Sil, Sulph, Sul-ac, Sulph-iod, Tub, Verat, Viol-o, Viol-t.*
Bluish — *Lach, Sulph.*
Groups, in — *Caust.*
On nose — *Calc-p, Cann-s, Caust, Psor.*
Chin — *Hydr, Verat, Viol-t.*
Forehead — *Ant-c, Ars, Aur, Bar-c, Bell, Calc, Caps, Carb-an, Carb-s, Carb-v, Caust, Cic, Clem, Hep, Kreos, Led, Nat-m, Nit-ac, Nux-v, Ph-ac, Psor, Rhus-t, Sep, Sil, Sulph, Viol-t.*
Lips — *Cadm, Caps, Hydr.*

Nose — *Ars, Calc-p, Caps, Cann-s, Caust, Graph, Selen, Sulph.*
Back eruptions, acne — *Carb-v*
Back eruptions cervical region — *Amph, Jug-r.*
Acne simplex : *Ambra, Ant-c, Ant-t, Ars, Ars-br, Ars-i, Ars-s-r, Asim, Aster, Bell, Bellis, Berb-ac, Bov, Calc-p, Calc-pic, Calc-sil, Calc-s, Carb-ac, Carb-an, Carb-v, Cic, Cim, Clem, Cob, Con, Crot-t, Echin, Eug-i, Granat, Graph, Hep, Hydrocot, Ind, Jugl-c, Jug-r, Kali-ars, Kali-br, Kali-bi, Kali-c, Kali-i, Kali-m, Lappa, Led, Lyc, Med, Nabul-s, Nat-br, Nat-m, Nit-ac, Nux-v, Oleland, Phos-ac, Psor, Puls, Rad, Selen, Sep, Sil, Staph, Sulph, Sul-i, Sumb, Thuj.*
From abuse of K.J. — *Aur*
From abuse of mercury — *Kali-i, Mez, Nit-ac.*
From cheese — *Nux-v*
From cosmetics — *Bov*
From syphilis — *Aur, Kali-i, Merc-s, Nit-ac.*
In anaemic girls at puberty with vertex, headache, flatulent dyspepsia, better by eating — *Calc-p*
In drunkards — *Ant-c, Bar-c, Led, Nux-v, Rhus-t.*
In fleshy young people with coarse habits, bluish red, pustules on face, chest, shoulders — *Kali-br*
In scrofulous — *Bar-c, Brom, Calc-c, Calc-p, Con, Iod, Merc, Mez, Sil, Sulph.*
In tubercular children — *Tub*
With Cachexia — *Ars, Carb-v, Nat-m, Sil.*
With gastric derangements — *Ant-c, Carb-v, Cim, Lyc, Nux-v, Puls, Robin.*
With glandular swellings — *Brom, Calc-s, Merc.*
With indurated papules — *Agar, Arn, Ars-i, Berb-v, Bov, Brom, Carb-an, Cob, Con, Eug-i, Iod, Kali-br, Kali-i, Nat-br, Nit-ac, Robin, Sulph.*
With menstrual irregularities — *Aur-m-n, Bell, Bellis, Berb-aq, Berb-v, Calc, Cim, Con, Eug-i, Graph, Kali-br, Kali-c, Kreos, Nat-m, Psor, Puls, Sang, Sars, Thuj, Ver-a.*
With pregnancy — *Bell, Sab, Sars, Sep.*
With rheumatism — *Leg, Rhus-t.*
With sexual excesses — *Aur, Calc, Kali-br, Ph-ac, Rhus-t, Sep, Thuj.*
With scars unsightly — *Carb-an, Kali-br.*
With symmetrical distribution — *Arn*
With blepharitis, from indulgence in high living or fat food — *Puls*

Centre of pustule depressed, leaves scars — *Kali-br*
With muddy complexion — *Sulph*
Like that of drunkard — *Ant-c, Ars, Bar-c, Carb-s, Crotalus, Kreos, Lach, Led, Nux-v, Puls, Sulph.*
In young growing girls — *Puls*
With sick headache — *Sulph*
Indurata — *Ant, Sul-aur, Ars, Bell, Berb, Carb-a, Carb-v, Con, Hep, Kali-br, Kali-iod, Led, Nux-v, Puls, Sil, Sulph.*
With displacement of uterus < before menses — *Sep*
Since menopause — *Tarent*
Punctata (Comedones) — *Abrot, Ant-c, Ars, Bar-c, Bell, Bor, Bry, Calc, Carb-s, Carb-v, Chel, Dig, Dros, Eug, Graph, Hep, Hydr, Kali-br, Lach, Lyc, Mez, Nat-a, Nat-c, Nat-m, Nit-ac, Petr, Plb, Psor, Sabad, Sabin, Sel, Sep, Sil, Sulph, Sul-iod, Sumb, Thuj, Tub.*
Ulcerating — *Dig, Selen, Tub.*
Chin — *Dros, Tub.*
And upper lip — *Sulph*
Nose — *Dros, Graph, Nit-ac, Sabin, Sel, Sulph, Sumb, Tub.*
Forehead — *Sulph*
Comedones with emaciation — *Abrot*
Suppurate and ulcerate — *Dig*
Acne rosacea, after sexual abscess — *Calc, Crotal, Jamb, Kali-br, Phos-ac, Sulph.*
In dispersed groups — *Caust*
Sebacea — *Con, Iod, Nat-m, Psor, Sulph.*
In young scrofulous persons — *Carb-ac*
Solare (Dysmenorrhoea) — *Graph*
After suppression, hyperaemia of retina — *Puls*
In urinary troubles — *Cop*
In young people — *Carbo-v*
In young fleshy people of gross habits — *Kali-br*

PIMPLES

Acetan, Acon, Aloe, Agar, Alum, Ambr, Am-c, Am-m, Anac, Ant-c, Ant-t, Aran, Arg-m, Arg-n, Arn, Ars, Ars-i, Aster, Aur, Bar-c, Bar-m, Bell, Benz-ac, Berb, Bov, Brom, Bry, Bufo, Calad, Calc, Calc-p, Calc-s, Canth, Caps, Carb-an, Carb-s, Carb-v, Caust, Cham, Chel, Chin, Chin-a, Cimic, Cina, Cist, Clem, Cocc, Cocc-c, Con, Crot-h, Crot-t, Cub, Cupr, Cycl, Dros, Dulc, Euphr, Fl-ac, Gels, Gamb, Graph, Hell, Hep, Iod, Kali-ar, Kali-br, Kali-c, Kali-chl, Kali-n, Kali-p, Kali-s, Kreos, Lach, Led, Lyc, Mag-c, Mag-m, Mang, Meph, Merc, Merc-c, Mez, Mosch, Mur-ac, Nat-a, Nat-c, Nat-m, Nat-p, Nat-s, Nit-ac, Nux-v, Op, Pall, Par, Petr, Ph-ac, Phos, Plb, Psor, Puls, Rhus-t, Ruta, Sabad, Sars, Sel, Seneg, Sep, Sil, Spig, Spong, Squil, Stann, Staph, Stront, Sulph, Sul-ac, Tab, Tarax, Tarent, Tell, Thuj, Til, Valer, Verat, Viol-t, Zinc.

Acuminated whitish, filled with watery fluid, commence with itching and burning, especially on abdomen, hands, and between fingers — *Ars*
Black — *Carb-v, Spig.*
With black heads — *Diosc*
Bleed easily when scratched — *Kob*
Bleeding — *Cist, Par, Rhus-t, Stront, Thuj.*
From degraded state of blood — *Crotal*
Like blotches, stinging, itching like nettles < rubbing — *Stram*
Brain affections of children — *Sulph*
Leaving brown liver spots — *Berb*
Brownish (syphilis) — *Nit-ac*
Burning — *Agar, Ars, Bov, Canth, Caust, Graph, Kali-c, Mag-m, Merc, Nat-s, Ph-ac, Rhus-t, Squil, Staph, Stront, Sulph, Til.*
Burning heat — *Mosch*
Burning with yellow crusts — *Merc*
Burning itching — *Agar.*
Close together — *Cham, Staph, Thuj, Verat.*
Coalescing into blisters size of a split pea filled with yellow watery fluid with intense itching < night after 12 P.M. > rubbing with something rough until blisters are open — *Rhus, Sang.*
Confluent — *Cic, Mur-ac, Ph-ac, Tarent, Valer.*
Conical, hard and red — *Thuj*
Copper coloured — *Kali-i*

Crusty in young people — *Hep, Merc-sol.*
Crusts with — *Calc, Merc, Squil.*
Crust with green — *Calc*
Dry — *Iod*
Dry, red, itching when exposed to heat — *Sars*
Dry, like confluent smallpox — *Hyos*
Drunkards in — *Kreos, lach, Led.*
Exuding moisture like an ulcer painful on external pressure *Spong*
Soon filling with whitish yellow lymph and then shrivelling — *Cycl*
Clawing, itching — *Ant-c, Ant-t, Caust, Mang, Nit-ac.*
Little hard, red like flea bites — *Agar*
Furunculous, with red areola and itching sensation — *Sul*
Caused by disturbed action of follicular glands — *Kali-m*
Hard — *Agar, Bov, Nit-ac, Rhus-t, Sabin, Valer, Verat.*
In groups — *Berb*
Surrounded by blue halo — *Lach, Merc.*
Hard — *Arum-t*
Hard with burning biting itching — *Rhus*
Small hard — *Therid*
Humid — *Thuj*
Inflamed — *Agar, Berb, Bry, Chel, Nit-ac, Petr, Stann, Sulph.*
Like small cutaneous indurations — *Gels*
Inflamed (Liver complaint) —*Chel*
Isolated — *Berb, Lyc.*
Itching — *Acon, Ambr, Am-c, Ant-c, Apis, Ars, Bar-c, Bov, Bry, Calc, Carb-an, Carb-s, Caust, Cham, Cocc, Con, Dulc, Graph, Hep, Kali-c, Laur, Lyc, Mag-m, Merc, Mur-ac, Nat-c, Nat-m, Nat-s, Nit-ac, Ph-ac, Psor, Puls, Sep, Sil, Staph, Stront, Sulph, Tell, Til, Zinc, Ziz.*
Isolated, red with circumscribed areola, depressed centres, became confluent where they were most dense, bleed when scabs come off — *Syph*
Itching when warm — *Caust, Sars, Tell, Til.*
Itching, burning — *Ars*
Itching excessively — *Ascl-t*
Itching inflamed painful to touch — *Sul*
Itching red — *Asim*
Itching like nettle rash — *Sil*
Itching arises singly with ailments — *Kali-s*

Itching covered with a crust around ulcers and suppurates — *Cham*

Itching with small vesicles — *Kali-m*

Itch like — *Bar-m, Kali-iod.*

Itch like with burning, itching and smarting after scratching — *Rhus*

Large, deep seated and irritable to touch — *Rhus*

During menses, which she fears will prove to be little snakes and turn and twist around each other — *Lac-c*

Irregular menses — *Lac. def*

Miliary with yellow tips — *Grat*

Like nettle rash with biting itching — *Rhus*

Worse at night — *Merc*

In onanists — *Phos-ac*

Moist — *Calc, Graph, Kali-c, Nat-s, Ol-an, Puls, Sil, Sulph, Thuj, Zinc.*

Painful — *Ant-c, Apis, Ars-m, Arn, Cist, Cocc, Con, Dulc, Graph, Kali-c, Kali-chl, Kali-i, Lach, Mur-ac, Nat-ac, Nit-c, Nux-v, Phos, Plb, Puls, Seneg, Spong, Squil, Staph, Sulph, Verat.*

Painful for some distance about the — *Jamb*

Painful sore — *Ind*

Painful to pressure — *Spong*

Painful suppurating feels as though pierced with a needle, skin red far around each — *Ind*

As large as peas, itch when scratched off, are moist and burn — *Staph*

Like Petechiae — *Led*

Perspiring parts, on — *Con*

Phlyctenoidal — *Kali-m*

Purulent contain fluid like varnish — *Thuj*

Pustulous — *Cham*

Pustulous with yellow scabs — *Chel, Cina, Kreos, Iod, Lachn, Rhus, Thuj, Variol, Zinc.*

Bright red, small, conical, hard, inflamed base, resembling lichen, itching — *Ant-t*

Bright red in constipation of sucklings — *Apis*

Bright red, here and there — *Apis*

Bright red, filling with pus — *Dulc*

Red with prominent centres, rough to touch — *Chel*

Clusters of red, with red areolae and small tips containing pus, changing to brown spots — *Berb*

Fine red, running together, presenting a red, swollen appearance alkaline fluid oozes out copiously, after subsiding cuticle comes off in fine scales, itches and stings, better formerly by cold water, lately by hot — *Kali-s*

Red, itching every summer (eczema solaris) — *Mur-ac*

Large red - Verbas, Zing

Red like miliaria - *Ananth*

Red filled with pus and covered with yellow crusts — *Sep*

Single red, itching — *Berb*

Red, small — *Rumex, Sep.*

Red, small, itching, tipped with pus burn after scratching — *Graph*

Red small rose like — *Bov*

Red small (secondary syphilis) — *Ars-n*

Bright red, small, formed vesicles of a pearly look, with depressed tips and surrounded by red areolae — *Vacc*

Very bright red, small sharply defined, with minute vesicles upon them, severe itching, day and night, mostly at night after going to bed — *Tell*

Red in syphilis — *Nit-ac*

Red in typhus — *Stram*

Red, like urticaria - *Ananth*

Red, most evident when warm — *Vacc*

Red with white tip, painful and stinging (hip joint disease) — *Merc*

With redness and swelling — *Kali-c*

Form scabs (impetigo) — *Carbo-s*

Rise after scratching, ooze, moisture keeping parts sore — *Sars*

Scurfy — *Mur-ac, Oleand.*

Scurfs, itching, when getting warm in bed — *Mur-ac*

Covered with scurfs ulcerating around ulcers — *Cham*

Sensation as if pimples were coming out — *Cinnab*

Sensitive to touch — *Calad*

Scratching after — *Am-c, Am-m, Ant-c, Bar-c, Bry, Caust, Chin, Cocc, Con, Cycl, Dros, Dulc, Graph, Hep, Kali-c, Laur, Merc, Nat-c, Nat-m, Nit-ac, Petr, Ph-ac, Phos, Puls, Rhus-t, Sabad, Sabin, Sars, Sel, Sep, Sil, Spong, Squil, Staph, Stront, Sulph, Verat, Zinc.*

Scratching after — *Agar, Ars, Bov, Bry, Ip, Sulph.*

Single with rash — *Kali-m*

Small — *Cub, Ictod, Iod, Kali-c, Sep, Vacc.*
Small spreading into large scarlet blotches, discharging yellow matter — *Kali-bich*
Small colourless containing serum — *Sars*
Small then desquamation — *Elaps*
Small dry reddish (run around) — *Bov*
Small flat semi-transparent — *Berb*
Small here and there with terrible itching, when undressing in evening — *Pallad*
Small round — *Arum-t*
Small discharge serous fluid become dry on scratching, leaving skin roughness with brown herpetic spots here and there (chloroses) — *Sep*
Smarting — *Agar, Bell, Calc, Cham, Coloc, Dig, Kali-c, Kali-n, Lyc, Merc, Teucr, Verat.*
Sore, as if - excoriated — *Alum, Arg-m, Bell, Bov, Calc, Clem, Guaj, Hep, Hyos, Jamb, Kob, Mez, Ph-ac, Rhus-t, Sabin, Sel, Spig, Stann, Teucr, Verat, Zinc.*
Sore smarting — *Hep*
Sore painful — *Hep*
Sore pressing pain when touched — *Zinc*
Sore discharge and form a scab, painful when touched — *Lac-c*
Sore to touch — *Arg-met*
Splinter, pain like a — *Arn, Hep, Nit-ac.*
Stinging as from a splinter when touched — *Arn*
On small red spot — *Cham*
Stinging — *Alum, Ananth, Ant-c, Arn, Bell, Calc-p, Canth, Caps, Caust, Cocc, Hell, Kali-c, Kali-n, Kreos, Nat-c, Petr, Squil, Staph.*
As from stings of insects — *Ant-c*
Suppressed, nervous palpitation — *Calc*
Suppurating — *Ars, Arund, Bar-c, Hep, Sars, Sulph, Tarax, Zinc.*
With sweat — *Con*
Swollen hard — *Calc-s*
Tearing — *Dulc*
Tips full of pus, surrounded by red areola — *Thuj*
Tensive — *Arn, Bov, Con, Mang, Nat-s.*
Tingling — *Canth*
Titillating — *Bell, Caust, Mag-m, Verat.*
Touch sensitive to — *Berb, Calad, Hep.*
Ulcerated — *Kali-c, Merc, Nit-ac, Ph-ac, Sabin, Sep.*

Ulcers, pimples, surrounded by — *Acon, Ars, Bell, Carb-v, Caust, Cham, Fl-ac, Hep, Lach, Lyc, Merc, Mez, Mur-ac, Nat-c, Petr, Phos, Puls, Ran-s, Rhus-t, Sep, Sil, Staph, Sulph.*

Like varicella — *Thuj*

Variola — *Bapt*

Small, develop at point of vaccination — *Vacc*

Watery fluid — *Lochr*

Discharge water when scratched — *Kali-n*

Water, suppurate forming scabs — *Tuber*

Varicose veins, pimples, covered with — *Graph*

White on red nose — *Nat-c*

Small white with small moisture after moderate wine drinking — *Zinc*

White suppurating with red areolae — *Calad*

White transparent, filled with acrid tumor, which form scab like those of scabies — *Con*

Head : Eruption — Pimples — *Act-sp, Agar, Alum, Ambr, Anac, Ars, Aur, Bar-c, Bov, Valc, Calc-s, Carb-s, Con, Crot-c, Cund, Cycl, Hep, Kali-bi, Kali-c, Kali-p, Kali-s, Led, Merc-i-r, Mez, Mur-ac, Nat-c, Nat-m, Nux-v, Olnd, Petr, Phos, Sec, Sil, Spig, Sulph, Tarent, Zinc.*

Margin of hair in front — *Nit-ac*

Occiput on — *Am-m, Bufo-s, Clem, Cycl, Kali-bi, Kali-n, Lyc, Merc, Sulph.*

Eyes-about the pimples — *Hep, Merc.*

Pimples minute — *Bar-c*

Eyebrows about pimples — *Kali-c*

Lids on pimples — *Alum, Chel, Guaj, Hep, Lyc, Merc-c, Nat-m, Rhus-t, Sec, Seneg.*

Eyelids pimples — *Bell, Hep, Lyc, Petr, Rhus-t, Sele, Sil.*

Upper — *Hep*

Right — *Canth, Lyc.*

Left — *Chel*

Lower — *Croc, Nat-m, Seneg.*

Right — *Alu*

Ear pimples — *Agar, Am-c, Berb, Calc-p, Calad, Cann-s, Cic, Coff, Kali-c, Kali-s, Kreos, Merc, Merc-c, Mur-ac, Nat-m, Petr, Phos, Psor, Sabad, Sel, Spong, Staph, Sulph.*

Behind ears pimples — *Alum, Calad, Calc, Cann-s, Canth, Caust, Dros, Graph, Ham, Mez, Nat-m, Nicc, Pall, Puls, Rhus-t, Sabad, Sel, Sulph.*

Burning on touch — *Canth*

Itching — *Rhus-t*
Lobes on pimples — *Lach, Merc.*
Meatus in — *Jug-r, Kali-p.*
Face eruptions pimples — *Agar, Alum, Am-m, Ambr, Anan. Anac, Ant-c, Apis, Ars, Ars-h, Ars-i, Arum-t, Aster, Aur, Bar-c, Bar-m, Bell, Berb, Bor, Bov, Brom, Calad, Calc, Calc-p, Calc-s, Carb-an, Carb-s, Carb-v, Caust, Chel, Chin, Cic, Clem, Coloc, Con, Crot-h, Cund, Diad, Dig, Dulc, Dros, Eug, Fl-ac, Gels, Glen, Graph, Hep, Hura, Hydr, Hydro, Hyper, Hyos, Indg, Iod, Jug-r, Kali-ar, Kali-c, Kali-chl, Kali-n, Kali-s, Kreos, Lach, Led, Lyc, Lyss, Mag-m, Meny, Meph, Merc, Mer-c, Mez, Mur-n, Myr-cer, Nat-a, Nat-c, Nat-m, Nat-p, Nat-s, Nit-ac, Nux-v, Ol-an, Pall, Par, Petr, Ph-ac, Phos, Psor, Puls, Rhus-t, Ruta, Sabin, Sanic, Sars, Seneg, Sep, Sil, Sol-t-ac, Staph, Sulph, Syph, Tabac, Tarax, Tarent, Thuj, Til, Tromb, Vinc, Zinc.*
Red (acne of alcoholics) — *Kreos, Lach.*
Pimples — night agg. — *Mag-m*
Bluish — *Lyss*
Burning — *Aphis-ac*
When touched — *Nat-s*
Cold air Agg — *Ars*
Confluent — Cic, Psor, Tarent.
Copper coloured — *Kali-i*
Elevated margins — *Verat*
Greenish — *Cupr*
Inflamed — *Bry, Chel, Stann, Sulph.*
Insects as from — *Ant-c*
Itching — *Ant-c, Asc-t, Caust, Con, Graph, Hep, Mur-ac, Ol-an, Pall, Psor, Sep, Til, Zinc.*
When warm — *Ant-c, Cocc, Til.*
Moist after scratching — *Graph*
Menses before agg — *Mag-m*
During — *Dulc, Eug, Graph.*
Purplish halo with — *Merc*
Warm room agg — *Mag-m*
Washing agg — *Nux-v, Sulph.*
Chin — *Alum, Ambr, Ant-c, Aster, Bor, Chel, Clem, Crot-h, Con, Dulc, Ferr-m, Mep, Kali-chl, Lyc, Merc, Nat-s, Nit-ac, Ph-ac, Psor, Rhus-t, Sars, Sep, Sil, Sulph, Thuj, Zinc.*
Forehead — *Agar, Alum, Ambr, Am-c, Am-m, Anac, Ars, Aur, Bell, Bov, Bry, Calc, Calc-p, Canth, Carb-v, Chel, Clem, Con,*

Cycl, Ferr-m, Graph, Hep, Hura, Indg, Kali-bi, Kali-br, Kali-chl, Kreos, Lach, Led, Mag-m, Meph, Mez, Mur-ac, Nat-c, Nat-m, Nat-p, Nit-ac, Olnd, Par, Ph-ac, Phos, Psor, Puls, Rhod, Rhus-v, Sep, Sol-n, Sulph, Tab, Tarent, Zinc, Ziz.

Burning — *Bell, Canth.*

Itching — *Alum, Calc, Sulph, Ziz.*

Painful — *Indg, Staph.*

Red — *Anac, Bell, Carb-v, Nat-m, Sol-n.*

Sore to touch — *Ph-ac*

Washed, smarting when — *Nux-v*

White — *Carb-v, Kali-br, Sulph, Zinc.*

Wine after — *Zinc*

Lips — *Ars, Am-m, Arn, Aur, Berb, Bor, Bov, Bufo, Calc, Carb-v, Ferr-m, Graph, Guai, Hep, Kali-c, Kali-chl, Kali-p, Merc, Mur-ac, Nat-c, Nux-v, Pall, Par, Petr, Ph-ac, Ruta, Sep, Thuj.*

Burning — *Aur*

Lower — *Nicc, Pall.*

Lips Upper — *Am-m, Ant-c, Arn, Bufo, Carb-v, Mang, Spig, Thuj, Zinc.*

Burning — Apis.

Sore to touch — *Zinc.*

Lower jaw — *Par, Sil.*

Mouth around — *Bar-c, Bov, Dulc, Mag-c, Mur-ac, Phos, Rhus-t, Sep, Sil, Zinc.*

Corners of — *Bar-c, Petr, Tarax.*

Nose — *Agar, Alum, Am-c, Anac, Arum-d, Aur, Bar-c, Bell, Bor, Brom, Calc, Caps, Cann-s, Carb-an, Carb-v, Caust, Clem, Dulc, Euphr, Fl-ac, Graph, Guai, Kali-c, Kali-i, Lach, Lyc, Mag-act, Mang, Merc, Nat-c, Nat-m, Ol-an, Ox-ac, Pall, Petr, Ph-ac, Phos, Podo, Plan, Plb, Psor, Rhus-t, Sars, Sel, Sep, Sil, Sulph, Syph, Teucr, Thuj.*

Burning — *Alum, Apis, Canth.*

When touched — *Canth*

Oozing — *Ol-an*

Red — *Ant-c, Aur, Calc-p, Plan.*

White — *Carb-v, Kali-c, Nat-c.*

About nose — *Par, Tarax.*

Dorsum on with inflamed base — *Fl-ac*

Inside — *Arn, Calad, Calc, Carb-an, Graph, Guaj, Kali-c, Ox-ac, Sil, Tub.*

Inside right nostril — *Apis, Ox-ac, Phos, Rat.*

Painful only when muscles of face and nose are moved — *Calc*
Inside left nostril — *Calc, Dulc, Graph, Kali-c.*
Root — *Caust, Led.*
Septum — *Arg-n, Asc-t, Calad, Chin, Nat-m, Ol-an, Teucr.*
Oozing — *Ol-an*
Side — *Aster, Sil.*
Side small and hard — *Agar*
Side right — *Alum, Euphr, Lach, Ox-ac, Sars.*
Tip — *Am-c, Asaf, Caust, Coc-c, Cund, Lyc, Nit-ac, Pall, Ph-ac, Spong.*
Tip sore — *Lyc*
Tip bleeding when pressed — *Pall*
Wings — *Bar-c, Chin, Nat-m, Tarax, Zing.*
Wings left — *Fl-ac*
Wings perforation size of a pea — *Fl-ac*
Temples — *Arg-m, Mur-ac, Nit-ac.*
Whiskers — *Agar, Ambr, Calc, Calc-s, Graph, Lyc, Nit-ac, Pall, Sulph.*
Mouth, pimples — *Caps, Dulc.*
Inner cheeks and lips — *Berb*
Red and painful — *Berb*
Gums — *Berb*
Palate — *Bapt, Dulc, Nux-v, Rumx, Thuj.*
Tongue — *Bell, Berb, Brom, Calc-p, Lyc, Manc, Nux-v, Plb, Tarax.*
Tongue painful — *Bell, Graph, Nit-ac, Nux-v, Sulph.*
Tongue bleeding — *Graph*
Tongue edges — *Apis, Arg-n, Hura, Nat-c, Nit-ac, Osm, Sulph.*
Tongue tip — *Bell, Caps, Hell, Kali-c, Nat-c.*
Throat pimples on uvula — *Kali-bi, Rumx.*
External throat pimples — *Agar, Ant-c, Berb, Bov, Canth, Cinnb, Clem, Hep, Jug-r, Kali-n, Lyc, Mez, Mur-ac, Nat-m, Ph-ac, Raph, Puls, Spong, Sulph, Thuj, Zinc.*
Abdomen pimples — *Agar, Aloe, Arn, Ars, Ars-b, Bar-m, Bry, Dulc, Fl-ac, Merc, Nat-c, Nat-m, Petr, Rhus-t, Staph.*
Itching — *Aloe, Bry, Dulc, Nat-c, Staph.*
Chest pimples — *Am-m, Ant-c, Arg-n, Ars, Berb, Bor, Bov, Calc, Cann-s, Canth, Chin, Cinnb, Cist, Cocc, Con, Dulc, Fl-ac, Graph, Hep, Hura, Hyper, Iod, Kali-ar, Kali-c, Lach, Led, Mag-m, Mez, Nat-a, Nat-c, Nat-p, Ph-ac, Plb, Puls, Rhus-t, Squil, Staph, Stront, Tab, Valer, Verat, Zinc.*

Chest acne — *Bar-c*
Angry — *Sep*
Bleed easily — *Cist*
Burning — *Agar, Bor, Staph.*
Elevated — *Valer*
Flattening — *Rhus-t*
Hard — *Bov, Valer.*
Hard under the skin — *Alum*
Indolent — *Cond*
Itching — Cann-s, Dulc, Gins, Mag-m, Nat-c, Tab.
Painful — *Cist*
Pointed with whitish semi-transparent vesicles on — *Bry*
Red — *Am-c, Apis, Arund, Bov, Cocc, Iod, Mez, Ph-ac, Plb, Stram, Zinc.*
Red evening — *Ph-ac*
Red like lichen simplex — *Ant-t*
White — *Valer*
White red areola with — *Bov*
Nipples, pimples — *Agar, Graph.*
Back pimples — *Agar, Alum, Agr-n, Ars, Bell, Berb, Bry, Calc, Cann-s, Carb-v, Cham, Chel, Chlor, Cocc, Coch, Con, Crot-h, Dig, Fl-ac, Hura, Hyper, Jug-r, Iod, Kali-bi, Kali-c, Kali-p, Lach, Led, Lyc, Mag-m, Mag-s, Meph, Nat-m, Nicc, Petr, Ph-ac, Psor, Puls, Rhus-v, Rumx, Sars, Sel, Sil, Squil, Staph, Stram, Tab, Sil, Vesp, Zinc.*
Evening — *Cocc, Fl-ac, Ph-ac, Rumx.*
Itching — *Arg-n, Asc-t, Calc, Cann-s, Carb-an, Crot-t, Fl-ac, Led, Mag-m, Mill, Rat, Rhus-t, Sel.*
After scratching — *Psor*
Sore pressing pain when touched — *Zinc*
Suppurating — *Chlor, Kali-bi.*
Nape, pimples — *Ars, Bell, Carb-v, Hep, Kali-c, Kali-n, Lyc, Sil, Staph.*
Cervical region — *Agar, Alum, Berb, Cann-s, Carb-an, Carb-v, Cinnb, Clem, Crot-t, Gels, Hep, Hyos, Jug-r, Kali-bi, Kali-c, Kali-n, Lyc, Meph, Nat-a, Nat-m, Nice, Pall, Petr, Ph-ac, Psor, Puls, Rhus-t, Sil, Staph, Sulph, Sul-ac, Thuj, Trom, Verb, Zing.*
Burning — *Am-c*
Confluent — *Tarent*
Deep seated — *Til*

Flattened — *Rhus-t*
Hard — *Crot-t*
Inflamed — *Sulph*
Itching — *Sil, Staph.*
Moist — *Clem*
Painful to touch; *Hep, Sulph.*
Scratching on — *Carb-an, Nicc, Puls.*
Suppurating — *Nat-c, Calc-p.*
Extending to scalp — *Clem*
Dorsal region — *Am-m, Berb, Cic, Cist.*
Scapulae — *Ant-c, Berb, Com, Con, Crot-h, Mag-m, Ph-ac, Rat, Squil.*
Lumbar region — *Ars-h, Calc, Chel, Chin, Clem, Kali-c, Nat-c, Nicc.*
Burning — *Lyc*
Inflamed — *Sulph*
Itching — *Lyc, Tab.*
Oozing when scratched — *Sulph*
Red at night on scratching, better morning — *Apoc*
Scratching after — *Chin, Nicc.*
Extremities, pimples — *Acon, Agar, Am-c, Am-m, Anac, Ant-c, Ant-t, Arg-n, Arn, Ars, Asc-t, Bar-c, Bar-m, Bell, Berb, Bov, Bry, Bufo, Calc, Calc-p, Calc-s, Cann-s, Carb-an, Carb-s, Caust, Chel, Chin-s, Cic-v, Clem, Cob, Con, Crot-c, Cupr-ar, Elaps, Fago, Fl-ac, Graph, Hura, Iris, Iris-i, Jatr, Kali-ar, Kali-br, Kali-c, Kali-chl, Kali-p, Kali-s, Kreos, Lac-ac, Lach, Lyc, Mag-c, Mag-m, Mang, Merc, Mez, Morph, Mur-ac, Nat-m, Nat-s, Nicc, Ol-an, Op, Osm, Ph-ac, Plan, Plat, Psor, Puls, Rat, Rhus-t, Rhus-v, Rumx, Sabad, Sars, Sel, Sep, Spig, Stann, Staph, Stront, Sulph, Tab, Tarax, Thuj, Til, Valer, Verat, Zinc.*
Joints, pimples — *Calc-p, Sep.*
Upper limbs pimples — *Acon, Agar, Am-c, Am-m, Anac, Ant-t, Arg-n, Arn, Ars, Arum-t, Asc-t, Bar-c, Bell, Berb, Bry, Bov, Bol-s, Calc-p, Calc-s, Cann-s, Canth, Carb-an, Carb-s, Carb-v, Caust, Chel, Chin, Chin-s, Cob, Com, Crot-c, Cupr-ar, Dulc, Elaps, Fl-ac, Hura, Jatr, Iod, Kali-ar, Kali-bi, Kali-c, Kali-chl, Kali-n, Kreos, Lac-ac, Lach, Lyc, Mag-c, Mag-m, Osm, Ph-ac, Plat, Psor, Puls, Rat, Rhus-t, Rhus-v, Sabad, Sars, Sel, Sep, Spig, Staph, Sulph, Tab, Tarax, Thuj, Til, Valer, Zinc.*
Bleeding when scratched — *Cob*

Burning — *Am-c, Bov, Mag-m, Nat-s, Rhus-t.*
Burning scratching after — *Canth, Carb-an.*
Hard — *Arg-n, Bov, Calc-s, Rhus-t, Rhus-v, Valer.*
Head black, with depressed — *Calc-s*
Indolent — *Chel*
Inflamed — *Calc-s*
Itching — *Acon, Am-c, Am-m, Asc-t, Bar-c, Cann-s, Carb-an, Carb-s, Caust, Hura, Kreos, Lyc, Mag-c, Mag-m, Merc, Sabad, Sel, Sulph, Ziz.*
Menses during — *Sulph*
Painful — *Kali-chl, Thea.*
Red — *Acon, Anac, Ars, Bov, Chel, Com, Elaps, Hura, Kali-chl, Mag-s, Rhus-t, Sulph, Til.*
Sensitive — *Calc-s*
Stinging — *Acon, Arg-n.*
White — *Til, Valer.*
Shoulder, pimples — *Ant-c, Berb, Chel, Cist, Cob, Cocc, Com, Fl-ac, Hura, Jug-r, Kali-c, Kali-chl, Mag-c, Mag-m, Puls, Sulph, Tab, Zinc.*
Bleeding when scratched — *Cob, Mosch.*
Boils like — *Zinc*
Burning — *Mag-m*
Indolent — *Chel*
Itching — *Hura, Mag-m.*
Painful — *Kali-chl, Thea.*
Red — *Chel, Com, Hura, Jug-r, Kali-chl.*
Upper arm pimples — *Anac, Ant-c, Ant-c, Arn, Carb-v, Dulc, Iod, Kali-c, Lach, Laur, Mang, Mosch, Sep, Sulph, Tax, Til, Valer.*
Bleeding after scratching — *Mosch*
Elbow, pimples — *Ant-c, Asc-t, Berb, Bry, Dulc, Hyos, Kali-n, Lach, Merc, Nat-c, Ol-an, Sabin, Sep, Staph, Sulph, Tarax, Thuj.*
Biting — *Kali-n*
Burning — *Kali-n*
On inflamed base — *Tarax*
Bend of elbow pimples — *Ant-c, Hyos, Hura, Ol-an, Phos, Sep, Thuj.*
Olecranon, pimples — *Berb*
Forearm, pimples — *Am-c, Am-m, Ant-t, Ars, Asc-t, Bell, Bov, Bry, Calad, Calc-p, Carb-s, Caust, Cit-r, Fago, Gamb, Iod, Kali-bi, Kali-n, Lach, Laur, Lyc, Mag-c, Mag-s, Mang, Merc,*

Nat-m, Nat-s, Ol-an, Osm, Ph-ac, Rat, Rhod, Sabad, Sars, Sulph, Tax, Thuj, Valer, Zinc.

Morning — *Mang*

Afternoon — *Mag-c*

Evening — *Am-c, Fago.*

Alternating with asthma — *Calad*

Burning — *Am-c, Calad, Mang, Nat-s.*

Itching — *Am-m, Calad, Carb-s, Caust, Gamb, Lyc, Nat-s, Sabad, Sulph, Zinc.*

Menses, during — *Sulph*

Scratching after — *Am-m*

Oozing — *Kali-n*

Washing from — *Mag-c*

Wrist, pimples — *Ant-t, Arg-n, Asc-t, Arn, Bar-c, Bry, Buf-s, Calc-p, Carb-an, Crot-c, Cycl, Elaps, Hura, Jatr, Mag-c, Op, Plan, Psor, Rhus-t, Rhus-v, Sep, Staph, Sulph, Tarax, Ziz.*

Burning after scratching — *Carb-an*

Exuding water — *Hura, Psor, Rhus-v.*

Exuding water on pressure — *Mag-c*

Hard base — *Arg-n*

Itching — *Bar-c, Carb-an, Mag-c, Ziz.*

Sore — *Sep*

Stinging — Arg-n

Hand pimples — *Acon, Agar, Am-c, Anac, Ant-c, Arg-n, Ars, Bell, Bov, Bry, Canth, Carb-s, Carb-v, Chin, Cic, Cupr-ar, Dig, Elaps, Hep, Iod, Kali-ar, Kali-chl, Kreos, Lac-ac, Lyc, Merc, Mur-ac, Nit-ac, Ol-an, Op, Psor, Rhus-t, Rhus-v, Sel, Sulph, Tarax, Zinc.*

Burning — *Bov, Rhus-t.*

Greenish — *Cupr-ar*

Hand — *Bov, Rhus-t, Rhus-v.*

Itching — *Acon, Am-c, Bov, Kreos, Lyc, Selen, Sulph.*

Itching periodically — *Sulph*

Itching warm in bed, when becoming — *Mur-ac*

Red — *Acon, Ars, Anac, Bov, Sulph, Til.*

Scurf forming — *Mur-ac*

Stinging — *Acon*

Suppurating — *Anac, Elaps.*

Hand back of pimples — *Acon, Agar, Am-m, Calc-p, Canth, Carb-s, Carb-v, Cic, Kali-chl, Zinc.*

Itching — *Am-m, Zinc.*

Palm, pimples — *Nat-s, Psor, Spig, Thuj.*

Hard, itching, discharging stony concretion — *Thuj*
Between the fingers pimples — *Ars, Lyc, Ph-ac, Puls.*
Between index finger and thumb, pimples — *Agar, Bry, Canth, Ham, Sulph, Thuj.*
Burning on touch — *Canth*
Itching — *Ars, Sulph.*
Third and fourth fingers, pimples — *Canth*
Fingers — *Anac, Ant-c, Arn, Ars, Bar-c, Berb, Canth, Carb-ac, Cycl, Elaps, Graph, Kali-c, Lyc, Mez, Mur-ac, Ph-ac, Sars , Spig, Tab, Tarax, Ther. Zinc.*
Tips of fingers pimples — *Elaps*
First finger pimples — *Sulph*
Thumb pimples — *Ant-c, Berb, Kali-c, Lyc, Ther.*
Beside the ball of — *Berb, Ther.*
Between index finger pimples — *Arn, Bry, Canth.*
Lower limbs pimples — *Agar, Am-c, Am-m, Ant-c, Arg-n, Arn, Asc-t, Bar-c, Bell, Berb, Bov, Bry, Calc, Calc-p, Cann-s, Cast, Chel, Chin-s, Clem, Con, Crot-c, Elaps, Fago, Fl-ac, Graph, Hura, Iris, Iris-f, Kali-bi, Kali-br, Kali-c, Kali-chl, Kali-s, Mag-c, Mang, Merc, Mez, Morph, Nat-m, Nat-p, Nicc, Petr, Ph-ac, Puls, Rumx, Sars, Sep, Sil, Stann, Staph, Stront, Sulph, Thea, Thuj, Til, Verat, Zinc.*
Bleeding — *Agar, Thea.*
Burning — *Mang*
Burning when scratched — *Staph*
Flat — *Ant-c, Plan.*
Hard — *Plan*
Indolent — *Chel*
Itching — *Asc-t, Bell, Elaps, Hep, Kali-bi, Mang, Petr, Ph-ac, Sel, Sep, Stann, Staph, Sulph.*
Itching after scratching — *Mag-c*
Painful — *Bry, Thea.*
Red — *Asc-t, Chel, Clem, Graph, Kali-c, Sars, Sulph, Thea, Til.*
White — *Plan*
Yellow — *Ant-c*
Nates, pimples — *Ant-c, Ars-h, Bar-c, Berb, Calc, Canth, Chel, Cob, Graph, Ham, Hura, Kali-n, Lyc, Mag-c, Mang, Meph, Merc, Nat-p, Nux-v, Petr, Plan, Rhus-t, Sel, Sulph, Thuj, Til.*
Itching — *Kali-n, Lyc, Til.*
Painful — *Ham, Sulph.*
Nates between, pimples — *Sulph*
Hip, pimples — *Hyper*

Thigh, pimples — *Agar, Ant-c, Asc-t, Bar-m, Berb, Bov, Bry, Calc, Cann-s, Cast, Chel, Clem, Cocc, Elaps, Fago, Fl-ac, Graph, Kali-c, Kali-chl, Kali-cy, Lach, Lyc, Mag-c, Mang, Meph, Merc, Mez, Nat-m, Petr, Phos, Plan, Rumx, Sars, Sel, Stann, Staph, Sulph, Thea, Thuj, Til, Zinc.*

Burning — *Mang*

Burning morning and evening — *Mang*

When scratched — *Staph, Til.*

Flat — *Ant-c, Plan.*

Indolent — *Chel*

Itching — *Asc-t, Stann, Staph, Sulph, Zinc.*

— **morning** — *Mang*

— **evening** — *Mang, Sulph.*

After scratching — *Mag-c*

Painful — *Bry, Thea.*

Red — *Asc-t, Chel, Clem, Graph, Kali-c, Sars, Sulph, Thea, Til.*

White — *Plan*

Leg-Pimples — *Agar, Am-c, Arg-m, Arn, Arum-t, Bell, Bov, Chin-s, Elaps, Fl-ac, Hura, Iris-t, Kali-bi, Kali-chl, Merc, Morph, Nat-m, Nicc, Puls, Sars, Sep, Staph, Stront, Sul-ac, Thuj, Verat.*

Bleeding easily — *Agar*

Itching — *Asc-t, Bell, Elaps, Kali-bi, Sep, Stront, Ziz.*

Moist — *Puls*

Red — *Iris-t, Kali-chl, Rumx.*

White — *Staph*

Leg-calf pimples — *Agar, Arg-n, Asc-t, Bov, Bry, Elaps, Hura, Kali-bi, Lach, Nat-c, Ph-ac, Puls, Rumx, Sabin, Sars, Sep, Staph, Zinc.*

Foot-Pimples — *Caust, Led, Mosch.*

Toe-Pimples — *Am-c, Bov, Sulph, Zinc.*

CHAPTER 14

Pyoderma

Pyoderma is a group name for pyococcal dermatoses which are generally purulent. In tropical countries, pyoderma is a common problem, particularly in the summer and the monsoon. The two important pyogenic organisms are : the staphylococcus aureus and the streptococcus pyogenes. The former is more important in skin infections than the latter. Follicular infections are mainly due to staphylococci; while erysipelas and cellulitis are caused by streptococci. Besides thése, other organisms occasionally come across in pyodermas are bacillus proteus, Pseudomonas and coliform bacilli. The following are, broadly speaking, the different conditions produced by them depending upon the causative organisms and the location of the lesions :

1. Epidermal — Impertigo pityroides.
Streptococcal intertrigo.
Impetigo contagiosa, pustular bactéride, granuloma pyogenicum, pyoderma gangrenosum, infectious eczematoid dermatitis, otitis externa.

2. Sub-epidermal — Erysipelas.

3. Follicular	—	Bockhart's impertigo, sycosis, furunculoses, carbuncle, stye, marginal blepharitis.
4. Seat glands	—	Ecorine-SudoriporaSuppurativa.
5. Dermis	—	Apocrine-Hidradenitis suppurativa. Cellulitis.
6. Subcutaneous fat	—	Panniculitis.
7. Lymphatics	—	Lymphangitis.
8. Blood vessles	—	Arteritis, capillaritis, vasculitis, phlebitis.

Impetigo Contagiosa

The causative organisms are mainly pyogenic staphylococci, less so streptococcus pyogenes; diminished local resistance leads to the development of this disease. Impetigo contagiosa leads to the development of this disease. Impetigo contagiosa can occur primarily as such, or secondarily, as a complicating factor in scabies, pediculoses, eczemas, seborrhoeic dermatitis and herpes simplex. To this second process we give the name, Impetiginization.

Impetigo contagiosa has a world-wide distribution. Though it can occur at any age, it is commonly a disease of childhood. Patients are usually undernourished or run down. Infection is transmitted by contact with any individual carrying pyogenic organisms, directly or through towels, handkerchiefs, etc. The sites of predilection are the exposed regions of the body, especially the face and scalp; though it can occur on any part of the body. The incubation period is two to three days.

Clinical Features : It starts as a superificial bulla containing seropurulent matter. The contents soon coagulate producing a thick, stuck-on, honey coloured crust. This characteristic crust is the most important diagnostic feature of impetigo. At the periphery of the crust may be seen the epidermal tags or the edge of the bulla. The removal of the crust reveals a moist glistening surface with copious serous secretion which is infectious to contiguous areas and to other persons. One or several lesions may be seen in one individual; usually, however, the lesions are multiple. Infection may spread to hair follicles in the scalp or beard region and set up folliculitis. In the tropics, bullous impetigo may be seen in adults.

The intervening skin is completely normal. Usually no pain or itching accompanies the condition. The regional glands are only slightly enlarged. Constitutional symptoms are noticeably absent, except in children and in extensive impetigo. There is no scarring. Sometimes impetigo lesions heal in the centre and spread at the periphery producing circinate lesions.

In cachectic and debilitated individuals, the impetigo lesions are rather deep, giving rise to epidermal necrosis, thereby producing shallow ulcers with dirty brown crusts and pus underneath. This condition is called Ecthyma; the legs are the sites of predilection. The lesions heal slowly; on healing it leaves permanent scars. Streptococci may produce streptococcal gangrene and fuso-spirochaetal infection may spread from the gingiva to produce extensive necrosis of the lips, mouth and face (Cancrum orisnoma).

Pyoderma gangrenosum is a hypersensitive reaction necrosis of the skin associated with trauma, coccal infection, ulcerative colitis, rheumatoid arthritis and drug addiction. Ulceration, deep necrosis, boggy violacus, undermined edge, surrounding red areola and rapid evolution are characteristic. Outlook is serious but has improved with steroids (systemic and local injections into the rim), antibiotics, rifampicin and better topical management. Precipitating causes must be properly managed.

Histopathology : The impetigo lesion is a superficial bulla, the roof of which is formed by the stratum corneum. The contents are seropurulent; later a crust is seen. The underlying epidermis remains intact. The upper corneum shows dilated capillaries and polymorphonuclear infiltration.

Impetigo neonatorum implies impetigo contagiosa of the newborn. The eruption is extensive and involves the limbs, trunk, face and neck. Palms and soles are spared. The bullae are tense, and contain clear fluid; rupture produces a superficial, raw surface with overlying epidermal tags. Crusting is not prominent. Toxaemia is marked by fever, emaciation and collapse. Infection is conveyed by an infected genital passage, infected nipple, attendants with infected wounds of throat, or from other impetigo cases in a maternity ward. The condition used to be dreaded in maternity hospitals because of its easy communicability and high mortality rate. Prophylactic measures are important in controlling the spread of disease.

Diagnosis: The diagnosis of impetigo is not difficult if the disease and its features are remembered. In persistent impetigo of the scalp, pediculoses must be suspected, and a search should be made for nits and parasites. Persistent, impetigo-like lesions on the body may be due to scabies and dermatitis herpetiformis. The former is characterized by intense nocturnal pruritus, burrows, a typical distribution of lesions and by a history which reveals that several members of the patient's family have been affected. Acarus and ova can also be demonstrated by skin shavings. Dermatitis herpetiformis is distinguished by the presence of chronic, symmetrical polymorphous lesions on the arms, scapulae and lower back accompanied by itching. Annular lesions need to be differentiated from tinea. In the latter, there are no bullae or honey-coloured crusts. On the other hand, it shows an inflammatory border of papulo-vesicles, accompanied by itching.

Impetigo is usually an acute condition. In chronic, crusted lesions, infective granulomas like syphilis, tuberculosis, and leishmaniasis must be borne in mind. A chronic history, underlying infiltration and associated accompanying features, a biopsy and bacteriological examination, help to distringuish them. Impetigo neonatorum is differentiated from syphilitic pemphigus by the presence in the latter of symmetrically distributed bullae on the hands, feet and face. The child is poorly developed and has a waxen appearance. Lesions develop within a few days of birth, and there is no history of a septic source of infection. Serological tests for syphilis are positive, both in the mother and the infant.

Prognosis: The disease usually lasts for 3 to 4 weeks. In some cases, particularly when it complicates other skin conditions, it may last for months. An average case can be cured in 6 to 10 days leaving behind no scars. being a contagious disease, it can spread to other parts of the body and to other people.

Homoeopathic Approach to Impetigo

The presence of impetigo in a patient indicates to us a dominant tubercular miasm. The suppurating tendencies that one frequently observes in homoeopathic practice is best seen in pyodermas and impetigo since they have a strong tendency to recur if inadequately treated, hence proper selection and administration of acute, chronic and inter-current drugs should be undertaken.

(1) After a detailed case-taking, evaluate the present stage that is :

(a) Whether it is the first attack?
(b) Whether the patient has recurrent attacks?
(c) Whether in the past suppressive measures were taken?
(d) Whether patient has come early or in late stage?

The above facts help us to select the type of remedy that has to be administered.

(2) It has to be remembered that patient with low susceptibility develop lesions deep enough, thereby producing epidermal necrosis and shallow ulcerations. Hence the basic duty of a homoeopath is to increase the susceptibility with the help of similimum so that suffering is at its minimum.

(3) Whenever these lesions heal they usually leave behind a permanent scar, hence proper precautions should be taken to prevent the same.

(4) Since streptococcus and staphylococcus are the commonest organism responsible, drugs like streptococcinum and staphylococcinum should be kept in mind. I would also like the student to read the provings of isopathic drug, e.g., Terramycin which in potentized form is an excellent drug for impetigo.

(5) The affected part must be kept dry, clean and covered. In children with extensive affection of the scalp, the hair must be shaved off.

(6) The crusts are removed with a warm solution of calendula and water mixed in the ratio of 1:2.

(7) Being a contagious disease, it can spread to other parts of the body. Hence patients, especially children, should be advised strictly not to scratch the lesion.

Selection and Administration of Homoeopathic Remedies

Enough clinical hints can be drawn by mere observation :

(a) location — face : Viola-t.
(b) type and character of the crust,e.g.,hard, soft, red, bloody, yellowish, greenish crust.
(c) discharge — thin, thick, offensive; bloody, yellowish, greenish.
(d) presence of itching with its characteristic modalities.

Keeping at the back of the mind, the patient's conceptual image and the sector totality of impetigo, the drug is selected.

The selection of potency is based on the resemblance of the patient's symptom with materia medica and the stage of the disease.

There are cases which are recorded where only nosodes have helped to clear the picture of an acute remedy like Viola-t has permanently cured the impetigo.

Kent repertory gives impetigo directly under the chapter "Skin — Eruptions-Impetigo". Many other rubrics also should be considered,e.g.,

Skin-eruptions-crusty.
Skin-eruptions-discharging moist.
Skin-eruptions-suppurating.
Skin-eruptions-pustules.

The reader is requested to read the chapter on eczema and refer its therapeutics along with the current chapter.

Alnus : Impetigo associated with gastric disturbances situated especially on the fingers, characterised by crusts and pustules. Impetigo that tends to ulcerate easily, angry looking impetigo associated with glandular enlargement.

Alumina : Alumina produces impetigo on the scalp. Eruptions are humid, scabby, scurfy, with gnawing itching sensation. They bleed easily when scratched < evenings; < alternate days; from heat of bed; at full and new moon; from eating potatoes; > open air (Baryta-c). Dry skin even in hot weather. Impetigo that appears periodically, especially in winter, skin feels as if the white of egg had dried on its surface.

Amm-Carb : Impetigo on bends of extremities; excoriation between the thighs and above the genitals, < wet application. Violent itching, after scratching, burning, blisters appear.

Impetigo in individuals with scrofulous diathesis who dislike washing.

Ant-Crud : Impetigo especially on face, genitals extremities, neck, chest and back.

Suppurating, yellow crusted eruptions, painful to touch and easily detached — a green serous pus oozes out from beneath. Thick, hard, yellow crusts, irritating the surrounding parts, itching violently < from application of poultices, bathing, working in water, alcohol and in the sun.

Impetigo in individuals who are gluttons in their eating habits and frequently suffer from gastric upsets.

Ant-Sulp-Aur : Impetiginous eruptions, especially on hands and feet. Typical pustular lesions are accompanied by itching. As with other antimony's there is disordered digestion, pasty mouth and taste in the morning. Respiratory affections like chronic bronchitis may act as a concomitant symptom.

Ant-Tart : Impetigo around the face, chiefly around the neck and shoulders, above the nose and behind ears with itching. Pustular eruptions like varioloids, as large as peas, with red areola and which afterwards form a crust and leave a scar. The eruptions leave a bluish red mark. It is indicated in individuals who have ailments from ill-effects of vaccination.

Ars-Alb : Impetigo mainly affecting the scalp and face extremities, genitals, margin of hair. Black pustules, filled with black blood and foetid pus. There is a painful sensation as from cutaneous ulceration; worse at night and from cold and touch; better from warmth. Eruptions bleed on scratching. Skin symptoms alternate with internal derangements like asthma.

Ars-Iod : Impetigo on the face, especially affecting the beard. Small vesicles which burst and discharge an acrid fluid with severe itching and burning, worse night; application of cold. Itching is so violent that patient scratches till it bleeds. Impetigo in individuals with tuberculous, scrofulous or syphilitic diathesis.

Arum-T : Impetigo affecting corners of mouth, face, fingers and toes. The appearance of the lesion is raw, red, beefy and bloody. There is presence of itching which on scratching leads to peeling of the skin. There is characteristic sensation of itching, burning and rawness in the affected part. The symptoms are aggravated at night.

Bar-C : Impetigo chiefly affecting the cold people and children. Moist vesicular eruption with formation of thick crust, itching burning, causes the hair to fall out; skin is humid and sore. Impetigo of fat dwarfish children with swollen lymphatics, enlarged tonsils who take cold easily.

Calc-C : Impetigo appears on the occiput and then spreads to the face. Impetigo on neck, around navel and flexures of extremities. On scalp, there is thick, large, yellow scabs with thick bland pus under the crust. Itching is not very intense but on awakening from sleep, person is apt to scratch his head till it bleeds. Impetigo during dentition. Eruptions aggravated by water.

Impetigo associated with cold feet as if damp stockings on them; sweat of forehead, chalky stool. Skin inclines to ulcerates.

Calc-Mur : Impetigo that chiefly affects the scalp, especially in infants. Impetigo associated with glandular enlargements and gastric disturbances.

Causticum : Impetigo chiefly affects nape of the neck, around the nipple, around the mouth. There is presence of itching worse night, evening, open air, with formation of thick crusts which tend to ulcerate. It is better from heat and warmth of bed. Indicated in persons where eruptions are suppressed by local application of Mercury or Sulphur.

Cicuta : Impetigo sparsa. Eruptions on scalp, chin, upper lip and cover part of the face. Eruptions which form thick yellow crusts, honey-comb like crusts, which fall off and leave a bright red smooth surface. There is no itching whatsoever with impetigo. Suppression of impetigo leads to disease of the brain.

Conium : Impetigo affecting face, arms and mons veneris. Seropurulent eruptions in the aged. Moist vesicles with bluish sticky discharge forming hard crusts. Itching is worse after scratching. Impetigo developing after being over heated. Impetigo in old, feeble persons with scrofulous diathesis.

Croton-Tig : Almost all parts of the body are affected, face, genitals, eye-lids, soles of feet, abdomen, temples and vertex. Pustular eruption upon an inflamed base with itching and stinging pain. There is presence of small vesicles which get clustered or may burst. There is violent itching and burning after eating; worse at night, better gentle scratching and after sleep.

Clematis : Impetigo occurring on occiput, forehead, nape of neck, root and sides of the nose, face and lower lips. Tender to touch. The eruptions itch violently with profuse desquamation, vesicular and pustular. Easily corrode the skin and ultimately develops flat eating ulcers with thick crusts. Eruptions change character during the changes of moon; worse in bed; when washed with cold water and towards morning. Impetigo developing after suppression of gonorrhoea with glandular enlargement.

Dulcamara : Affects the scalp, forehead, cheeks, chin, extremities. Itching vesicles that pass into suppuration and become covered with a thick brown or yellow crust. The discharge corrodes the skin causing loss of hair. Itching of the skin diminishes after formation of crusts but remains sensitive to contact and bleeds after scratching. The impetigo tends to become worse before menses.

Euphorbia Lath : Impetigo starts on the face and spreads all over the body. The eruptions are characterized by itching, burning and smarting sensation. Worse by touch, in cold air and better by sweet oil application. When the impetigo is scratched it forms deep ragged ulcers.

Graphites : Folds of skin, vertex, scalp, ears, extremities, around anus, are some of the common places where the graphites impetigo develops. Scabby eruptions with excessive oozing around mouth and nose or the whiskers; hair fall out. Foul acrid gluey discharge; it mats hair together and leads to formation of deep rhagadeswith ulceration. Eruptions bleed easily on scratching. The skin is dry and sensitive to cold. Eruptions are worse from heat and are better by cold. Impetigo of fat, blonde women with scanty menses and an inability to perspire.

Gun-powder : Gun-powder contains nitre, sulphur and charcoal. Hence it has symptoms which resemble that of sulphur and carbo-veg. When the suppuration sets in impetigo with very offensive discharge and there are no indications of healing, this remedy should be thought of.

Hepar-S : Impetigo after mercurialism. Sites affected are the scalp, genitals, folds of scrotum and thighs. Presence of foul moist eruptions with a tendency to ulcerate. They are very sore and sensitive to touch. Humid scabs and pustules upon the head oozing a foetid substance; there is a presence of thin, acrid, offensive discharge from the eruptions. Impetigo in individuals with coldness of palms and soles.

Iris : Impetigo capititis, Pustular eruptions associated with gastric complaints, nausea and vomiting. Impetigo with nightly itching.

Jug-C : Impetigo especially on lower extremities, sacrum and hands. There is presence of itching and pricking when heated. Worse when heated. Itching is associated with burning and redness. Impetigo associated with dyspepsia and bronchial irritation and scrofulous swelling.

Kali-Bi : Eruption starts on the ear and spreads over the ear with formation of greenish crusts which oozes whitish thick matter. Eruptions tend to ulcerate. There is a sensation of itching which is worse from heat and hot weather. Impetigo, gastric complaints and rheumatism alternate with each other. Impetigo developing in individuals with suppressed catarrh.

Kreosote : Painless, pustular eruption all over the body. Violently itching, moist or scrufy impetigo on eyelids, face, joints, back of hands. Sticking pains. Mentally the patient is sad and weeping; worse in open air.

Lyco : Impetigo arising after abuse of mercury. Eruption on the head, face and also on the hands. Itching and suppurating eruptions which form thick crusts that bleeds easily, oozing of foetid moisture. There is presence of violent itching; worse from 4-8 P.M.; from getting overheated, from poultices and the patient gets relief from cold air or uncovering the parts. Impetigo that is associated with urinary, hepatic and gastric disorder. Impetigo in individuals who have a tendency to develop blood boils and abscess.

Merc : An important remedy for impetigo, eruptions are humid, foetid with thick yellow discharge or yellow crust formation. Moist scabs with excoriation of scalp and destruction of hair. These eruptions are surrounded by irregular margins. Itching in worse from warmth of bed with pain from scartching and tendency to bleed. Excessive odorous viscid perspiration, worse at night. Complaints increase with perspiration and rest. Also associated with a great deal of weariness and prostration.

Mezereum : Impetigo affects especially those parts of the skin which are deficient in fat. There is intolerable itching, compelling patient to scratch and change his position. Eruption moist and full of serous exudation, especially on nose and back. Deep inflammatory redness of face. Ichor from scratched places which excoriates other parts.

Itching is better in bed, from touch, burning and change of position after scratching. Scurf like fish scales on back, chest, thigh and scalp. Scabs thick, lamellated like rupia with blood secretion beneath. They look like chalk and spread to brows, nape and throat. Crusts above mouth and cheeks, worse from undressing. They ulcerate and form thick scabs under which purulent matter exudes. There is marked thirst and scrofulous tendency.

Nat-Carb : Inclination to perspire easily. The skin is dry, rough, cracked. Itching as if fleas all over the body. Eruptions on finger tips, knuckles and toes. Vesicular eruption in patches and circles. Impetigo on dorsum of hands, the soles of feet are raw and sore. Worse from summer heat; mental exertion, changes of weather, sun, least draught. Great debility caused by summer heat.

Nat-Mur : Affects the margins of the hairy scalp, flexures of skin, knuckles, skin behind the ears and covers mouth and eyelids. Persons with oily, dry, harsh, unhealthy skin who are always worse when at sea-shore. Impetigo in persons who are in the habit of eating too much salt. Raw, red inflamed Impetigo.

10 a.m. to 11 a.m., in warmth and during exercises.

Nit-Ac : Affects anus, vertex, temples; genitals, auditory meatus. The eruptions bleed easily when scratched and there is a pricking, splinter-like pain. Impetigo of the anus with long lasting pain in rectum after stool. Pustular eruption on face with large red margins and heavy scabs. Adapted to person with gouty diathesis and person who crave for sweets.

Rhus Tox : Vesicular crusty impetiginous eruptions, more around the genitals. Small pustules on a black base; greenish pus with violent itching at night. Itching is worse in the hairy parts. Humid eruptions with thick scabs on face and head, destroying the hair. Burning eruptions with a tendency of scale formation. The eruptions alternate with dysentery. Impetigo worse on change of weather, during wet weather and in winter. The skin is sensitive to cold air.

Rhus-Ven : Vesicular eruptions with intense itching which is relieved by application of hot water; and is worse at night. Dry eruptions on back of hands during winter which disappears in spring.

Sarsaparilla: Affects persons with emaciated shrivelled skin which lies in folds. Eruptions which come in summer and spring; also after abuse of mercury. The base of the eruption is inflamed. Crusts get separated in open air and the adjoining skin gets chapped.

Sepia : Acts on face, vertex, occiput, bends of joints. Eruptions during pregnancy and lactation. Itching vesicles and pustules with soreness of skin. Eruption is dry or moist and discharges copious purulent matter which when dries, cracks and exfoliates. Itching is worse in the open air and better in a warm room. Itching changes to burning when scratched.

Silicea : Acts on skin behind ears, skin of scrotum, hands, scalp and neck. Itching, burning offensive eruptions ending in scabs discharging pus. Violent itching of scalp. Moist scald head. Skin is sensitive to cold, Patient wants to wrap up warmly. Unhealthy skin — every injury suppurates.

Staphysagria : The Impetigo is characterised by thick scabs that itch violently. The person changes the place of itching on scratching. Impetigo alternates with joint pains. There is presence of early ulceration once the scabs are removed. Eruptions extremely sensitive to touch. Impetigo developing in individuals with ill-effects of anger and insults; sexual excess and abuse of Mercury.

Sulphur : Dry, thick, yellow scabs on scalp with profuse discharge, great itching which is relieved by scratching. Purulent eruptions on elbows.

Thuja : Eruptions all over the body; itching and shooting, especially at night. Pustular eruptions about the knee; better from gentle rubbing.

Viola-Tricolor : Good for acute cases. Pustular eruptions and scabs upon face with burning and itching and discharging foetid pus; worse at night. There is a sensation as of tension of the integument of face. The patient has a horribly offensive smelling urine-like discharge like that of cat's urine.

THE HOMOEOPATHIC HERITAGE
Page No. 217 - Case No. 977

Impetigo - Sepia 30

June 25th 1872. A little girl — 3½, fleshy leucophlegmatic, for three years has had impetigo, consisting of a thick, putrid smelling, pustular eruption covering the scalp like a skull-cap, surrounding the eyes, on the face, and appearing on the genitals. A papular eruption is scattered all over the body, with pustules here and there. Much itching. After scratching the scalp it bleeds. The hair is agglutinated. Excretion probably albuminous. Urine putrid when first voided. The impurities of the blood seek an outlet through the skin and kidneys. Bowels regular. *Sepia* 30. July 1st — Better every way. July 15th— General improvement; urine normal; scalp smells less putrid; face and genitals healed. August 19th — Profuse scalp-sweat and impetigo. *Calc. carb* 85m. Impetigo soon afterwards disappeared and the child was well.

In this case, the putrid urine and offensive impetigo indicated the putrescent state of the blood. On constitutional grounds *Calcarea carb.* was first prescribed without apparent benefit, the case growing worse, as it did previously without medicine. Afterwards the putridity of the urine suggested *Sepia* which nearly cured the patient. Finally the occurrence of profuse head-sweat indicated the appropriate time for administering *Calcarea carb.*, which completed the cure.

Eruptive disease, are called skin diseases on account of their location. But they originate in certain diseases of the blood of which they are symptomatic and they are occasioned by the elimination from the blood of various impurities through the skin.

CHAPTER 15

Angular Stomatitis

Synonym : Perleche

It implies bilateral linear cracks at the angles of the mouth. It is a clinical entity which can be brought about by several causes, viz. Malnutrition particularly deficiency of riboflavin, monilial infection, low-grade pyogenic infection, as a feature of seborrhoeic dermatitis, or as a complication brought on by an ill-fitting or a sensitizing denture, or by pipe smoking. It is rarely seen as an evidence of secondary syphilis.

Clinically, it is seen as erythema and as a crack covered by a yellowish crust.

Perleche is usually a chronic condition. The prognosis depends upon the cause; unless the cause is corrected, the patient cannot be helped very much. So in every case of angular stomatitis, instead of relying on vitamins, the attending physician should examine the patient thoroughly.

Homoeopathic Approach

First of all the homoeopathic physician has to decide whether the person is well-nourished or not. If a person is ill-nourished, then dietetic advice and vitamin supplement has to be given. If the patient is well-nourished, then one must try and find out the exact cause like monilial infection, seborrhoeic dermatitis etc. Since the lesions are characterised by deep cracks, it indicates a dominant syphilitic miasm. The crusts formed in the lesion should be gradually removed with the help of a solution prepared by mixing calendula and water in ratio of 1:2. And on the raw surface, calendula ointment should be applied. The above application is only meant for the protection of the raw surface from the environment. The rest of the approach remains same as that of Impetigo.

Kent's Repertory should be referred for the therapeutic utility. See : Face - cracked - corners of the mouth.

Drugs :

Antim Crud : Ant crud has got cracks at the corners of mouth. They are small, sore with presence of thick yellow crusts on top. The tongue is coated thick white and the patient is extremely thirstless. The cracks are associated with gastro-intestinal disturbances.

Condurango : The cracks are extremely painful to slightest touch. They are associated with digestive disturbances. Presence of angular stomatitis in cancerous diathesis.

Graphites : There is presence of rawness in the cracks. They bleed easily and ooze out a gluey moisture which turns into a crust. The cracks are usually associated with eczema. There is a sour foul odour from mouth and there is a sensation as if a cobweb is present on the face. The cracks are associated with gastric and menstrual disturbances.

Nit-Ac : Angles of lips are raw, cracked and scabby. The cracks are very painful; pricking pain like a splinter is a characteristic symptom which is worse when touched; at night. The cracks turn into ulcers which oozes acrid, then bloody, offensive, dirty brown discharge. The tongue is also fissured or mapped. Presence of apthous stomatitis in individuals who have history of abuse of mercury.

Silicea : The cracks are indurated, situated at the corners of lips. Cracks are also present on the lips. The cracks suddenly become painful and they suppurate easily. There is presence of itching sensation in the cracks. Cracks are present in individuals with scrofulous diathesis.

CHAPTER 16

Furunculosis

It is a condition familiar to every one. A furuncle or boil is a deep-seated septic affection of the hair follicle in which the hair root is completely destroyed and comes out as the core of the boil. Multiple boils are given the name of furunculoses. A carbuncle is a big conglomeration of boils, the inflammation spreading from one follicle to another under the epidermis. The intervening corium is destroyed, and pus is discharged through multiple holes.

Etiology.: The causative organism in these conditions is staphylococcus aureus, less frequently other staphylococci. Furunculosis is a common skin problem, very prevalent in the tropics. It is more common in the summer, especially the monsoon season. Maceration of the skin, dusty and dirty environments, and the ingestion of too many carbohydrates, predispose to furunculosis. The eating of too many mangoes has a similar effect (mango boils). A stye is a boil around an eyelash. When one deals with chronic furunculosis, the following predisposing causes must always be kept in mind.

Constitutional

1. Diabetes mellitus.

2. Chronic nephritis.

3. Poor general health — malnutrition, worries, anxieties etc.

4. Seborrhoeic diathesis.

5. Ichthyosis.

Environmental

1. Oily occupations or dusty jobs.

2. Friction or changing at work or by rough garments.

3. Scabies pediculoses,etc.

In acute furunculoses, the pain is intense, replaced by uncomfortable itching when the condition becomes chronic.

Homoeopathic Approach

Furuncles or boils is one of the commonest conditions that every homoeopath has an opportunity to treat. Patients present to us either during the acute stage or with recurrent tendency to develop furuncles.

(a) When one is dealing with chronic tendency to boils, one must improve the general state of health by making necessary dietary changes and encouraging the patients to eat fresh fruits and plenty of green leafy vegetables.

(b) Worries and anxieties are known culprits that predispose an individual to develop recurrent boils.

(c) Investigations to rule out diabetes mellitus, and chronic nephritis should be advised.

(d) Seborrhoeic diathesis if present should be tackled accordingly.

(e) Overall hygiene and cleanliness should be maintained.

(f) Eating excessive amount of carbohydrates and fatty foods, e.g., chocolates, mangoes should be strictly avoided as they predispose individuals to develop boils.

(g) Local application of magnesium sulphate paste should never be encouraged.

For selecting the right remedy, the following points should be considered :

(i) Note whether boils are matured or not.

(ii) Whether there is more inflammation than suppuration or vice versa.

(iii) The overall look of the boil that is red, pale, yellow, dark red; blackish, etc.

(iv) The type of pain with its modalities should be inquired.

(v) In chronic conditions, itching becomes an important symptom and hence it has to be thoroughly analysed.

(vi) The lower potencies are to be selected to enhance the suppuration. Higher potencies are selected to abort the suppuration.

Staphylococcus Aureus is the causative organism most commonly cultured from the discharge of the furuncle. Hence the use of staphylococcinum in recurrent and chronic cases should be employed.

Finally, in obstinate cases, I have found encouraging results when patients are exposed to :

(a) Sea bathing;

(b) Bathing in natural sulphur spring baths.

Therapeutics

Abrotanum : Tendency to boils in marasmic children. The skin develops purplish discoloration after the boil heals. The emaciation progresses with good appetite.

Aethusa : Boils associated with enlargement of lymphatic glands. The skin is cold and covered with cool clammy sweat. It is specially useful in children during dentition who have tendency to develop summer boils.

Anantherum : It is one of the remedies which is full of suppuration. The patient has tendency to develop boils, abscesses and ulcers. The important concomitant symptom is offensive foot sweat and disease deformed nails.

Anthracinum : Whenever there is purulent focus this drug should be thought of. There is tendency to develop succession of boils. The boils have an angry look, they may be discoloured, black or blue at a later stage. There is terrible burning sensation with great prostration.

Antimony-Crud : It is suitable to individuals who have a tendency to grow fat. Boils are associated with gastric derangement. There is itching and burning sensation which is worse at night. The skin is extremely sensitive to cold bathing.

Arnica-Montana : The tendency to small painful boils one after another which are extremely sore. Small boils in crops. The most important observation to make before prescribing Arnica is that the pain is more than the swelling (opp. Rhus-tox).

Ars-Alb : Chief remedy for furunculosis with burning, as if coals of fire were put on the affected part. Cutting and burning pains, worse after midnight and better with warm fomentation. Indicated when anthracinum fails.

Belladonna : When the boils are red during the stage of inflammation there is throbbing pain without formation of pus. Blood boils.

Bellis Per : Boils all over the body. Sensitive to touch. The boil begins as a small pimple with burning pain and then gradually turns into a dark fiery purple colour furuncle. When boils rupture it liberates acrid pus which destroys the surrounding hair. The pain within the boil is worse by application of heat and better by application of cold.

Calc-Carb : Skin is cold, unhealthy, flaccid. Blood boils which are recurrent in nature. The skin is extremely unhealthy and every injury tends to suppurate. The characteristic observation is that boils appear big but when rupture, liberate too little pus. Tendency to develop boils in emaciated children with big head, big belly who sweat easily and are extremely sensitive to cold.

Calc-Hypophos : Suited to persons who become pale, weak, with violent drenching sweat, rapid emaciation with extreme debility due to suffering from continued abscesses having reduced the vitality.

Calc-Picrata : A remedy of prime importance in recurring or chronic boils, particularly when located on parts thinly covered with muscle tissue, as on skin bones, coccyx, auditory canal. The boils appear to be small but compared to its size they are excessively painful.

Calc-Sulph : Abscesses slow to heal after rupture, with a continuous discharge of yellow pus. Patient desires the open air but sensitive to drafts. Tendency to the formation of furunculosis. Purulent exudations in or upon the skin. The discharge when it gets dried it forms scabs of various colours like green, brown or yellow.

Carbo-Veg : Tendency to furunculosis. The skin is blue in colour moist with hot perspiration. Sensation of burning within the furuncles. Discharges are offensive, pus smells like asafoetida. Tendency to develop furuncle with systemic illnesses like typhoid, cholera, septicemia, etc.

Carbo-Ac : Furuncles on the lumbar region with diabetes. Pus discharge with a very foul odour from several openings. Severe prostration is almost always associated. The most characteristic concomitant is intensely foul breath.

Echinacea : Recurring furunculosis. This remedy helps in correction of blood dyscrasias and hence it is useful in septic conditions like furunculosis. The discharge from the furuncle is extremely offensive. Due to presence of septic condition there is pyrexia with chills and sweat. The important concomitant symptoms are (a) Patient feels weak and tired with aching in muscles. (b) Nausea with chilliness.

Ferr-Iod : Crops of boils develop in individuals who are anaemic, emaciated and have tendency to develop goitre. There is presence of debility following drain upon vital forces.

Gun-Powder : A remedy introduced by Dr. Clarke is extremely useful for blood poisoning and septic states. Acts as a protective against wound infection. Gun-powder consists of a combination of Nitre with sulphur and charcoal; therefore one may get symptoms suggestive of sulphur, carbo-veg. and kali-nitricum.

Hepar-Sulph : In early stage of pus formation. Excessive sensitiveness of the part with sharp sticking pains. It helps to stop the formation of pus or aids in its abortion. If there is oozing of pus, then it is indicated when the pus is thick, yellow and the patient is sensitive to touch. Patient is chilly yet feels better in wet weather. The skin is unhealthy; every little injury suppurates.

Hippo-zaeninum : This nosode was introduced by Dr. Garth Wilkinson. It promises useful service in the treatment of Pyaemic states with lympatic involvements. The boils fail to heal and gradually progress to ulceration.

Icthyolum : Its action on the skin is prompt and useful. Crops of boils associated with itching. Tendency to develop boils in individuals with uric acid and tubercular diathesis.

Lachesis : Boils or furuncles surrounded by bluish areolae. They are usually surrounded by small pimples, and are extremely sensitive to touch. The discharge from the lesion is bloody, foul pus containing dark particles like charred straw. There is burning, throbbing, constricting pain in furuncle which is worse at night, during sleep, heat of summer and slightest touch and pressure. The patient feels better in open air; local application of heat. However the striking modality is that patient feels better when the boil ruptures and free flow of discharge sets in.

Ledum : Development of boil or furuncle after injury with a sharp needle. There is accumulation of foul pus within the boil. Patient feels locally better by cold fomentation.

Lycopodium : Boils which do not mature but remain blue. Tendency to develop blood boils. Sites of old boils indurate and form nodules that remain long. The discharge from the boil is thick yellowish offensive. Boils are associated with urinary gastric and hepatic disorders.

Myristica : It is a remedy of great antiseptic power. It hastens suppuration and shortens its duration. Furuncles which develop on end of fingers and phalanges.

Morbilinum : Recurrent boils in the external auditory meatus with terrible pain, having past history of measles.

Oleum Myristicoe : A remedy for boils and furuncles to be used in obstinate cases.

Operculina Turpethum : Furuncles that are associated with G. I. T. upset. The lymphatic glands are enlarged and indurated. It is an excellent remedy when boils and furuncles suppurate very slowly.

Phos-Acid : Tendency to develop boils and furuncles, especially after fever. The discharge is horribly offensive. Furuncles that develop on buttocks. Furuncles that proliferate deep into soft tissues and affect the bony structure producing ostitis and periostitis.

Phytolacca : The patient has inherent disposition to develop boils and furuncles, associated with swelling and induration of glands. The pus is watery, foetid and ichorous. Furuncles and boils which penetrate deep into the soft tissues thereby affecting bones and joints.

Presence of furuncles and boils in an individual with syphilitic dyscrasia.

Picric Acid : Tendency to develop abscesses and boils during summer. Furuncles that chiefly affect nape of neck. It is chiefly indicated in grave and serious conditions, e.g., toxaemia, uremia, pernicious anaemia, after burns. There is presence of tired heavy feeling all over the body, especially in the limbs which is worse on slightest exertion.

Secale-Cor : Presence of furuncles in thin, scrawny feeble individual of cachectic appearance. There is a burning sensation in furuncles which is better by local application of heat. The discharge is very offensive, bloody and greenish. The abscess matures very slowly.

Silicea : Presence of boils and pustules practically on each and every part of body. They are painfully sensitive. The discharge is highly offensive, purulent, bloody. The patient gets improvement by applying local heat. The furuncles have tendency to corrode the soft tissue and spread deep in the bones.

Stramonium : Chronic abscesses with severe pain characterized by shiny red flush. Hip joint is chiefly affected.

Sulphur : Unhealthy skin that develops furuncles everywhere which refuse to heal. The skin is dry, rough and wrinkled. Presence of voluptous itching worse at night, and in bed. The suppuration is characterised by presence of air bubbles in it. There is severe burning sensation in the furuncle which is worse by local application of heat.

Tarentula Cubensis : A useful remedy in toxic and septic condition where the progress of symptoms is rapid with alarming prostration with atrocious burning and sharp stinging pain. Furuncles are extremely painful with bluish, black, purplish discoloration. The symptoms are worse at night.

JOURNAL OF THE AMERICAN INSTITUTE OF HOMOEOPATHY
Vol. 62 — Nos. 7 - 9 (1969)
Page No. 161 - Case No. 4

A woman of 30 years suffered from boils in the ears, alternating from one ear to the other. Chemotherapy helped to clear up the boils but did not stop recurrence. She had no freedom from boils for more than a week or two at a time. The following symptoms were present : Dislikes consolation, could not weep, even when she lost her mother who died from cancer of the uterus. Nausea and vomiting at the beginning of her periods. Dragging down at M.P. Headache before a thunder-storm. Tired in the morning, better in the evening. Profuse offensive axilliary perspiration. *Nat-mur* and *Gelsemium* have sadness but cannot weep. Sepia, however, which contains *Nat-mur*, seemed to be much more indicated. The patient was given *Sepia* 30, 200, 1 m, 10m, which was followed by three weeks freedom, after which another relapse. *Carcinosin* 30, 200, 1m was given. It was followed by a severe aggravation lasting about a week and then has been followed by complete freedom for three years.

A lady of 39 years of age; a very successful person in life, working as a P.A. to the top most boss of a reputed company; well respected and feared. She had a injury on her toe and developed a sore, which would bleed easily with the slightest injury. When she had been to London, she had it removed by surgery. She was told that the name of the disease is *Pyogenic Granuloma*; its benign in nature, so she should not worry.

After sometime she developed a red mass on upper lip, which would also bleed on slightest injury. She was told that this was recurrence of her old complaint, only difference being that now it has come up on the face, and advised excision.

This difference was nothing to the advising doctor, but it made a hell of a lot of difference to the patient. Advice of best doctors in India and abroad was taken. All were unanimous in their opinion "Get it operated. You need not fear, though, because it is a harmless condition; but may keep, on recurring even after operation". But its appearance on lip made a lot of difference to the patient.

So she wanted to try Homoeopathy at this stage, but she had no time to come and see me. She sent her brother only with the news that she has "Pyogenic Granuloma", and I should give some medicine for her. I asked her brother to ring her up from my clinic and I talked to her. The symptoms which I got were as follows; over and above the ones narrated above :

The patient has had vaccination, all sorts of vaccinations many times, as she has to travel a lot.

Fond of warm drinks : Desire for milk but it disagrees, gives flatulance in abdomen and diarrhoea; so she adds coffee in it. Desire for sweets, very fond of chocolates.

Chilly person : Has to sit in an air-conditioned office but is uncomfortable in it. She covers herself properly when in the office. When at home she does not want breeze or fan.

I asked the brother about her mental attributes. He could not say anything which could be of help; but he said, "She is very fastidious; fastidious in office work, fastidious in what she wears; and fastidious at home, finding fault with little things."

The meaning of fastidious in the dictionary is — Squeamish, scrupulous, critical.

So the following rubrics were selected from the *Kent's Repertory* :

Conscientious : p. 16; Desires, warm drinks : p. 486

Censorious : p. 10; Desires, sweats : p. 486

Eruptions, bleeding : p. 1309

Eruptions, bleeding after scratching : p. 1309

Tumours, excrescences : p. 1324

Vaccinations : p. 1410 ... Desire, milk : p.485

Heat, vital, lack of : p. 1366-7 — Milk disagrees : p. 1363.

Treatment was started with *Sulphur* 30 T.D.S. for 3 months. No change. *Sulphur* 200 T.D.S. for another 3 months.

50% improvement. Repeat. Altogether *Sulphur* was given for 8 months. When the tumour was gone, the patient was asked to continue medicine for two months more. No recurrence.

THE HOMOEOPATHIC HERITAGE - 1982
Page No. 192 — Case No. 2

Mrs. B. age 30 years, had large suppurating pustules on the hands, particularly near the ends of the fingers. Has had eight or ten within a few weeks, and several more forming at present. Itching of body, particularly while in bed. *Psorinum* 30 in repeated doses of which some half dozen were given during a few days, preventing the development of those just beginning, and healing those which were suppurating within ten days.

THE HOMOEOPATHIC HERITAGE, 1982
Page No. 192 — Case No. 3

B. age 3 months; pustules and boils on head, particularly on the scalp; scalp had a dirty look and emitted an offensive colour; fine red eruption on the body, forming small white scales. Pustules on the hands. *Psorinum* 30. Odour removed in 24 hours. Eruption began to improve in a few days. Heard from the child several weeks later; quite well and skin in much better condition; pustules and boils had disappeared; rash still on neck and one arm; later reports show continued improvement.

THE HOMOEOPATHIC HERITAGE
May 1983
Page No. 230 — Case No. 983

Abscess

January 3rd, a woman 55 years age, came to hospital because of an abscess in left axilla; just starting to discharge. She was given *Tarentula cub* CM, three doses and a compress of *Hypericum*. Two days later it was well. No pain; no discomfort; no induration; a slight redness round, and a scrap of dressing adhering to the actual spot where it had discharged. People seemed rather surprised.

Seen again January 19th. Slight recurrence three days ago and very slight discharge. Dry now, but a tiny area of induration and two reddish spots that might be a threat of more, so *Tarentula cub* was repeated.

HOMOEOPATHY 1934-42
Vol. IV - No. 1
Page No. 22 - Case N. 3

Boil

One of our doctors reports, "About a week ago saw a girl with large boil on cheek, with hard centre and bluish discoloration. Gave *Tarent. cub.* and heard a few days later that it had disappeared with discharging."

HOMOEOPATHY AND COMPARATIVE MEDICINE
October 1956
Page No. 189 - Case No. 1

Abscess on Face

A middle-aged gentleman had an abscess on the side of the face just in front of the ear. Suppuration was advanced and the fluctuation was marked. *Silicea* had done some good, as it has controlled the pain. The cavity was aspirated by a surgeon several times, but it continued to refill. After three weeks there was no abatement. The integument took on a new feature, becoming bluish, mottled, with great burning and sharp cutting pains. The hardness was extending and opening gave out a bloody thin excoriating fluid of foul smell. He was chilly and nauseated and had symptoms of pyaemia. After one dose of *Tarentula cubensis* 12x, an immediate change for the better took place, no more pus formed, and he was well in ten days. The discoloured localization became a bright red and then faded to the natural colour. The nausea and general pyaemic symptoms were greatly relieved within twelve hours. No more medicine.

HOMOEOPATHY AND COMPARATIVE MEDICINE
Page No. 190 — Case No. 3

Carbuncle on the Back of the Neck

A lady aged about thirty, suffered greatly from a carbuncle on the back of the neck. She had applied many domestic medicines and obtained no relief. The tumefaction seemed destined to suppurate. It was mobbled bluish, and the pain was intense, knife cutting and burning. She felt terribly sick even to vomiting and at night she was delirious. Her eyes were staring, and she had fever; the tongue was foul and breath fetid. There was great tension in the scalp and muscles of the face. She begged for morphine to stop that burning and cutting.

Tarentula cubensis 12x, one dose produced improvement quite immediately, and the angry looking tumefaction failed to complete its work; it did not suppurate. The discoloration was gone in two days and the hardness soon disappeared. She regained her normal state very rapidly and she said to me a short time ago, that she never had her old headaches since that swelling left her, showing how deeply the medicine affected her whole system. If the part is mottled bluish, growing dark, with those symptoms, *Tarentula cubensis* must be the most appropriate remedy.

You see, therefore, that *Tarentula cubensis* is not a specific for an abscess, bubo or carbuncle, but only when it is bluish, mottled with great burning and sharp cutting pains. When you have these you cannot go wrong.

BOILS AND FURUNCLE

Abrot, Aeth, Agar, Aloe, Alum, Alumn, Am-c, Am-m, Anac, Anan, Anth, Ant-c, Ant-t, Apis, Arn, Ars, Ars-i, Aur, Bar-c, Bell, Bellis, Bov, Brom, Bry, Bufo, Calc, Calc-hypophos, Calc-picr, Calc-p, Calc-s, Carb-an, Carb-s, Carb-v, Chin, Chin-a, Cist, Cocc, Coc-c, Colch, Colo, Con, Crot-h, Dulc, Echin, Elaps, Euph, Ferr-i, Gels, Graph, Grat, Ham, Hep, Hippoz, Hydras, Hyos, Ichth, Ign, Ind, Iod, Iris, Jug-r, Kali-ars, Kali-i, Kali-m, Kali-n, Kreos, Lach, Laur, Led, Lyc, Mag-c, Mag-m, Med, Merc, Merc-c, Mer-i-r, Mez, Mur-ac, Nat-a, Nat-c, Nat-m, Nat-p, Nit-ac, Nux-m, Nux-v, Ol-myr, Operc, Op, Petr, Ph-ac, Phos, Phyt, Pic-ac, Plb, Psor, Ptel, Puls, Rhus-r, Rhus-t, Sars, Sec, Sep, Sil, Spong, Stann, Staph, Stram, Sulph, Sulph-i, Sul-ac, Tarent, Thuj, Tub, Zinc, Zinc-ox.

Aborting, leaving induration — *Cinch, Lach, Sil.*
Blind Fago — *Lyc*

Blood boils — *Alum, Arn, Aur-m, Bar-c, Bell, Bry, Calc, Cypr, Euph, Hep, Hyos, Iod, Iris, Kali-bi, Lach, Led, Lyc, Mag-c, Mag-m, Mur-ac, Nat-m, Nit-ac, Phos, Ph-ac, Sec, Sep, Sil, Sulph, Sul-ac, Syph, Thuj.*
Blood boils instead of asthma — *Calc*
Blood boils, large — *Hyos*
Blood boils during new moon — *Calc*
Blood boils pricking when touched — *Mur-ac*
Blood boils after abuse of sulphur — *Bell*
Blood boils after abuse of sulphur — *Bell*
Burning with — *Anthr, Ars, Carb-v, Tarent.*
Blue — *Anthr, Bufo, Crot-h, Lach.*
Body all over — *Viol-t.*
Crops of — *Echi, Sil, Sul, Syph.*
Dark bluish red — *Lach, Sec.*
Debilitating — *Ars, Sec.*
Greenish pus — *Sec*
Impotency with — *Pic-ac*
Injured places — *Dulc.*
Inflamed — *Bell, Merc.*
Inflammation and pain predominates — *Tarent*
Large — *Ant-t, Apis, Bufo, Crot-h, Hep, Hyos. Lach, Lyc, Merc, Nat-c, Nit-ac, Nux-v, Petr, Phos, Sil, Viol-t.*
Large red borders, near small of back — *Thuj*

Many openings with — *Hep, Lyc, Nit-ac.*
Mature do not, but remain bliud— *Lyc*
Maturing slowly — *Hep, Sil, Sulph.*
Mature and heal slowly — *Sec*
Mature do not — *Sanic.*
Multiple — *Arn, Ars, Nux-v, Sulph.*
Menses at — *Merc*
Menses during — *Med*
Painful — *Ars, Hep.*
Painful small — *Kali-bi*
Painful, small, indolent — *Sep*
Painful to touch — *Spong.*
Painless — *Nat-c*
To eradicate predisposition — *Calc*
After pus has formed — *Merc*
Periodical — *Ars, Hyos, Iod, Lyc, Merc, Nit-ac, Phos, Phyt, Sil, Staph, Sulph.*
Phagedenic — *Bov.*

Receding — *Lyc*
Recurring — *Ant-c, Arn, Ars, Ast-r, Berb-v, Calc, Calc-mur, Calc-p, Calc-pic, Echin, Hep, Hydr, Iod, Kreos, Lyc, Merc, Nat-m, Nat-s, Nux-v, Rhus-t, Sec, Sulph,Sulph-i, Tub.*
Returns periodically — *Lyc*
Sequelae of itch — *Calc, Sulph.*
Scars leave — *Kali-i*
Small — *Arn, Bar-c, Bell, Dulc, Fl-ac, Grat, Hydras, Iod, Kali-i, Lyc, Mag-s, Mag-c, Mag-m, Nat-m, Nux-v, Sulph, Tarent, Ust, Viol-t, Zinc.*
Small and sore — *Arn, Lapp, Pic-ac, Sec, Tub.*
Small frequent — *Fl-ac*
Small spometimes stinging on touch — *Sars*
Spring in the — *Bell, Crot-h, Lach.*
Small, suppurating, often leaving scars — *Kali-i*
Scarlet red — *Ap, Bell.*
Sore to contact — *Hep*
Stinging, burning — *Ap*
Stinging when touched — *Mur-ac, Sil.*
Stringing when touched on chin — *Sil*
To hasten suppuration — *Berb, Hep, Merc.*
Successions of — *Anthr,. Arn, Sulph.*
Several small ones unite — *Nux-v*

Ulcers, boils from — *Calc-p*

Head eruptions : boils — *Anac, Arn, Bar-c, Bell, Calc. Hep, Kali-bi, Kalic, Kali-i, Led, Mag-m, Meg, Mur-ac, Nit-ac, Psor, Rhus-t, Sulph.*

Occiput — *Kali-bi, Lyc, Nat-c.*

Temple right — *Mur-ac.*

Boils on lids — *Ant-t, Arg-m, Carb-s, Lyc, Merc, Sep, Sil, Sulph, Tell.*

On canthi — *Bell, Bry, Calc, Kali-c, Lach, Lyc, Nat-c, Petr, Puls, Sil.*

Left inner — *Stann.*

Margins — *Arg-m, Puls, Sep.*

Ear eruptions : boils — *Kali-c, Sil, Spong, Sulph, Syph.*

Ear eruptions boils before — *Bry.*

Ear eruption boils behind ears — *Ang, Bry, Calc, Carb-an, Caust, Con, Nat-c, Phyt, Staph, Sulph, Thuj.*

Ear-eruption boils in front of — *Bry, Carb-v, Laur, Sulph.*

Ear eruption boils lobes on — *Nat-m.*

Ear eruption boils meatus in — *Bell, Bov, Calc-pic, Crot-h, Ferr-pic, Kali-c, Merc, Pic-ac, Puls, Rhus-t, Sil, Sulph.*

Ear eruption boils on external — *Nat-m, Spong.*

Face eruption : boils — *Alum, Am-c, Anan, Ant-c, Bar-c, Bell, Bro, Bry, Calc, Calc-s, Carb-v, Chin, Cina, Coloc, hep, Hyos, Iod, Iris, Kali-ar, Kali-br, Kali-i, Lappa, Laur, led, Mez, Mur-ac, Nat-c, nat-m, Nit-ac, Pic-ac, Rhus-t, Rhus-v, Sars, Sil, Sulph.*

Blood boils, small — *Alum, Iris, Sil.*

Painful — *Hep.*

Chin — *Am-c, Caust, Cob, Hep, Lyc, Nit-ac, Sil.*

Chin under — *Carb-v.*

Chin right side of — *Cob.*

Forehead — *Am-c, Led, Mag-c, Phos, Sep.*

Above the eyes — *Calc-s, Nat-m.*

Lips — *Hep, Lach, Nat-c, Petr.*

Mouth corner of — *Am-c, Ant-c.*

Nose — *Acon, Alum, Am-c, Anan, Cadm, Carb-an, Con, Hep, Mag-m, Phos, Sars, Sil.*

Nose inside — *Alum, Am-c, Carb-an, Sep, Sil, Tub.*

Nose tip — *Acon, Am-c, Anan, Apis, Bon, Carb-an.*

Temples — *Mur-ac.*

Boils Gums — *Agn, Anan, Arn, Aur, Carb-an, Carb-v, Caust,*

Chel, Euph, Jug-r, Kali-chl, Kali-i, Lac-c, Lyc, Merc, Mill, Nat-m, Nat-p, Nat-s, Nux-v, Petr, Ph-ac, Phos, Plan, Plb, Sil, Staph.

Small, near left upper canine, painful to touch — *Agn*

External throat and neck—blood boils — *Arn, Caust, Sep.*

Vessels distended — *Aran, Ars, Canth, Hydr-ac, Lach, Nux-v, Op, Thuj.*

Throbbing in — *Bell, Glon, Hep, Lac-ac, Old, Op, Spong.*

External throat eruptions : boils : side of neck — *Caust, Coloc, Graph, Kali-i, Mag-c, Nat-m, Nit-ac, Phyt, Rhus-v, Sep.*

Abdomen : boils — *Phos, Rhus-t, Sec, Zinc.*

Abdomen inguinal region — *Ars, Merc, Nit-ac, Phos, Rhus-t, Stram.*

Rectum boils in anus — *Calc-p, Carb-an, Caust, Petr.*

Boils near anus — *Caust*

Perineum : boil — *Ant-c*

Genitalia boils on pubes — *Apis*

Boils on mons pubis — *Rhus-t*

Chest eruptions boils — *Am-c, Chin, Hep, Kali-i, Lach, Mag-c, Phos, Psor, Sulph.*

Back eruptions boils — *Caust, Coloc, Crot-h, Graph, Kali-bi, Kali-i, Lach, Mur-ac, Ph-ac, Phyt, Sanic, Sulph, Sul-ac, Tarent-c, Thuj, Zinc.*

Blood boils — *Carb-an, Caust, Graph, Hep, Iris, Kali-bi, Sul-ac, Thuj.*

Groups in — *Berb*

Cervical region — *Calc, Carb-an, Coloc, Crot-h, Cypr, Dig, Graph, Hep, Indg, Kali-i, Lach, Nat-m, Nit-ac, Petr, Phos, Rhus-v, Sec, Sil, Sulp, Thuj, Ust.*

Scapular region — *Am-c, Am-m, Bell, Led, Lyc, Nit-ac, Zinc.*

Dorsal region — *Ars, Caust, Fl-ac, Graph, Hep, Iris-v, Kali-bi, Lach, Mur-ac, Nat-m, Sec-c, Sulph, Sul-ac, Thuj, Zinc.*

Shoulders between — *Iod, Tarent-c, Zinc.*

Lumbar region — *Hep, Psor, Rhus-t, Thuj.*

Sacrum — *Aeth, Thuj.*

Extremities eruption boils — *All-c, Am-c, Apoc, Ars, Aur-m, Bell, Brom, Calc, Carb-s, Clem, Cob, Elaps, Graph, Guare, Hep, Hyos, Iris, Kali-bi, Kali-n, Lyc, Merc, Mez, Nat-m, Nit-ac, Nux-v, Petr, Ph-ac, Psor, Rat, Rhus-t, Rhus-v, Sec, Sep. Stram, Sulph, Thuj.*

Upper limbs boils — *Aloe, Am-c, Ars, Bar-c, Bell, Brom, Calc, Carb-an, Carb-v, Cob, Coloc, Elaps, Graph, Guare, Iod, Iris, Kali-n, Lyc, Mag-m, Mez, Petr, Ph-ac, Rhus-t, Sil, Sulph, Syph, Zinc.*

Shoulder boils — *Am-c, Am-m, Bell, Hydr, Kali-n, Lyc, Nit-ac, Ph-ac, Sulph, Zinc.*

Blood boils large — *Calc, Jug-r, Lyc, Zinc.*

Upper arm boils — *Aloe, Bar-c, Carb-v, Coloc, Crot-h, Iod, Jug-r, Mez, Sil, Zinc.*

Forearm boils — *Calc, Carb-v, Con, Iod, Lach, Lyc, Mag-m, Nat-s, Petr, Sil.*

Wrist boils — *Iod, Sanic.*

Hand boils — *Calc, Iris, Lach, Led, Lyc, Psor.*

Back of hand boils — *Calc.*

Fingers boils — *Calc, Lach, Sil.*

Finger joints — *Calc.*

Thumb joints — *Hep, Kali-n.*

Eruption lower limbs boils — *All-c, Am-c, Apoc, Ars, Aur-m, Bell, Carb-s, Clem, Hep, Hyos, Kali-bi, Nat-m, Nit-ac, Nux-v, Petr, Ph-ac, Phos, Rhus-t, Rhus-v, Sec, Sep, Sil, Stram, Sulph, Thuj.*

Nates boils — *Agar, Alum, Am-c, Aur-m, Bar-c, Cadm, Calad, Graph, Indg, Hep, Lyc, Nit-ac, Ph-ac, Phos, Plb, Psor, Rat, Sabin, Sars, Sec, Sep, Sil, Sulph, Thuj.*

Blood boils — *Aur-m.*

Thigh-boils — *Agar, All-sm Alum, Am-c, Apoc, Aur-m, Bell, Calc, Carb-s, Clem, Cocc, Hep, Hyos, Ign, Kali-bi, Lach, Lyc, Mag-c, Nit-ac, Nux-v, Petr, Ph-ac, Phos, Olb, Rhus-t, Rhus-v, Sil, Sil, Thuj.*

Thigh boils right — *Calc, Hell, Kali-bi, Kali-c, Rhus-v.*

Knee boils — *Am-c, Calc, Nat-m, Nux-v.*

Leg boils — *Anan, Anthr, Ars, Calc, Cast-eg, Mag-c, Nat-m, Nit-ac, Nux-v, Petr, Rhus-t, Sil.*

Blood boils — *Mag-c.*

Calf boils — *Bell, Sil.*

Ankle boils — *Merc.*

Foot boils — *Anan, Calc, Led, Sars, Sil, Stram.*

Sole of foot boils — *Rat.*

Heel boils — *Calc, Lach.*

Itching lower limbs boil, at the side of a previous — *Graph.*

Toes — *Cocl.*

FURUNCLES

Suppuration furuncles — *Abrot, Alum, Anac, Apis, Ars, Calad, Calc-s, Cina, Merc, Sil, Sulph.*

Near anus, with fistula — *Berb*
Commence with small blisters — *Cist*
Chronic, could not sit of tie — *Apis*
In diabetes — *Ph-ac, Sec, Tarent*
As if it would form — *Ars*
Relieve head — *Chin-a*
From indigestion — *Mag-c*
With functional derangement of liver — *Sep.*
Malignant, painful, turn blue and spread — *Lach*
Periodic — *Lyc*
Small — *Ars*
Small, on places formerly injured by concussion — *Dulc*
Small particularly in ears — *Pic-ac*
Sudden appearance — *Hep.*
Sudden appearance, with day blindness — *Sil*
After vaccination — *Ant-t*
Form ulcers — *Calc-p*

CHAPTER 17

Syphilis

hilis derived its name from a poem written by Girolomo :astorius in 1530 about "Syphilus". a shepherd who blas-med against the sun god and was punished by an attack of rrible disease. Though world-wide in distribution, it is fairly mon in the tropics.

duction

ilis is a specific, highly contagious disease, caused by the chaete, Treponema pallida; found all over the world; ned only to the human race of all ages and both sexes es more than females); with a high morbidity but low direct ality rate; acquired usually by sexual intercourse, and times accidentally, and also capable of congenital transmis- systemic from the outset; capable of involving almost all tures in the body; distinguished by florid manifestations years of complete latency, capable of stimulating many dis- ; transmissible to certain laboratory animals; and treatable to a point of demonstrable cure by penicillin.

gy

lis is caused by a spiral organism, Treponema pallidum, ered by Fritz Schaudinn and E. Hoffmann on March 3, The organism is corkscrew shaped, 0.25 micron in diameter, the length varying from 6 to 14 micron, with an average of 7 micron (the thickness of a red blood corpuscle) having usually, about 6 to 14 spirals). It can be seen only under the dark-field microscope as a shining, silver corkscrew, against a dark background, with characteristic movements of propulsion, rotation on its own axis and angulation.

Mode of Infection

There are four modes of infection, namely :

1. Direct
2. Indirect
3. Accidental
4. Congenital

The most common way in which infection sets in is throug direct contact (90-95 per cent), and this is usually by sexua intercourse. Kissing and fondling the genitalia can produc extra-genital chancres, on the lips, fingers and nipples. Indire infection occurs through improperly cleaned vessels used fc eating and drinking, and through toilet articles on which th secretions containing the spirochetes have not dried. Accident infection is seen commonly amongst doctors, nurses an midwives, and sometimes, takes place through blood tran fusion. Congenital infection occurs through the transplacent route.

Syphilis is usually associated with poverty and immorality. It prevalent mostly in the poorer strata of society; posititutes, ca girls and society women being the biggest source of dissem nation.

Course of Untreated Syphilis

The spirochaetes usually enter the body through minute abr sions in the body, either on the skin or mucous membrane; th are also capable of penetrating the unbroken skin or muco membrane. They invade the perivascular lymphatics and rea the regional lymph glands within a few hours after infection. T spirochaetes then enter the circulation, multiply and lodge the selves in different tissues.

While the spirochaetes invade the body, local reaction occ at the site from which the spirochaetes made their entrance. T is called the primary lesions or chancre. The disease passes through the following stages. Early syphilis consisting of the primary, secondary and the early asymptomatic infection is known as latent syphilis. Latent syphilis denotes all the other manifestations of syphilis occuring after more than four years of infection.

The course of untreated syphilis, as studied by Brusgaard, showed that 28 per cent of the cases did not show any complications of syphilis 20 to 25 years after the infection. Though this is good from the patient's point of view, from the public health point of view these cases should be viewed, with the same seriousness as those with complications, as they are equally liable to spread the disease when in the active stage.

Course of Syphilis

Early	*Late*
Primary	1. Latent
Secondary	2. Benign late syphilis affecting the skin, mucous membranes, muscles, joints, bones, etc.
Latent	3. Visceral syphilis. 4. Cardiovascular syphilis. 5. Neuro-syphilis.

Not every case of syphilis passes through all these stages. The primary stage may be skipped (Syphilis D'Emblee), or may pass unnoticed by the patient, e.g., meatal chancre; this feature is quite common in females due to the anatomical structure of the genital organs. As such, during the examination and investigation of the patient having either secondary or late manifestations of syphilis, one should be careful in eliciting the history.

Pathology

The typical histopathology consists of peri-vascular infiltration with plasma cells, lymphocytes and histiocytes; the other features vary with the stage and lesion.

General Diagnosis

After eliciting a history of exposure (usually illicit) and the subse quent development of primary lesion occurring after the charac teristic incubation period, a thorough clinical examinatio should be made.

1. ***The Dark-ground Illumination Test*** for treponema pa lida in the serum from the sores.

2. ***V.D.R.L. Test*** on the blood serum, or cerebro-spinal flui

The Dark-ground Illumination Test : It is performed with th help of the special objective and a special dark-ground co denser attached to the microscope by means or which th spirochaetes are viewed against a dark background. Care shou be taken to use only thin slides (1 mm. thick) and No. coverslips.

The serum taken for the examination should be clear or with little blood as possible. For this, the serum should be obtain from the deeper parts, near the margin of the sore, by applyi a steady continuous pressure with the thumb and forefinger the hand and mopping up the blood that comes out first. T serum is taken on the special cover-slip (No. 1) which is carefu placed on the thin glass slide. This is placed on a blotting pap and the cover-slip pressed evenly to squeeze out the ex amount of fluid leaving a thin film. Vaseline is applied around t cover-slip, to prevent air currents during examination, and slide is seen under the dark-ground illumination microscope treponema pallida.

Treponema pallida is seen against the black background as silvery-white corkscrew with its characteristic movement already described.

The V.D.R.L. Test (Venereal Disease Research Laboratory Test) : T V.D.R.L. test is used for the sero-diagnosis of syphilis.

The V.D.R.L. test is a microflocculation test using cardioli antigen. A simple test, it requires only two ingredients its performance, thus helping to establish the diagnosis i much shorter ume than the other tests. This has made it v popular, both for routine hospital work and mass screening. The exact method is as follows :

> The blood of the patient is taken and centrifuged. The serum is inactivated in a water-bath at 56 degrees C for 30 minutes. 0.05 cc. of the serum is dropped into the depressions of a special slide. To it is added one drop of the freshly prepared antigen emulsion. The slide is subjected immediately to a shaking movement for 4 minutes and the test read without delay. As a control, known positive, weak positive and negative sera are always included.
>
> The test is read under a low power objective (X 100) of a microscope. The positivity is interpreted depending on the size of the clumps formed.
>
> 1. No clumps or slight roughness .... Negative
> 2. Small clumps............................ Weak positive
> 3. Neduyn and large clumps .... Positive
>
> Quantitative tests are performed on diluting the serum with saline (from 1:2, 1:4, 1:8, 1:16, 1:32 etc.) and tested as for the qualitative test described above.

Serological tests for syphilis (S.T.S.) become positive about 8 to 10 weeks after exposure. So they may be negative in primary syphilis, but are usually positive in secondary (95-100 **per cent**) and tertiary syphilis (80 **per cent**). Sometimes these tests become positive in leprosy, malaria, yaws etc. Therefore, one must be careful in interpreting them. The problem of biological false positive reaction obtained with V.D.R.L. has been considerably solved by the introduction of specific treponemal antigen. The various tests in vogue are : the treponema pallida immobilization test (T.P.I.); the treponema pallida agglutination test (T.P.A.); The treponema pallida immune adherence test (T.P.I.A.), the fluorescent antibody test (F.T.A.) and the treponema pallida complement fixation test (T.P.C.F.).

Synonyms : Chancre, Hunterian chancre, primary chancre or sore, hard chancre.

Incubation period : It is the period between the inoculation of the spirochaetes at the time of exposure and the manifestation of the sore. The usual period being 2 to 3 weeks; it can range from 10 to 90 days.

Clinical features : Chancre is usually the first recognisable sign of syphilis. It starts as the point of inoculation as a macule and then develops into a papule, the surface of which becomes eroded and ulcerated. The chancre usually starts on an eroded point, balanitis, or on lesions of herpes and scabies. It is usually single, ham-coloured, relatively painless, with an indurated base and pink areola, discharging serous fluid; with an indurated base and pink areola, discharging serous fluid; with a painless, characteristic, bilateral enlargement of the regional lymph glands which are shotty, discrete and painless. It usually occurs on the genitalia (about 95 per cent) and rarely extra-genital (about 5 per cent). The common sites in the male are the coronal sulcus, prepuce, glans, frenulum, meatus, etc., and in the female, the cervix, labia majora and minora, fourchette, urethra, clitoris etc. The extra-genital chancres are seen usually on the lips, tongue, tonsils, anal region, fingers, breasts, eyelids, and may occur on other parts of the body also.

Secondary Syphilis

The manifestations of secondary syphilis occur, usually, within six months after the primary stage. The primary sore may not be present. But the V.D.R.L. test is always positive. This stage is characterized by a rash, adenitis and constitutional symptoms which are manifested usually, as general malaise, fever, headaches, vague pains and arthralgia which is worse at night. The manifestations of secondary syphilis affect, most commonly, the skin and the mucous membranes; the other structures are involved less frequently.

The common characteristic features of skin lesions in secondary syphilis are :

1. A rash which is generalized and bilaterally symmetrical in distribution.

2. Reddish or coppery in colour (difficult to make out in dark skinned people).

3. Pleomorphic appearance, i.e., different varieties of skin lesions occurring at the same time.

4. Induration and infiltration.

5. Itching is characteristically absent.

6. Accompanying adenopathy.

7. The presence of treponema pallida in the dark-ground preparations.

8. On healing, they leave faint stains. There is atrophy and scarring only in advanced cases.

Macular Syphilide

It is a generalized, faint rash occurring on the trunk, extremities, palms of the hands and soles of the feet. It fades on pressure. The macules vary in size from about ½ to 1 cm. This rash, when viewed from an oblique angle, is very apparent.

Maculo-papular Syphilides

These are a transition between macular and papular lesions, the papules being situated at the centre of the macule.

Papular Syphilides

They affect the trunk, extremities, palms of the hands and soles of the feet. On the face, they have a special predilection to be present along the hair margin; they go by the name of corona veneris. On the palms and the soles, they may assume a pigmentary appearance, or present themselves as maculo-papules or squamous patches with infiltrated edges. Annular syphilides are arranged in circles, as the name indicates. The lesions have a special predilection for the face, neck and genitalia. Corymbose syphilides consist of a large central papule surrounded by small satellite lesions.

Condylomata lata are usually large, hypertrophic, papular syphilides with a moist, greyish plaque, situated in moist areas like the genitalia, crural and anal regions and the axillae.

Mucous patches are oral lesions found on the lips, cheeks, tongue, palate, tonsils and fauces. These are oval or circular, slightly raised patches, covered by a greyish sodden membrane. Superficial ulcers in the form of snail-track ulcers are occasionally seen.

Affections of the Bones and Joints

Bones, joints and the surrounding structures may be affected. A common feature is localized periosteitis, affecting usually the anterior surface of the tibia which exhibits itself as a painful and tender swelling. Other features are : vague oesteoscopic pains with nocturnal exacerbations and bilateral arthralgia. Other rarer manifestations are : tenosynovitis and bursitis.

Affections of Hair and Nails

Alopecia : The loss of hair during secondary syphilis is patchy, giving rise to a moth-eaten appearance, particularly over the back and sides of the scalp. This has to be distinguished from alopecia areata in which patches, completely denuded of hair, are present. Another condition to be excluded in tinea capitis, in which well-defined, circular patches of alopecia, with dull, greyish scales and dull, broken hair are seen.

Onychia and Paronychia : Syphilitic nail changes are not so common. They occur as onychia in association with paronychia and dactylitis.

Affections of the Central Nervous System

Neuritis of the eighth nerve with tinnitus may occur. Basal meningitis with the concomitant symptom of headache, and sometimes, with the involvement of the nerves, particularly the seventh, are observed. The cerebrospinal fluid. If examined at this stage, shows definite changes.

Ocular Affections

Iritis occurs during the secondary stage of syphilis; it is more common in inadequately treated cases. The usual signs and symptoms are : circumcorneal congestion, photophobia, pain and dimness of vision; later, the condition gives rise to irregularity of the pupil. Neuro-retinitis also occurs, but is usually diagnosed only on routine fundus examination, as the patient does not complain, and the condition disappears under routine treatment.

Relapse in Syphilis

A relapse usually occurs within two years, particularly in irregularly or inadequately treated cases of syphilis. The relapse may take any of the following forms :

1. **Serological relapse** : the blood V.D.R.L. test becoming positive in higher titres than before.

2. **Muco-cutaneous relapse** : recurrence of the chancre in its original place called the Chancre Redux, or recurrence of mucocutaneous lesions, both showing treponema pallida in the serum.

3. **Osseous relapse** : occurrence of osteitis and periosteitis.

4. **Neuro-relapse** : in the form of asymptomatic neurosyphilis of neurorecurrence.

5. **Ocular relapse** : occurring as iritis, irido-cyclitis or neuroretinitis.

6. **Visceral relapse** : as hepatitis.

7. An apparently healthy mother with negative serology giving birth to syphilitic child; or infection in the sex partner, without any clinical or serological relapse in the patient.

Latent Syphilis

Latent syphilis may be described as the asymptomatic stage of syphilis in a patient with a definite history revealing the contraction of the disease, but exhibiting only a reactive serology, after all causes of biological false positive reactions and other manifestations of syphilis have been excluded by a thorough clinical, radiological and cerebrospinal fluid examination. These would help to exclude any external manifestation, affection of the heart and the vessels and any changes in the cerebrospinal fluid respectively.

Latent syphilis may be either early or late; and it may either progress and develop signs and symptoms of late syphilis, or persist as latent syphilis, or have a spontaneous cure, as reported by Brusgaard.

Late Syphilis

The late or tertiary stage of syphilis is manifested by the appearance of lesions of benign late syphilis of the skin, mucous membranes, bones, joints, tendons and viscera and/or of the cardiovascular and nervous system.

As time passes, the number of spirochaetes is reduced greatly due to the tissue reaction and the natural defences of the human body coming into action, and state of allergy may be established between the tissues and the spirochaetes giving rise to the various types of lesions. These lesions generally occur four or more years after the infection has been contracted, depending on the structure affected.

Classification : The lesions may be classified as follows :

1. Benign late syphilis.
2. Visceral syphilis.
3. Cardiovascular syphilis.
4. Neuro-syphilis.

Benign Late Syphilis

This may affect the skin, mucous membranes, bones, joints, muscles, tendons and bursae etc. The tertiary skin lesions are characterized by their asymmetry, by the occurrence of a single or few lesions which are indolent, indurated and arranged in an arciform manner; with or without ulceration; with a tendency to central healing and peripheral spread and hyperpigmentation. On healing, the lesions leave thin, papery, atrophic scars.

Cutaneous Lesions : They may manifest themselves in any of the following forms : nodulo-cutaneous, nodulo-ulcerative, gummata, juxta-articular nodes.

The nodulo-cutaneous type is characterized by non-ulcerated, gummatous infiltrations of the skin which do not breakdown. The nodulo-ulcerative type consists of nodular lesions mixed with ulcerated ones which are relatively deep. A gumma is either cutaneous or subcutaneous swelling, which may subside under treatment or develop a central softening discharging thin pus, and later, leaving an ulcer with its characteristic punched-out margin and a "wash-leather" slough covering its base. Juxta-articular nodes are usually multiple, fibrous, painless, slow-growing subcutaneous nodules of varying sizes, found commonly over the knees, elbows, and hips. They may also be found over the other joints.

Mucous Membrane Lesions : The common lesions are the gummata found in the mouth, pharynx and nose. They occur mainly over the palata, fauces, posterior pharyngeal wall, nose, tongue, lips and the inside of the cheeks. Ultimately, the gummata may lead to ulceration and performation. The perforation of the palate may result in regurgitation of fluids, and may also produce a nasal twang in the voice. One other late manifestation of syphilis is leukoplakia of the angles of the mouth and tongue.

Lesions of Bones, Joints, Muscles, Tendons, Bursae etc.

Bones : The common lesions are : periosteitis, osteitis and osteomyelitis affecting the long bones, the skull and the shoulder girdle. Clinically, a perforated palate, saddle nose (depressed bridge of nose) and bossy thickening of the cranial and leg bones are some of the typical features.

Joints : Arthritis and synovitis may occur in late syphilis. But the most common lesion is the Charcot's joint of tabes dorsalis. This is a neuropathic condition usually affecting the larger joints such as those of the knees, hips, ankles, shoulders and elbows. It is a painless, hypertrophic, osteoarthritic affection, with triple displacement of the affected joint. An X-ray will show destruction of the bones with areas of rarefaction and hypertrophy, along with loose bodies in the joint described as "bag of bones".

Muscles, Tendons and Bursae : Affection of these is not common, except of the prepetaller bursa, which is sometimes observed.

Visceral Syphilis

Lesions are seen more frequently on the liver and testes than on the other viscera.

Liver : The common type is gummata of the liver, and the less common type is interstitial fibrosis. The gummata are of varying sizes : secondary fibrosis and scarring give rise to the characteristic "Hepar lobatum". This is to be differentiated from secondary carcinoma, hepatic abscess, cirrhosis of the liver and hydatid cyst of the liver.

Testes : Late syphilis manifests itself as gumma of the testes, and diffuse interstitial fibrosis. The diffuse interstitial fibrosis is characterized by an increase in the size and weight of the testes, accompanied by the complete loss of testicular sensation. Gumma of the testes is less common; it may be associated with diffuse interstitial fibrosis. It produces a localized swelling which becomes adherent to the scrotum, and breaks down, resulting in gummatous ulceration.

Cardio-Vascular Syphilis

It usually occurs 10 to 30 years after the initial infection. It is more common in males than in females. Physical exertion seems to make people more prone to develop cardiovascular lesions. The blood serology is positive in about 80 per cent of cases.

The most common affection is that of the aorta, in the form of aortitis, aortic regurgitation and aneurysmal formation. The heart muscle may also be affected. The veins are rarely affected. The prognosis of cardiovascular syphilis is, as a general rule, bad.

Neuro-Syphilis

The central nervous system is invaded by the treponema pallidum during the generalization stage of infection; this forms one of the most important causes of the organic disease of the nervous system. Males are affected more than females. Irregular and inadequate treatment may increase the incidence of neurosyphilis. The most common period for the onset of the signs and symptoms is from 10 to 15 years after infection has been contracted.

Patients having symptoms like ataxia, headaches, lightning pains, paraesthesias, visual disturbances, bladder symptoms and speech defects, have to be carefully examined. A thorough clinical examination should be carried out, along with the V.D.R.L. test, cerebrospinal fluid examination and Lange's colloidal gold curve.

The common neurological affections are : tabes dorsalis, general paralysis of the insane, optic atrophy and meningo-vascular syphilis.

Congenital Syphilis

Syphilis acquired by the foetus in utero from the mother is called congenital or prenatal syphilis.

The foetus is infected via the transplacental route by treponema pallida, usually after the fourth month. The chances of infection are greatest in early syphilis, diminishing with time.

The clinical features of syphilis tend to become less severe during pregnancy. Repeated miscarriages, still births, premature deliveries and neonatal deaths are good indications of syphilitic infection.

The only means of diagnosing syphilis in a pregnant woman, in the absence of clinical signs, is by a routine blood serological examination during the early and late stages of pregnancy. An early diagnosis followed by adequate treatment is the only effective way of preventing congenital syphilis.

Signs : They may be classified as *early*, occurring before the age of two and *late*, occurring at a time later. As a general rule, the early manifestations resemble the lesions of secondary syphilis, and the late ones, those of the tertiary stage.

The cutaneous lesions of congenital syphilis are very characteristic. Within the first seven days of birth, a bullous eruption (Syphilitic pemphigus) may develop. It consists of bullae distributed bilaterally and symmetrically on the front of the wrists, palms, ankles and soles; later, bullae develop on other parts of the body. Other features of congenital syphilis are usually present. The differential diagnosis is made from impetigo contagiosa in which the eruption develops at a later age, the history reveals contact with an infective case and the lesions are asymmetrical and the child is quite healthy to begin with.

Later, a maculo-papular rash may develop all over or on the buttocks, where it may resemble napkin rash. Even condylomata lata may be found. The palms of the hands and the soles of the feet are usually shiny, and may also show a maculo-papular eruption.

In the late type of congenital syphilis, nodulo-cutaneous and gummatous lesions are found.

Diagnosis : In the early stages, diagnosis is established by a careful examination followed by the demonstration of treponema pallida in the lesions, and by serological tests of the parents and child.

Immediately after birth, the diagnosis is assisted by an examination of the placenta, which shows characteristic features, viz., it is pale, greasy and bulky (weighing more than one-fourth of the foetal body weight). Treponema pallida can be demonstrated in a smear from the umbilical vein.

An X-ray examination of the long bones reveals characteristic features.

Late cases are diagnosed with the assistance of a carefully elicited history, clinical manifestations, serological findings and examination of the parents. The X-ray examination of the parents. The X-ray examination of the long bones and the unerupted incisors gives conclusive evidence.

Types of Congenital Syphilis

Early (Within Two Years)	*Late (After Two Years)*
Wasting, irritability, fever	Saddle nose
"Old man" facies.	Sabre tibia
Macular, papular and bullous lesions of the skin.	Periosteitis and osteitis (8-10 years).
	Clutton's joints
Snuffles.	**Teeth**
Rhagades.	Hutchinson's incisors
Laryngitis (cracked aphonic cry).	Moon's molars

Early (Within Two Years)	*Late (After Two Years)*
Onychia	**Eye**
Adenopathy	Iritis
Periosteitis, osteochondritis	Interstitial keratitis
(Parrot's pseudoparalysis)	Choroiditis
and osteitis.	Optic atrophy
Dactylitis	**Ear**
Cranio-tabes	Suppurative otitis media.
Parrot's nodes	Eighth nerve deafness
	Vertigo and tinnitus
Nervous system	**Nervous system**
	Meningitis
Basal meningitis	Hydrocephalus
Hydrocephalus	Epilepsy
	Mental deficiency
Visceral	Vascular lesions
	Parenchymatous lesions
Enlargement of liver and	Juvenile paresis
spleen. "White pneumonia".	Juvenile tabes

Homoeopathic Approach

The approach for the management of syphilis has to be extremely systematic before one starts treating a case of syphilis, One has to know in detail, the clinical aspects of syphilis. Also cases of syphilis should not be hidden by an inexperienced homoeopathic physician. It is advisable to consult an experienced homoeopathic physician so that chances of error in management should be minimum. Given below are the steps :

(1) Know the syphilis i.e. the clinical picture, prognosis investigations, etc.

(2) Confirm syphilis through various tests that are mentioned in the chapter.

(3) A detailed homoeopathic case taking should be done and here the staging of the illness should be done so as to suggest the prognosis. In cases of primary syphilis,

the chancre has to be described in detail. In cases of secondary syphilis, the rashes and other eruptions have to be described with peculiar modalities etc.

(4) Selection of remedy should always be based on totality of symptoms. However, referring the therapeutics of syphilis given below makes the task simple.

The role of homoeopathy in preventing syphilis is as important as the role of a dermatologist or a medical social worker. Early detection and treatment of cases of syphilis reduces the infectivity and hence could be stopped from spreading further in society.

It is very essential for a homoeopathic physician to know that homoeopathy can cure syphilis only in its initial stages i.e. primary and early secondary stage. The congenital and latent variety cannot be cured because in such cases irreversible, structural changes have taken place. Hence such cases can only be palliated. Also while treating a case of primary syphilis, all sexual contacts made by the patient in the last four-eight weeks must be identified, examined, and investigated, since the incubation period is about 4 weeks. A person whose morals are too low and who frequently has illicit intercourse should be advised to wear condom during and to wash his genitalia with calendula soap and water after every intercourse.

Whilst treating a case of syphilis homoeopathically, a homoeopath is strictly advised to assess the case clinically with the parameters given below :

(1) Rendering the contagious lesion into non-contagious lesions.

(2) All cases of syphilis should be watched regularly for at least 2-3 years. During this period, the blood serological examination should be performed once in 3 months for one year, and once in 6 months for 2 years.

A C.S.F. examination should be performed in 6 months, and then again in two years after finishing the therapy.

Syphilis — Drugs

Anacardium : Syphilitic patients who often suffer from an impaired memory, depression and irritability, usually a diminution of the senses of smell, sight and hearing is also observed. There is a sensation of burning in glans penis during and after urination. The patient has increased sexual desire with dribbling of the prostatic fluid during stool.

Arsenicum : Phagedenic chancres, usually a livid hue in colour, with an intense burning. And occasionally even sloughing. Chancres, after mercury, with very florid granulations. Margins of the ulcers are hard and bleed at the least touch. Such ulcers exude a thin, offensive discharge.

The inguinal glands are swollen, indurated and very painful. There is an indescribable feeling of weakness, occasionally accompanied with dropsy and malignant ulceration.

Asafoetida : Tertiary syphilis, especially after the abuse of mercury. Ulcers, especially when affecting the bones, discharging an ichorous, foetid, thin pus and extremely sensitive to touch.

Syphilitic iritis and intra-ocular inflammation with ciliary pains and boring, throbbing pains at night.

Syphilitic caries and necrosis with foetid and bloody discharge. Patients with hysterical and hypochondriacal manifestation, intolerably nervous and oversensitive.

Aurum Met : Infantile and secondary syphilis, especially after the abuse of mercury and the potassium salts.

Iritis, with a tense feeling and much pain around the eye, as if in the bones. The pain extends from without inward and is much worse by touch.

Boring pains in the mastoid process with caries of the nasal bones. Skull bones are painful when lying on them. There is a putrid smell from the mouth with caries of the palate along with offensive and ichorous discharge.

Syphilitic cerebral or meningeal tumours.

Mental state of great melancholia and sleeplessness due to the excessive pain. Every opportunity is sought for self-destruction as he does not want to live.

All pain better in open air.

Aur-Mur : Chancre on the prepuce and scrotum; bubo in left groin. Snuffles of children suffering from hereditary syphilis, with flat ulcers on the scrotum secreting a foetid ichor; secondary syphilis with exostoses and bone pains in both skin-bones.

Melancholy with diminished vitality.

Vaginitis and gonorrhoeal discharge, with swelling of both groins.

Badiaga : Syphilis of infants who present themselves with glandular enlargements. The patient develops buboes and chancres with violent burning pain in the night. It affects those individuals where chancres have been suppressed by mercurial ointments leaving elevated discoloured cicatrices. The patient is emaciated and his skin is full of freckles and rhagades. Also it is indicated in those cases of cancer especially of breast, who in the past, had a history of maltreated syphilis.

Belladona : Syphilitic buboes which are large and painful with an intense inflammation of the integuments. These present with a deep-red hue, extend over large surfaces. Eruptions are very painful.

Phlegmonous phimosis or paraphimosis; erysipelatous balanitis.

Benz-Ac : Syphilitic spots and marks. Syphilitic rheumatism; with very painful nodes. Warts around the anus, appearing after suppression of a chancrous gonorrhoea.
Urine usually repulsively offensive.

Carbo-An : Constitutional or tertiary syphilis. Coppery-red blotches on the skin, particularly on face. Glands enlarge slowly and painfully and become indurated. Bubo, which is hard as a stone, especially if maltreated, opened or cauterised soon. They present with large, terrible ulcers with callous edges, and secrete an offensive ichor. Buboes are usually on the left side, indurated with lancinating and cutting pains. When they begin to suppurate, they are extremely sensitive to touch. Nasal syphilis.

Carbo-Veg : Syphilitic ulcers with high edges. These ulcers tend to become more irritable after some local treatment.
Sores, with sharp, ragged and undermined margin, with a thin acrid and offensive discharge. They are painful and liable to bleed very freely when touched.
Vesicles and blisters on prepuce; burning pains of labia.

Causticum : Vesicles under the prepuce which change into suppurating ulcers. Watery, greenish corroding discharge with jerking pains. Chancre with fungus excrescences.
Even buboes secrete an acrid, corrosive ichor, with various systemic complication, such as scurvy or gout.

Cinnabaris : Chancres that are indurated or neglected. They appear fiery red, inflamed, swollen, hard, discharging thin pus. The chancre is not so sensitive to touch and pressure. It is very useful in those cases where *Merc-sol* apparently well indicated fails. It is also a good drug for syphilitic iritis. The important concomitant symptoms are : (a) corner of the mouth chapped, (b) small fiery red ulcers on roof of mouth and on tip of the tongue.

Corallium Rubrum : Prepared from red coral. The syphilitic ulcers resemble the coral. There is presence of red, flat ulcers on glans of inner surface and prepuce, with profuse yellow, ichorous discharge which emits an offensive odour. The ulcers are extremely sensitive to touch. The important concomitant symptom is presence of constant trickling of mucus from posterior nares into fauces and smooth, copper-coloured spots on palms of hand and fingers.

Fluoric Acid : It has a wide spectrum of use in cases of syphilis, to start with it has signs and symptoms suggestive of congenital syphilis accompanied by ulcerations in mouth and throat. The bones are prone to caries, the one that are affected the most are temporal and mastoid, the pain is characterised by burning and boring sensation, the discharge from the caries is thin, acrid and corrosive. Psychologically patient has increased desire for sex and is extremely ill-humoured and fault finding, full of imaginary fears.

Hepar Sulph It is an important anti-syphilitic remedy where the patient has chancres which are extremely sensitive to touch with splinter-like pain. They are disposed to bleed easily, the margins of the ulcer are elevated and spongy looking, without granulations in their centre. The most characteristic symptom over here is that chancres are painless.

The buboes on the other hand are extremely painful and are prone to easy suppuration, when it ruptures, it liberates cheesy offensive matter.

Bones especially of nose, face, skull are inflamed and necrosed as a result nose is flattened or destroyed with offensive ozaena.

Jacaranda : The chancre is surrounded by itching pimples. The prepuce is painful and swollen. It is indicated in syphilitic arthritis with morning stiffness and soreness of muscles.

Kali-Bich : The syphilitic ulcers of *Kali bich* affects the root and glans penis. Margins are indurated and they perforate quite deep. The edges are punched out. The ulcer secretes thick jelly-like yellow discharge. There is presence of constrictive pain at the root of the penis which is worse at night. There is formation of depressed round scars after healing of the syphilitic ulcers. Syphilitic coryza affecting mucous membrane, mouth, nose and throat. Perforating ulcers in mouth and throat. Offensive and destructive ozaena with thick yellow nasal discharge.

Kali-Iod : Potassium iodide was once used as an antisyphilitic remedy. It has presence of ulcers on genitals which secrete acrid, thick foul discharge. There is presence of exostosis, especially in the skull and tibia. Syphilitic rheumatism that chiefly affects phalanges of fingers and toes. There is presence of excoriating syphilitic coryza which forms blisters on nostrils and mouth. There is boring pain which is worse by local application of heat, night and after abuse of mercury. Extremely useful remedy for syphilitic headache.

Kreosotum : Extremely useful remedy for congenital syphilis which is characterized by falling of hair, hot acrid smarting tears, deafness chronic catarrh from the nose, very rapid decay of teeth with putrid odour from mouth; foul breath. The urine and stool are offensive.

There is a presence of burning sensation in genitals. The corners of mouth are ulcerated and cracked.

Lach : It covers all three stages of syphilis. In the primary stage, syphilitic chancre are present which are extremely sensitive to touch. There is a burning sensation. The ulcer is surrounded by bluish purple areolae. The ulcer bleeds on slightest friction. During the secondary stage, there is a presence of syphilitic endocarditis which is characterised by restlessness, anxiety about the heart. The pulse is weak, intermittent, slow and irregular. There is a sensation as if the heart is hanging by a thread. In tertiary phase, there is presence of buboes with offensive dark black purulent and bloody discharge. The buboes chiefly affect the left side. In syphilitic affection of meninges there is a presence of headache with burning in vertex. The patient does not want his head to be touched. Also there are nocturnal bone pains which are worse after sleep. This ultimately develops into caries of bones, especially tibia. The guiding symptom being that the surrounding area is sensitive and livid.

Merc-Cor : Chancres that are situated on corona glans with excessive pain, swelling and inflammation. It bleeds very easily and the part surrounding the chancre is oedematous. The ichor with the chancre is adhering very firmly to the bottom of the ulcer that it cannot be removed by washing, the discharge leaves the stain on linen as from melted tallow.

Merc-i-R : This preparation of mercury is used for chancres that are painless and have no tendency to suppuration. The chancres remain indurated for a long time.

Merc-Sol : An all sufficient remedy in uncomplicated cases where mercury has not been previously employed. Sores present indurated bases and margins, secreting thin, offensive ichorous fluid or are covered with dirty tenacious matter. Chancres, bleed readily, are very painful and secrete a yellowish-white foetid pus. The most characteristic objective sign to be observed is the inverted red edge of ulcer, cheesy flow with lardaceous base. The edges resemble raw flesh. It is one of the principal remedies to be used in initial stage of syphilitic periostitis when bone pains are very severe towards the night.

Nitric-Acid : It is very useful in cases maltreated with penicillin or mercury. Chancres with raised edges and tendency to bleed easily and profusely and where no signs of central granulation are present. The discharge is thin, serous and bloody. The ulcer is inclined to spread more in circumference than in depth. The common sites for ulcers are throat, vagina, urethra, penis, oral cavity, etc. There is constant stitching pain which is worse at night and better by local application of heat. There is presence of offensive odour from urine, sweat and breath. There is also presence of syphilitic melancholia.

Mezerium : There is presence of syphilitic periostitis, especially shafts of the cylindrical bones are inflamed and swollen. The affected parts feel sore, as if ulcerated which is worse at night, least touch is unbearable to the patient.

Phosphoric Acid : It has special affinity for ends of long bones where patient complaints of severe nocturnal pain with sensation as if bones were scraped with a knife.

The chancres are characterised by raised rounded and prominent edges with presence of pale granulation tissue. The inguinal lymph nodes are enlarged but they are painless.

Phytolacca : It is indicated in syphilis for ulcers and bone pains. The bone is affected at three places viz. (a) Periosteum, (b) the attachment of muscle, (c) middle of the long bone. The pain is tearing, shooting and shifting, worse at night and in damp weather. The ulceration occurs in the throat and on glans penis. The ulcers appear as if punched out, with lardaceous bottom associated with weakness and prostration.

Sabina : Used for exostoses, especially when disease affects the hollow bones, particularly of hands and feet and attended with lancinating or drawing tearing pains.

Sepia : The syphilitic chancres of Sepia resemble indolent ulcers characterised by burning, itching sensation and having a very foul odour.

Stillingia : It is a remedy having scrofulous diathesis with syphilitic affection introduced in Homoeopathy by Dr. Hale. It affects genito-urinary organs, pharynx, trachea, mouth, head and bones. It has dry, spasmodic, syphilitic cough. Also it affects periosteum, especially tibia by producing syphilitic painful nodes that burn and pain violently. They are more at night. It has a popular repute in preventing nasal caries in patients suffering from syphilis. There is also the presence of syphilitic headache which is characterised by persistent dull pain on vertex.

Silicea : It is used for inflamed, painful chancres, with raised edges and thin bloody discharge. There is formation of unhealthy granulation tissue. Also it is indicated in cases of phagedenic chancres when the discharge is excessive, foetid, discoloured, bloody and thin. In suppuration of glands as in bubo it hastens the process of suppuration and prevents formation of ugly looking scars. Syphilitic affection of bones, especially jaw and vertebral column when suppuration and necrosis set in. The pus is thick, offensive and bloody. It is invaluable when the dead portion of the bone is still adherent to the living part or when it becomes loose and the discharge of pus and ichor is excessive.

Staphysagria It has beneficial action in cases of exostosis syphilitic gumma involving the bone, also syphilitic periostitis comes within its domain. The part affected feels sore, with tearing pain. Ultimately the bone develops caries and necrosis with abundant suppuration.

Thuja : It is an equally important remedy for syphilis as it is for gonorrhoea. Its characteristic mental symptoms like fixed ideas, flurried nature, lack of concentration with poor memory can become an important indication in cases of syphilitic dementia. For meningo vascular syphilis characterised by typical syphilitic headache. The most important symptoms are as follows : (a) pain as if pierced by a nail, (b) headache worse sexual excess, from tea better by bending head backward. In cases of syphilitic iritis the patient complains of a sensation as if cold air was streaming out of head through eye. Syphilitic ulceration of nasal bones with presence of thick bloody scabs. The teeth decay at the edge of gums. There is presence of apthous stomatitis. On genitals one has chancres with pain as from a splinter sticking, the edges are hard and indurated. The vagina is very sensitive so as to prevent coition. There is presence of syphilitic gumma which emits foul odour. It itches and burns violently. The patient feels worse from cold bathing.

Viola-Tric : Chancroid ulcer on posterior surface of fauces and soft palate; painful pustules on the labia and mammae, in axilla; syphilitic hoarseness.

SYPHILIS

Aethiops, Alnus, Am-c, Anac, Anag, Anan, Ant-c, Ant-t, Apis, Arg-i, Arg-m, Arg-n, Ars, Ars-i, Ars-s-fl, Asaf, Asc-t, Aur, Aur-ar, Aur-m,, Aur-m-n, Bad, Bapt, Benz-ac, Berb, Calc-i, Calc-s, Calop, Carb-an, Carb-v, Caust, Cean, Chim-umb, Cinnb, Clem, Cond, Con, Coryd, Cor-r, Crot-h, Cund, Echin, Fl-ac, Francis, Gels, Graph, Guaj, Hekla, Hep, Hippoz, Hydrc, Iod, Iris, Jacar, Jacea, Kali-ar, Kali-bi, Kali-chl, Kali-i, Kali-m, Kali-s, Kreos, Lac-c, Lach, Laur, Led, Lonic, Lyc, Merc, Merc-c, Merc-d, Merc-i-f, Mez, Nit-ac, Osm, Petr, Ph-ac, Phos, Phyt, Psor, Sang, Sars, Sep, Sil, Staph, Still, Sulph, Sulph-i, Syph, Thuj.

Alopecia — *Ars, Aur, Carb-v, Cinnb, Fl-ac, Graph, Hep, Kali-i, Lyc, Merc-i-f, Merc-v, Nit-ac, Phos, Sulph.*
Bones affected — *Ars, Asaf, Aur, Aur-m, Calc-i, Fl-ac, Hekla, Kali-i, Merc, Nit-ac, Phos-ac, Phyt, Sil, Staph, Still, Sulph.*
Inflamed, swollen especially shafts of cylindrical — *Mez*
Brain complications — *Arg-n, Crotal, Merc, Ph-ac, Pic-ac, Sil, Staph, Zinc.*
Buboes first stage — *Ars-i, Bell, Bufo, Kali-i, Merc, Merc-i-f, Nit-ac, Sil, Thuj.*
— **later stage** — *Aur, Bad, Carb-an, Staph, Sulph.*
Maltreated with mercury — *Carb-an, Hep, Kali-i, Phyt.*
— **becomes vast** — *Aur-mur*
— **inguinal glands suppurate** — *Aur, Aur-m.n, Bad, Bufo, Carb-an, Lac-c, Lach, Merc, Merc-c, Nit-ac, Phyt, Syph.*
Stony hard large in right — *Hep*
— **hard, large, inflamed** — *Sulph*
— **in left large as a hen's egg, stony hard** — *Canth, Hep.*
Painless, large in right opened and discharged freely — *Syph*
Ulcerating with fistulous openings — *Kali-i*
Chancre — *Apis, Ars, Aur, Bad, Cinnb, Con, Coral, Cupr-s, Kali-i, Lac-c, Lyc, Merc, Merc-c, Merc-i-f, Mygale, Nit-ac,*

Ph-ac, Phyt, Sep, Sil, Thuj, Viol-t.
— **bleeds readily** — *Hep, Merc.*
— **with burning** — *Ars-m*
— **chancroid with gonorrhoea** — *Merc*
— **on corona** — *Merc-c*
— **on corona, watery discharge** — *Ars-m*
— **discharge corrosive** — *Nit-ac*
— **discharge fetid** — *Hep*
— **discharge thin bloody** — *Sil*
— **discharge thin, offensive, corrosive, ichorous** — *Kali-i*
— **discharge torpid watery** — *Iod*
— **discoloured** — *Sil*
— **deeply ulcerating** — *Kali-bi*
— **eating through fraenum** — *Merc*
— **edges deep, hard** — *Kali-i*
— **edges elevated** — *Cinnb, Lyc, Nit-ac, Ph-ac, Sil.*
— **edges hard** — *Cinnb, Kali-i.*
— **edges, lardaceous** — *Hep*
— **thick edges, rounded and prominent** — *Ph-ac*
— **gangrenous** — *Ars, Crotal, Kali-i, Lach.*
On glans — *Nit-ac*
On glans indolent — *Sep*
On glans, round, deep — *Merc*
— **with gonorrhoea** — *Merc*
— **indistinct granulations** — *Sil*
— **granulation pale and flabby or absent** — *Phos-ac*
— **hard** — *Carb-an, Cinnb, Kali-bi, Kali-i, Merc, Merc-i-f, Merc-i-r.*
— **hard of long standing** — *Con*
— **with boardlike hardness of red and swollen prepuce** — *Sulph.*
— **hard on middle of penis** — *Cinnb.*
Hunterian — *Aur, Jacar, Merc-i-r.*
Hunterian with lardaceous bottom — *Merc, Merc-c.*
— **increasing fast and bleeding easily** — *Nit-ac*
Indolent — *Merc-i-r.*
Inflamed — *Sil*
Irritable — *Sil*
— **large, easily bleeding, lardaceous** — *Staph.*
Mercurialized — *Hep*
Neglected — *Cinnb*
Neighbouring parts oedematous, hot and painful — *Merc-c*

— painful — *Merc, Sil.*
Pain as of splinters — *Nit-ac*
Painless with swelling of inguinal glands — *Merc*
— from centre to circumference — *Lac-c*
On prepuce red — *Merc*
On prepuce studded — *Bor*
On prepuce, yellowish, fetid discharge spreading and deeply penetrating — *Merc*
Phagedenic — *Ars, Cinnb, Hydr, Lach, Merc-c, Nit-ac, Sil.*
Pricking — *Sulph*
— abundance of budable pus — *Aur-m*
Pus : corrosive — *Kali-i*
Pus : curdy — *Kali-i*
Pus : thin — *Cinnb, Kali-i.*
Pus thin leaving stains on linen as from melted tallow — *Merc-c*
Recent cases — *Eucal*
Red — *Cinnb*
Round deep on glans — *Merc*
- on scrotum — *Aur-m*
Secondary — *Merc*
Sensitive to touch — *Coral*
Small with cheesy bottom and inverted edges — *Kali-m, Merc.*
Soft — *Coral, Merc, Nit-ac, Thuj.*
Soft in gonorrhoea — *Merc*
Soft margins dark red, painful and easily bleeding — *Merc-c.*
Soft painful — *Coral*
Soft in weakly, scrofulous subjects — *Nit-ac*
— with pain, as from splinters — *Thuj*
Suppurating, slow, difficult, curdy after abuse of mercury — *Kali-i*
Swollen — *Cinnb*
Like an indolent ulcer — *Ph-ac*
Urethral ulcer — *Lac-c*
Contact of urine which causes tearing, affecting whole organism — *Jacar.*
— with warts — *Ph-ac*
Figwarts — *Ph-ac*
Pointy warts on corona — *Kali-m*
— with fungous excrescences — *Caust*
Whitish with hard edges — *Thuj*
Third in 2 years all on one spot — *Syph*
In children (infantile) — *Aethiops, Ars-i, Ars-m, Aur, Bad, Calc,*

Calc-f, Calc-i, Coral, Ferr-i, Fl-ac, Hell, Hep, Kali-i, Kali-m, Kreos, Lach, Merc, Merc-d, Merc-v, Mez, Nit-ac, Phyt, Psor, Sang, Syph, Thuj, Viol-t.

— **glandular swellings** — *Bad*

Chronic — *Calc-s, Kali-m.*

Suppuration and induration — *Sil*

Congestion intense to parts — *Merc, Sulph.*

Constitutional — *Ars, Asc-t, Aur, Benz-ac, Clem, Coral, Crotal, Cund, Euphor, Ferr-i, Fl-ac, Guaiac, Kali-bi, Kali-i, Merc, Merc-c, Merc-d, Merc-i-r, Mez, Nit-ac, Petr, Phos, Ph-ac, Phyt, Sars, Sil, Still, Sulph, Syph, Thuj.*

— **hereditary keratitis parenchymatosa** — *Merc*

Mercurial — *Aur-m-n, Daph, Kali-i, Lach.*

Mercurial - scrofulous — *Apis*

— **large doses of mercury (deafness of left ear)** — *Petr*

— **mothers to prevent disease in offspring** — *Aur-m-n*

Prosopalgia — *Phyt*

Erosions : exuding a thin, badly smelling ichor — *Coral*

Exostoses — *Calc-fl, Fl-ac, Hekla, Merc, Phos.*

Glands - indolent swollen — *Kali-i*

Gonorrhoeal — *Aur-m, Cinnb, Thuj.*

Gonorrhoeal of a torpid character with suppurating bubo — *Merc*

Gout — *Caust*

Gummata - nodes — *Asaf, Aur, Berb, Calc-f, Carb-an, Condur, Coryd, Fl-ac, Iod, Kali-bi, Kali-i, Merc, Mez, Nit-ac, Phyt, Sil, Staph, Still, Sulph, Thuj.*

Hair - falling out — *Ars-m, Aur, Hep, Kali-i, Lyc, Nit-ac, Petr, Phos.*

Mercuris (abuse of mercury) — *Aur, Aur-m.n, Cinnb, Hep, Iris, Kali-i, Lach, Nit-ac, Ph-ac, Sars, Staph, Still, Sulph.*

— **with morbus brightii** — *Kali-i*

Mucous patches — *Asaf, Aur, Calc-f, Calop, Cinnab, Condur, Fl-ac, Hep, Iod, Kali-bi, Kali-i, Kali-m, Merc-c, Merc-d, Merc-nit, Merc-pr, Merc, Nit-ac, Phyt, Rub, Sang, Staph, Still, Thuj.*

Nails : paronychia, onychia — *Ant-c, Ars, Graph, Kali-i, Merc.*

Nervous lesions — *Anac, Asaf, Aur, Iod, Kali-i, Lyc, Merc-nit, Merc-phos, Mez, Phos.*

Pustular, chiefly in cachetic persons — *Kali-i*

Red — *Phyt, Sars, Sulph.*

Scrofulosis in children — *Still*

Spots — *Benz-ac*

Squamous — *Ars*

Secondary stage — *Arg-n, Ars-i, Aur, Aur-m,* **Berb-aq.** *Calop, Carb-v, Chel, Chion-v, Cinnb, Fl-ac, Graph, Guaic, Hep, Iod, Jaca, Kali-bi, Kali-i, Lac-c, Lach, Lith, Lyc, Merc-br, Merc-c, Merc-i-f, Merc-i-r, Merc,* **Merc-v,** *Mez, Nit-ac, Osm, Petr, Phos, Ph-ac, Phyt, Rhus-t, Rhus-gl, Sars, Sep, Still, Sulph, Sul-ac, Syph, Thuj, Ustil.*

Secondary rash — *Kali-i, Merc-c.*

Pyaemia — *Crotal*

— **especially after mercury and iodide of potassium** — *Hep*

— **especially after abuse of mercury or with scrofula** — *Kali-i*

— **all symptoms worse towards night** — *Syph*

— **with deposits in throat** — *Kali-i.*

Stomatitis - mercurial — *Nit-ac*

Sore — *Nit-ac*

Stricture — *Arg-n, Berb, Clem, Iod, Kali-i, Merc, Nit-ac, Thuj.*

Tertiary — *Ars-m, Kali-i, Stictca, Syph.*

— **with ulceration of skin** — *Iod*

Tuberculosis — *Cinnb*

Tubercular — *Aur, Graph, Kali-i, Lyc.*

Extremities : eruptions : hand, back of psoriasis — *Aur, Ars. Phos, Merc.*

Eruptions hand palm — *Ars, Ars-i, Aur, Phos, Merc, Sel.*

Pain drawing wrist - Syphilitics in — *Asar*

Ulcers : upper limbs — *Phyt, Rhus-v.*

Rheumatism — *Benz-ac, Fl-ac, Kali-bi, Kali-i, Kalm, Merc, Nit-ac, Phyt.*

Skin - eruptions - Pustules — *Kali-bi*

Skin - eruptions — *Ant-t, Arg-n, Ars, Ars-i, Aur, Bad, Calc-i, Caust, Cund, Dulc, Fl-ac, Guaj, Graph, Hep, Kali-bi, Kali-chl, Kali-i, Kreos, Lach, Lyc, Merc, Merc-c, Merc-i-f, Merc-i-r, Nit-ac, Petr, Phyt, Plat, Rhus-t, Rumx, Sang, Sars, Sep, Sil, Staph, Still, Sulph, Syph, Thuj.*

— **in cachetic persons, squamosis** — Kali-i.

— **itching** — *Nit-ac*

Syphilitic neuralgia — *Syph*

Prickling — *Nit-ac*

Pustular syphiloderma — *Kali-bi*

— **resembling psoriasis after mercury, pustular** — *Ant-t, Kali-bi, Sulph.*

Eruptions : tubercles — *Ars, Ars-i, Dulc, Fl-ac, Hep, Kali-bi, Kali-i, Merc, Nit-ac, Phyt, Sil, Thuj.*

Mucous : tubercles — *Crotal, Staph.*

Excrescences — Condylomata -- *Aur, Aur-m, Aur-m-n, Cinnb, Euphr, Kali-i, Merc, Plat, Nit-ac, Nat-s, Sab, Staph, Thuj.*

Fibrous : Cauliflower — *Ars, Ars-i, Aur, Aur-m, Aur-m-n, Iod, Lach, Manc, Merc, Merc-c, Nit-ac, Staph, Sil, Thuj.*

Psora complications with — *Coral, Psor, Sulph.*

Scars — *Asaf, Carb-an, Fl-ac, Graph, Iod, Kali-bi, Kali-i, Lach, Sulph-ac.*

Ulcers — *Anan, Ars, Asd, Aur, Aur-m, Aur-m-n, Carb-v, Chim, Coral, Cund, Cist, Crot-c, Hep, Iod, Iris, Jacea, Kali-bi, Kali-chl, Kali-i, Lac-c, Lach, Merc, Merc-c, Merc-i-r, Mez, Nit-ac, Petr, Phyt, Rumx, Sang, Sars, Staph, Still, Stram, Syph, Thuj.*

Warts — *Aur, Aur-m, Aur-m-n, Caust, Cinnb, Hep, Merc, Nit-ac, Ph-ac, Sabina, Sep, Staph, Thuj.*

Ears : deafness — *Kreos, Nit-ac, Petr.*

Ears : deafness hereditary — *Lac-c*

Eye : inflammation : Syphilitic — *Arg-m, Arg-n, Ars, Asaf, Aur, Aur-m, Aur-m-n, Cinnb, Clem, Graph, Hep, Kali-i, Lyc, Merc, Merc-c, Merc-cy, Merc-i-f Nit-ac, Phos, Phyt, Staph, Syph, Thuj.*

Corneal ulcers — *Asaf, Thuj.*

— **iritis** — *Arg-n, Ars, Asaf, Cinnb, Kali-i, Merc, Merc-c, Merc-i-f, Nit-ac, Nux-v, Petr, Staph, Syph, Thuj, Zinc.*

Retinitis — *Crotal, Merc.*

Nose - Syphilis of — *Asaf, Aur, Hep, Lach, Merc, Nit-ac, Sulph, Thuj.*

Nose - Caries - Syphilitic — *Kali-bi, Sil.*

Nose Ozaena — *Aur, Aur-m, Asaf, Crot-h, Hep, Kali-i, Merc, Nit-ac, Phyt, Sil, Syph.*

Face : discoloration : yellow, syphilis — *Lach, Merc-c, Nit-ac.*

Face : eruption : rash syphilitic — *Syph*

Face : eruptions : syphilitic — *Ars-i, Aur, Cinnb, Fl-ac, Hep, Kali-bi, Kali-i, Kreos, Lach, Lyc, Merc, Merc-c, Nit-ac, Phyt, Sep, Sil, Sulph, Syph.*

Mouth : Patches syphilitic — *Hydro, Kali-i, Merc, Merc-c, Merc-i-r, Nit-ac, Sang.*

Mouth - of — *Aur, Carb-v, Kali-bi, Lach, Merc, Nit-ac, Phos, Ph-ac, Thuj.*

Mouth ulcers : syphilitic — *Aur, Aur-m, Fl-ac, Hep, Hydr,*

Kali-bi,Kali-i, Lach, Merc, Merc-i-r, Phyt, Syph.
Toothache — *Phyt*
— when mercurialized — *Clem*
Mouth ulcers palate - Syphilitic — *Aur, Aur-m, Hep, Kali-i, Syph.*
Mouth ulcers tongue — *Fl-ac, Kali-bi, Kali-i, Merc, Nit-ac, Phyt.*
Throat — *Aur-m, Hydras, Kali-bi, Kali-i, Kalm, Lach, Merc, Mez, Nit-ac, Phyt, Syph.*
— fauces affected — *Kali-m*
Throat - ulcers uvula — *Aur, Chel, Fl-ac, Iod, Kali-bi, Kali-i, Lach, Merc, Merc-c, Nit-ac, Phyt, Syph.*
Larynx : laryngitis — *Ars-i, Hep, Iod, Merc, Merc-i-r, Nat-ac, Pod, Phos, Still, Sulph, Viol-t.*
Tubercular sore throat — *Phyt*
Genitalia - eruptions — *Ars-i, Merc, Nit-ac, Scrotum.*
— hard, brown nodules, suppurating — *Nit-ac*
Back - eruptions maculae — *Syph*
Kidney - complicated — *Crotal*
— in Bright's disease — *Kali-i*
Liver - complicated — *Crotal*
Urethra - gonorrhoeal syphilitics in — *Aur-m, Cinnb, Merc, Merc-c.*
Urine - albuminous - syphilitics in — *Aur, Aur-i, Aur-m, Aur-m-n, Kali-bi, Kali-i, Merc-c, Nit-ac, Sars.*
Convulsions - syphilitic — *Nit-ac*
Vertigo syphilitic — *Aur*

HOMOEOPATHY AND COMPARATIVE MEDICINE
Page No. 189 - Case No. 2

Bubo in the Left Groin :

A young man came to me with a Bubo in the left groin. He had been disappointed, in that he had not obtained relief from the treatment used.

His bones ached, his tongue was loaded, and his breath smelled badly. The mortification was hard and painful, bluish and mottled, with great burning and sharp cutting pains. It spread some distance around and the heat was intense. He took *Tarentula cubensis* 12x (there and then), one powder, saying that he was poisoned. He complained of a wild feeling in his brain and a drawing sensation in his scalp and muscles of his face. He was in a great state of mental anxiety, and said he felt as if he was going to loose his reason. Mental restlessness was marked in his countenance. He could not keep quiet, even after I assured him that he was in no danger. His primary symptoms had nearly gone, and the bubo had lost its bad colour. The next day he was much improved in a general way, and the bubo had nearly disappeared. I saw him again in three days, and the improvement was going on rapidly. The chancre healed rapidly, and in one month, he told me he had never been so well.

CHAPTER 18

Chancroid

Synonym : Soft chancre, soft sore.

It is an uncommon venereal disease compared with syphilis or gonorrhoea. Nevertheless, one comes across it quite frequently, chancroid being the third most common venereal disease.

The incidence of this disease is greater in tropical countries than in countries that have temperate or cold climates. The people most commonly affected are usually those whose economic status is low and those negligent of personal hygiene. The disease is very common among males. Very few females cases are seen, although such cases have been known to act as asymptomatic carriers of infection.

Etiology : The causative organism is Ducrey's bacillus which is a gramnegative strepto-bacillus, 1.5μ by 0.5μ, found in small groups or chains, usually outside the cells. Infection is transmitted by sexual contact in the great majority of cases, although accidental infection by infected material is possible.

Clinical Features : In the male, the lesions usually appear near the frenum (junction of the prepucial skin with the glans), on the corona, the undersurface of the prepuce, glans penis and on the external urinary meatus. In the female, the infection rarely shows lesions; but when present, ulcers are seen on the labia, or in the fold between the inner surface of the thigh and the groin. Occasionally, the urinary meatus may be affected. The incubation period is 3 to 5 days, may be as short as 24 hours.

Chancroid starts as a small papule, which increases in size and becomes a pustule. This pustule breaks down to form a shallow ulcer with ragged, irregular margins; its floor is raw, of pale red colour, and has a typical sieve like appearance. The ulcer is always free of induration and bleeds freely on friction with clothes or physical manipulation.

Many more such lesions develop on the surrounding areas as described above, by the process of **auto-inoculation.** These multiple lesions present a rosette appearance. They may fuse with each other forming large ragged areas. An extra-genital spread is uncommon.

The constitutional symptoms consist of acute pain and tenderness in the affected areas; occasional headaches, and slight pyrexia, especially when superadded infection with pyogenic organisms takes place; this also results in spreading the local lesions.

Complications : The disease may take an uneventful course and subside after a few weeks; but with the spread of infection, local irritation, secondary infection with pyogenic organisms, the following complications may set in :

1. **Inflammatory phimosis** : Due to oedema of the prepuce causing difficulty in retraction. Haemorrhage from the frenal artery may also occur.

2. **Bubo formation** : It is the usual sequela of the disease. The bubo starts firstly, as a painful enlargement of the inguinal glands usually in one groin. The swelling is smooth, globular and tender to touch. After a few days, softening and fluctuation occur, and finally ulceration takes place with the rupture of the overlying skin by a single opening (cf. L.G.V. bubo which has multiple

openings). The ulcer formed has, once again, ragged margins and a dirty, sloughy base; it continues to discharge sero-sanguineous and purulent material.

3. Balanitis and balano-posthitis which are particularly common amongst non-circumcised persons.

4. **Phagedena** : This is the most dreaded complication. It results from secondary infection with micro-organisms like Vincent's spirilla and fusiform bacillus. The lesion becomes very ugly and foul smelling and the margins almost black, and spreads rapidly.

Diagnosis : The diagnosis is arrived at by :

1. The typical clinical features.

2. A history of exposure, and the appearance of sores within the incubation period.

3. A smear examination of material taken from the deeper parts of the margin of the ulcer and by staining this with Gram's stain.

4. A culture examination by a swab rubbed on a suitable medium in which defibrinated rabbit blood is added.

5. **The Ito-Reenstierna test** : This is done by an intradermal injection of 0.1 to 0.2 cc of vaccine prepared from the pus of an infected case. A positive reaction is indicated, if after 48 hours the site that has been injected with vaccine shows a papule of 5 mm diameter with erythema all around.

6. **The Dark-ground Illumination Test:** For spirochaetes of syphilis, and also a serological test for syphilis should form a routine diagnostic procedure to rule out any concomitant infection.

Differential diagnosis : It is to be made from all diseases causing an inflammatory genital lesion (a sore), viz., primary sore of syphilis, herpes progenitalis, dermatitis resulting from irritants or medicines, epithelioma, granuloma venereum and lymphogranuloma venereum (for distinguishing features, refer to Table 18.1). In scabies, secondary pyoderma may produce boils and pyogenic ulcers, but features like nocturnal pruritus and burrows are obvious.

Treatment : The treatment resolves itself into :

(a) Local applications.
(b) Internal medication.
(c) Treatment of complications.

Local Applications

The affected parts should be washed with a warm antiseptic, calendula.

Homoeopathic Approach

Kindly refer to the Chapter on Syphilis.

Table 18.1

Lymphogranuloma Venereum Bubo	*Chancroid Bubo*
1. The primary lesion is absent or healed.	1. The primary lesion is always present.
2. Slow evolution.	2. Quick evolution
3. Involvement of several glands.	3. Involvement of a single gland only.
4. Illiac adenopathy is invariably present.	4. Illiac adenopathy is absent.
5. Multiple areas of fluctuation	5. Single fluctuant swelling.
6. The skin is thickened and rugose. The bubo retains its shape after rupture.	6. The skin is thin and collapses when the abscess bursts.
7. The pus is sterile. The elementary bodies may be demonstrated by special staining.	7. Ducrey bacilli may be demonstrated in the pus, or scraping from the wall of abscess.
8. Frei test is positive	8. Ito-Reenstierna test is positive.
9. Complaint fixation test for L.G.V. is positive.	9. Complement fixation test for L.G.V. is negative.
10. Hyperglobulinemia is a constant feature.	10. No change in the serum proteins.

Granuloma Venereum

Several confusing synonyms exist; but it is always preferable to know one name and be sure of it. It is a chronic, mildly contagious disease, caused by Donovania granulomatis (distinct from Leishman — Donovan bodies, which cause leishmaniasis). They are gram-negative, encapsulated bodies present mostly inside the mononuclear cells. The disease is transmitted either through sexual contact with an infected individual or by infected vectors. It is mostly venereal in origin.

Incubation period. It varies from 8 to 60 days.

Clinical features : The lesions occur mainly on the genitalia. In the male, the prepuce and glans penis, and in the female, the labia are the sites of choice. The disease begins in the form of a papule which soon becomes a nodule; this progresses slowly to take the form of an ulcer or a papillomatous and vegetative nodule. Lesions in granuloma venereum are characteristically raw, red and beefy in appearance. Elephantiasis of the labia, penis or scrotum may also occur. The mucous membranes and viscera are usually spared. The regional lymph glands are not involved but pseudo-bubo may be seen. The course of the disease is slow and prolonged in the absence of modern treatment; the prognosis, though, has improved remarkably since antibiotics have come into use.

Diagnosis : It is confirmed by the demonstration of Donovan bodies in the lesions. Cultures and animal inoculations are, generally speaking, not helpful; serological tests for syphilis, however, should always be carried out to exclude syphilis, the most important of the venereal diseases. Sometimes, it may resemble epithelioma, hence careful examination is necessary.

Treatment : It is specific and consists of

(1) A course of streptomycin 1.0 gm. twice a day inframuscularly for 10 days. When administering streptomycin, what must be remembered are the toxic symptoms produce, like giddiness, tinnitus, deafness and dermatitis.

(2) Locally, antibiotic creams like bacitracin are helpful.

(3) Gloves should be worn while dressing the affected part. Penicillin and sulphonamides have no action.

Very good results have been reported with the systemic use of chloramphenicol and tetracycline. Since these are also successful against lymphogranuloma venereum, chancriods, gonorrheea and even syphilis, all venereal diseases, they hae become particularly important in treatment.

Lymphogranuloma Venereum

It is a contagious, venereal granuloma differing from granuloma venereum in one important aspect; it rapidly involves the lymphatic system. It is caused by chlamydia which is similar to chlamydia trachomatis organism, of 0.25 x 0.5 μ size.

Mode of infection. Infection is transmitted by sexual intercourse. Medical practitioners, nurses and laboratory workers can accidentally pick up the disease by handling infected material.

Usually young adults are affected; but no age is exempt. Localization of the disease differs in the two sexes; in the female, the genital and/or the ano-rectal regions are predominantly involved; in the male, the inguinal region. This is because of the difference in lymphatic drainage in the two sexes. Females are often asymptomatic carriers of the disease.

Incubation Period. It is ordinarily about a week.

Clinical features. The primary lesions is frequently not noticed by the patient. The most common type of primary lesions is the superficial, painless vesicle wich lasts a short while, and heals without scarring. In a small percentage of cases, the initial vascular lesions progress into an ulcer or a bacterial urethritis. In the male, the primary lesions usually occur on the corona and prepuce; in the female, the lesions are seen usually on the fourchette, the posterior half of the labia majora and the posterior wall of the vagina. Often, the primary lesions may be unnoticed.

One to three weeks after the primary lesions (on the average about two weeks after exposure), subacute inguinal adenitis develops. The adenitis is usually unilateral. To begin with, the glands are painful, tender, swollen and elastic. Soon they become matted and begin to soften, producing suppuration (bubo).

Less commonly, the adenitis becomes chronic and indolent. The pelvic and iliac glands may also be involved, but they rarely suppurate. The adenitis is accompanied by constitutional disturbance. The patient feels weak and feverish, suffers from headache and loss of appetite.

The adenitis is followed later by chronic genital and anorectal manifestations produced by hyperplastic or ulcerative changes or such as result from interference with the lymphatic system. Elephantiasis of the genitalia (esthiomene), rectal and vaginal strictures and chronic ulceration are the common late effects.

Manifestations of lymphogranuloma venereum are rarely seen extragenitally. One sometimes comes across an erythema-multiforme-like rash. The eyes, lungs and the meningeal membrane of the brain are rarely involved.

Prognosis : Lymphogranuloma venereum is a slowly progressive disease, resulting in considerable mutilation of the genitalia, anus and rectum and hence, causes a great deal of misery. Delay in treatment results in disfiguring and troublesome sequelae left by the healed lesions. So, a quick diagnosis and immediate treatment are essential. The outlook is good if treatment is given in time and corectly.

Diagnosis : It is confirmed by :

1. The demonstration of elementary bodies in the smears of bubo pus by Giemsa's stain. A microscopic examination helps to rule out related venereal diseases like chancroid.

2. **The Frei's Intradermal Test** : Pus from the lymphogranuloma bubo is used as the antigen, being intradermally injected on the flexor surface of the forearm. The result is read 48 hours later. An infiltrated papule is seen in positive cases.

3. The complement fixation test is usually positive.

4. The blood shows an increased level of serum globulin. An S.T.S. should be done to exclude any concomitant infection with syphilis. But biological false positive reactions may also be seen.

Gonorrhoea

Gonorrhoea is one of the most common sexually transmitted diseases all over the world. This is caused by Neisseria gonorrhoeae, which is present throughout the world. Since several strains of N. gonorrhoeae have developed penicillin resistance due to the production of betalactamase the disease increased in frequency and distribution. Due to altered sex practices the manifestations have extended to several areas in the body.

Gonococci attach themselves to cells with the help of pili before initiating infection. The organisms are ingested by polymorphs and they survive within the cells for variable periods, being protected from adverse environment. Four types can be distinguished by cultural characteristics. Types T_1/T_2 are virulent whereas T_3/T_4 are not.

Pathology : Gonococci affect columnar and transitional epithelium mainly, and infection is initiated in the urethra, anal canal, conjunctiva pharynx, and endocervix. Pus is produced locally. Direct extention from the site of infection leads to complication such as endometritis, salpingitis, peritonitis, and bartholinitis in the female, and periurethral abscess, epidi-dymo-orchitis, and prostatitis in the male. Ocular conjunctiva is affected. Metastatic spread of the organisms leads to arthritis, dermatitis, endocarditis, meningitis, myopericarditis, and hepatitis.

Clinical features : In the male the onset of the disease is more smart and acute than in women. Incubation period is usually 3 to 5 days.

Gonorrhoea in the male : In over 90% of cases urethritis presents with a constant burning sensation in the penis and discharge of infective pus which teems with the organisms. Meatal inflammation and penile oedema may be obvious. Variable amounts of pus can be milked from the urethra. Micturition is painful and the patient is severely distressed. Other adnexal structures like epidydymis, testes; and spermatic cord become inflamed. Rarely inflammation of the Tyson's gland and the medien raphe of the scrotum may develop. Gonococcal prostatitis and seminal vesiculitis are seen but they are rare. If left alone, the acute manifestations subside over a period of weeks or months even without treatment. Exacerbations occur frequently as a result of sexual indulgence, alcoholism, or undue exertion. Ultimately the anterior and, posterior urethra develop stricture. Periurethral abscesses may develop at times. Extention of suppuration into the periurethral tissues and scrotum result in fistulous openings discharging urine from multiple sites (water-can scrotum). In 10% of subjects the lesion may be asymptomatic and has to be detected by examination.

The rectum is an important site of ulceration in persons who are habitual catamites in homo-sexual relationship. The rectum and anal canal are ulcerated and show blood-stained mucopurulent discharge. The condition may present as proctitis and may be mistaken for other ulcerating lesions of this region.

Gonorrhoea in the female : In a good number of women gonorrrhoea may remain asymptomatic. Symptoms include leucorrhoea, dysuria, menstrual abnormalities and features of pelvic inflammation.

Rectal lesions develop in about 40% of affected women due to contamination by cervical discharges.

The gonococci may pass up from the endocervix leading to acute salpingitis and oophoritis. Chronic salpingo-oophoritis and tubo-ovarian masses may develop. Exacerbations occur during menstrual periods or one or two weeks thereafter. Gonococcal salpingo-oophoritis is a common cause of sterility.

Gonococcal infection in the newborn : Inoculation of gonococci into the baby's eyes from the maternal genital passages leads to ophthalmia neonatorum. This presents with purulent conjunctivities which may result in blindness. The infection can also disseminate to other tissues and result in arthritis in the newborn.

Disseminated gonococcal infection : This occurs in upto 30% of infected patients, 80% of them being females. Bacteremic spread occurs. Manifestations include cutaneous lesions, septic arthritis, septicemia, endocarditis, myocarditis, and rarely pericarditis and meningitis. Risk of dissemination depends on the type and virulence of the organism. Dissemination is more common from silent foci in the pharynx, rectum, or endocervix. The cutaneous lesions take the form of vesicles and pustules which do not usually ulcerate.

Dorpharyngeal infection : Pharyngitis and tonsillitis result, from oral sex and may affect both sexes. In the majority of cases symptoms are not severe enough to seek medical care. Strong clinical suspicion and microbiological investigations are required to make the diagnosis. Gonococcal pharyngitis may give rise to dissemination.

Diagnosis : Gonorrhoea should be suspected in all clinical situations where there is purulent urethral discharge, leucorrhoea in women, a typical oropharyngeal ulceration, proctocolitis and ophthalmia neonatorum. Bacteriological diagnosis is established by demonstrating Gram-negative diplococci inside polymorphonuclear cells in the exudates. The organism can be indentified by culture and further studies. Culture of cervical discharge is required in women with late manifestations to establish the diagnosis. On rare occasions purulent material may have to be collected by culdocentesis or laparoscopy. Fluorescent antibody techniques help in making quick diagnosis where such facilities exist. Complement fixation text is useful in selected cases of chronic gonorrhoea with systemic manifestations.

Homoeopathic Approach : Patients suffering from gonorrhoea can present to a homoeopath with multiple symptoms.

1. Acute Gonorrhoea.

2. Chronic Gonorrhoea (Sycosis) : (i) Gonorrhoeal stricture, (ii) Gonorrhoeal prostatitis, (iii) Gonorrhoeal cystitis, (iv) Gonorrhoeal opthalmic, (v) Gonorrhoeal, (vi) Rheumatism, (vii) Chordae. (Gonococcal), (viii) Disseminated gonococcal infection.

It is essential to know the philosophy of chronic miasm before one handles serious illnesses like gonorrhoea. After the disappearance of the discharge (under any non-homoeopathic treatment), the disease is in 90% of cases not cured, but remains latent, not only locally but constitutionally, what we commonly call as Sycotic constitution the ignorant patient remains in dark for quite a long time till the symptoms of sycosis come to the surface in the form of (a) poor general health, (b) sterility, (c) rheumatic troubles, (d) cauliflower like excrescences, etc.

Whenever a patient comes to a homoeopath with symptoms which resemble sycotic trait and there is a past history of gonorrhoea then he should be treated with anti-sycotic remedy till the previous discharge from the urethra has been brought back, then only in true sense we can label the person to be cured.

To achieve the right selection of anti-sycotic one has to jump two hurdles: (1) Recognition of the sycotic state by detailed case taking: (ii) Interposing intercurrent remedy like Medorrhinum, Sycotico and Thuja rationally whenever the cases demand.

Whilst taking the history the following points should be paid attention to carefully :

(1) Note down carefully the patients presenting symptoms chronologically and then evaluate the complication, chronicity and type of gonorrhoea (disseminated genital, oropharyngeal) etc.

(2) Review the previous investigation reports and confirm your clinical diagnosis.

(3) Whilst writing the symptoms, stress should be on the following points:

   (a) Characteristic of discharge.
   (b) The local appearance of genitalia.
   (c) Sexual history including erections.
   (d) Symptoms related to testes.
   (e) H/O previous treatment.
   (f) Special sensation in relation to urethra and bladder. *Example* — Drop running up and down in the course of urethra.

   Sensation of dryness in urethra.

The principal remedy often called for in the treatment of gonorrhoeal affection with the leading characteristics is as follows :

Agave Americana	: Extremely painful erections. Great difficulty in passing urine, accompanied by heat, pain and tenesmus at neck of bladder. Chordee. Drawing in the spermatic cords and testicles, extending to thighs, so violent that he wishes to die.
Agnus Castus	: Testes cold, swollen, hard; penis small, flaccid. Impotence with gleet, especially with those who have frequently had gonorrhoea. Yellow, purulent discharge from the urethra, especially in old sinners; or after inflammation has subsided. Disagreeable and uneasy feeling in back part of urethra with frequent desire to urinate. Sexual desire almost lost. Penis so relaxed that voluptuous fancies excite, no erection.
Argentum Nitricum	: Frequently indicated in acute gonorrhoea. Ulcerative pain in the middle of urethra, as from a splinter. Urging to urinate; urine passes less easily and freely. Urine burns while passing, urethra feels as if swollen, with feeling as if the last drops remained behind, causing a sensation of internal sore swelling. Towards the end of urination, sensation, as if the urethra was knotted or closed. Itching and tickling in the urethra. Chordee. Stricture of the urethra.
Camphora	: Gonorrhoea, with constant sticking together of the meatus.

Chordee.
Retention of urine; stranguary.
Stranguary from stricture following gonorrhoea, urine passes in a thin stream, and is very acrid.

Cannabis Indica: Burning and scalding, or stinging pain in the urethra, before during and after urination. Urging to urinate with much straining, but cannot pass a drop, or has to wait some time before urine flows.
Priapism.
The urine dribbles out after the stream ceases.
White glairy mucus may be squeezed from urethra.

Cannabis Sativa: Discharge from urethra thin, watery, of disagreeable odour.
Discharge of pus from urethra.
Burning when urinating , but especially just after; stream forked.
Great swelling of prepuce, phimosis.
Meatus inflamed and painful to touch.
Penis sore, as if burnt, when walking, walks with legs apart.
Stranguary.
Swelling of the prostate.
Urine bloody.
Pressing, dragging sensation in the testicles, when standing.
Dark redness of glans and prepuce.
In females : Cutting pain in the labiae during urination; urethra plugged with pus.

Cantharis : Violent pains in the bladder with frequent urging, intolerable tenesmus.
Violent burning-cutting pain in neck of bladder extending to fossa navicularis, worse before and after urinating.
Fruitless effort to urinate.
Constant burning, desire to urinate,

passing only a few drops at a time, often mixed with blood.
Yellow or bloody discharge.
Retention of urine and tenesmus vesicae when discharge is suppressed by injections.
Retention of urine with pain.
Before, during and after urination, cutting pains in urethra.
In females : "Burning heat of the external parts. Swelling of the vulva and vagina with itching, burning, and a thick white discharge." (Carleton)

Capsicum : Discharge from urethra; purulent; bloody; urethra painful to touch; discharge cream-like.
Prepuce swollen.
"Burning biting, cutting pains in the urethra, between acts of urination, most marked at the meatus."
Strangury, tenesmus of the neck of the bladder; he has urging to frequent, almost ineffectual urination.
Painful erection at night.
Especially indicated in the fat and indolent, with lax fibre.

Chimaphila Umbellata : Stricture, difficult urination.
Urine contains large quantity of ropy mucus.
Tensesmus of the bladder.
Acute and chronic cystitis.
Inability to pass urine without standing with the feet widely separated.
Acute inflammation of the prostate, with a feeling, as if a ball in the perineum.
Urine is highly coloured with a bloody, greenish or reddish sediment.

Cinnabaris : Gonorrhoea on a sycotic base or complicated with syphilis, of very long-standing, with much soreness and pain during micturition.

Warts on the prepuce, bleeding from the slightest touch, with swelling and itching, soreness on urinating.
Violent itching of corona glandis, with profuse secretion of pus.

Clematis : Painful, inflamed and swollen testicles.
Induration of testicles, which are as hard as stone.
Right spermatic cord sensitive, testicles drawn up.
Pain and burning while urinating, most severe at commencement.
Mucus in urine, but no pus.

Digitalis : Burning in urethra with purulent discharge, thick and bright yellow.
Glans inflamed with copious secretion of thick pus over its surface.
Inflammation of the neck of bladder.
In the right testicle the pain, as if contused.
Chordee.
Dropsical swelling of prepuce.

Gelsemium : "At the very beginning of Urethritis (Acon) with great pain and scanty discharge or little pain with much heat, urine voided in sufficient quantities, rather frequent, with smarted at meatus."
Whitish discharge.
Genitals cold, relaxed; dragging in testicles.
Suppressed gonorrhoea; followed by rheumatism or orchitis.
Gleet with stricture of urethra; sensation as if something remained behind when urinating, stream stops and commences again.
Constant dribbling of urine from muscular weakness.

Hydradtid : Acute of chronic form.
In second stage, copious, persistent discharge without pain or soreness in

urethra, discharge being thick, yellow, tenacious.
Gleet with copious, painless discharge and debility.
Feeling of debility and faintness after stool.

Kali Bichromicum : Gleet with profuse stringy or jelly-like discharge.
Pain across back with red urine.
After micturition, burning in back part of urethra, with sensation, as if one drop had remained behind, with unsuccessful effort to void it. Perforating sycotic ulcers about glans and prepuce.

Medorrhinum : "Burning in meatus during urination, feeling of soreness in urethra, and after urination feeling, as if something remained in urethra; profuse, yellow, purulent discharge, most copious in morning gumming up orifice; frequent calls to urinate." (Lilienthal)

Merc-Sol : Gonorrhoea with phimosis or chancroids.
Greenish discharge, worse at night.
Lips of meatus red and inflamed.
Glans penis dark red and hot, with burning, stinging, itching pains in urethra.
Stranguary.
Tenesmus.
Painful erections.
Glans and prepuce inflamed; Phimosis.
In female: Inflammation of vulva, which is swollen red and hot.
Aggravation from cold air.
Gonorrhoeal Cystitis.
Urine turbid.

Mezereum : A drop of gluey, albuminous liquid appears at times at the orifices of the urethra.
Discharge of watery mucus, increased by exercise.

Itching of the prepuce.
Heat, swelling and titillation along the course of the urethra.
Perineum sore and tender to touch.
Gleet with green discharge in the absence of any other remedy.

Natrum-Mur : Chronic Gonorrhoea, after injections of Silver nitrate.
Clear, sometimes yellowish discharge in gleet.
Cutting pain in urethra after urination.
Itching, crawling sensation at the corona glandis.

Nitric Acid : Gonorrhoea with chancres and warts.
Small blisters on orifice of urethra and inner surface of prepuce.
Bloody mucous or purulent discharge.
Pricking pain in urethra.
While urinating, smarting, burning in urethra.
Ulcers in urethra.
Urine very offensive.
Gleet.
Phimosis.
Itching, swelling and burning in vulva and vagina.

Pareira : Violent pain in urethra, with stranguary:
Violent pain in glans penis, with straining.
Severe pain when passing urine.
Discharge of mucus from urethra.

Pulsatilla : Discharge from urethra thick, muco-purulent, yellow or yellowish-green.
Gonorrhoeal rheumatism.
Orchitis and prostatitis.
Suppressed gonorrhoea causes orchitis.
Itching, burning on inner and upper side of prepuce.

Sarsaparilla : Rheumatism from suppressed gonorrhoea.
Severe pain at conclusion of urination.
Severe tenesmus of bladder.
Gonorrhoea checked by cold, wet weather, or by Mercury, followed by rheumatism.

Sepia : Gleet, no pain; discharge only during the night, a drop or so staining the linen yellowish.
Urine turbid and offensive.
Condylomata, from suppressing. Gonorrhoea with astringent injection.
Chronic cystitis.
Urine is so offensive that it must be removed at once.
Foetid urine, with reddish, clay-coloured sediment adhering to the chamber.

Sulphur : Burning in orifice of urethra, during micturition.
Bright redness and inflammation of orifice of urethra.
Discharge thick and purulent, or thin and watery.
Phimosis; prepuce inflamed and indurated. (Digitalis — not indurated.)
Phimosis, with discharge of fetid pus.

Terebinthina : Gonorrhoea with strangury, tenesmus of bladder, smarting in urethra; Chordee, painful; urination every ten minutes, better by micturition.
Haematuria.
Gonorrhoeal rheumatism.
Gleet.

Thuja : Discharge thin and greenish or yellow, with scalding pain during urination.
Urethra swollen stream of urine forked; after urination, sensation as if a drop remained behind; titillation, as though a drop of urine was passing along urethra;

urging to urinate frequently and hastily stream interrupted; red erosions on glans.
Perspiration on genitals, especially on scrotum, sweet smelling like honey.
Warty growths on genitals.
Articular rheumatism, especially of knee-joint after checked gonorrhoea.
Checked gonorrhoea causes prostatitis;
Sycosis; impotence.
Paresis-like weakness in extremities.
Sleeplessness.
Falling off of hair.
Urine clear when passed, but becomes cloudy on standing.

GONORRHOEA

Acon, Agar, Agn, Aloe, Alum, Alumn, Am-m, Amyl, Anag, Ant-c, Apis, Arg-n, Ars, Ars-s, Aur-m, Baros, Bar-m, Benz-ac, Bor, Bism, Calc, Calc-p, Calc-s, Camph, Cann-i, Cann-s, Canth, Caps, Caulo, Cedr, Cham, Chel, Chim-ump, Cinnb, Clem, Cochl, Cob, Cap, Cub, ***Cupr-ar, Dig, Dory, Echin, Equis, Erig, Ery-a, Eucal, Euphorb-pil, Fabiana, Ferr, Ferr-i, Ferr-p, Fl-ac, Gels, graph, Guaiac, Ham, Hep, Hydras, Hydrocot, Ichthy, Jacar, Kali-brom, Kali-chl, Kali-i, Kali-m, Kali-s, Kreos, lac-c, Led, lachn, Lyc, Lith, Med, Merc, Merc-c, Merc-i-r, Merc-s, Merc-v, Methyl-br, Mez, Millef, Nat-m, Nat-s, Nit-x, Nux-v, Naph, Ol-sant, Pareira, Petr, Petrosel, Phos, Ph-ac, Phyt, Pichl, Pin-c, Plb, Psor, Puls, Rhod, Sabad, Sabal, Sabina, Salix-n, Sars, Senecia, Sep, Silm, Stigm, Stilling, Sulph, Trarent, Tereb, Thuj, Tritic, Tassil, Zing.***

Acute, inflammatory stage — *Acon, Arg-n, Atrop, Can-s, Canth, Caps, Gels, Petros.*
Adenitis, lymphangitis — *Acon, spis, Bell, Hep, Merc.*
Bubo — *Aur-m-n, Bad, Bufo, Carb-an, Lac-c, Lach, Merc, Merc-c, Nit-ac, Phyt, Syph.*
Burning during urination — *Carb-an*
Chordee can only be subdued in cold water — *Caps*
Chordee with frequent priapism — *Petrosel*
Chordee in 2nd stage — *Kali-m*
Chordee — *Acon, Agare, Anac, Arg-n, Bell, Berb, Camph, Cann-i, Cann-s, Canth, Caps, Clem, Colch, Cop, Dig, Eryng,*

Fl-ac, Gels, Jacar, Hyos, Kali-br, Kali-m, Merc, Mygale, Nit-ac, Oenanthe, Ol-sant, **Petrosel,** *Phos, Pic-ac, Pip-m, Puls, Salix-n, Still, Tereb, Tussil, Thuj, Yohimb, Zinc.*

Chronic, subacute stage — *Arg-n, Can-s, Cop, Cub, Erig, Hep, Hydr, Kali-s, Merc-c, Merc-i-r, Merc, Naph, Nat-s, Ol-sant, Pin-c, Psor, Puls, Rhad, Sabal, Sep, Sil Stigm, Sulph, Thuj.*

Coition — renewed by — *Thuj*

Cowperitis — *Acon, Can-s, Gels, Hep, Merc-c, Petros, Pichi, Sabal, Sil.*

Constitution in anaemic persons, chronic — *Calc-p*

— in blonde men of light temperament — *Puls*

— in dark, irritable vindicative men — *Nit-ac*

— in elderly men, difficult urination — *Agar*

— in gleet of old sinners — *Agnus*

Sanguine, full-blooded — *Acon*

— with scrofula — *Hep*

— in strong men, particularly of hydrogenoid constitution in timid nervous men, acute — *Gels*

Discharge — night — *Merc, Merc-c, Sep.*

Discharge night only — *Sep*

Discharge chronic — *Alum, Alumn, Arg-m, Brom, Calc, Calc-p, Calc-s, Chim, Chlor, Cinnb, Colch, Cub, Cupr, Ferr, Hydr, Kali-s Med, Mygal, Myric, Nat-m, Nat-s, Petr, Petros, Plb, Psor, Sep, Sil, Sulph, Thuj.*

Discharge — acrid, exceriating — *Arg-n, Aur-m, Caps, Cop, Gels, Hydr, Kreos,* **Merc-c, Sars, Thuj,**

Discharge albuminous, yellow — *Petrosel*

Discharge black — *Nat-m*

Discharge bloody — *Ant-c, Arg-n, Calc-s, Canth, Cap, Cub, Ham, Merc-c, Millef, Nit-ac, Puls.*

Discharge — bloody, watery slime — *Millef*

Discharge clean transparent — *Mez, Nat-m, Phos-ac.*

Discharge constant — *Ars-s-f*

Discharge copious — *Ars-s-f*

Discharge creamlike — *Caps*

Discharge fetid — *Benz-ac, Carb-v, Puls, Sil.*

Discharge free and mucoid — *Merc-i-r*

Discharge folliculitis — *Caps, Hep, Merc-s, Sep, Sil.*

Discharge green — *Cann-s, Merc, Mer-c, Nit-ac, Thuj.*

Discharge green painless — *Merc*

Discharge purulent, worse at night — *Merc*

Discharge yellowish green thick — *Cannb, Nat-s.*
Lumpy — *Calc-s*
— **increase after having decreased** — *Bry, Lil-t, Sep, Sulph, Thuj.*
Milky — *Cop, Lach, Petrosel.*
Milky, glairy, mucus — *Cann-i, Cann-s, Cop, Cupr-ars, Graph, Hydr.*
Mucous — *Caps, Ferr, Kali-bi, Nat-m, Petr, Puls, Sep.*
Muco — purulent — *Benz-ac*
Muco - purulent yellowish green — *Agn, Alum, Arg-n, Baros, Cann-s, Canth, Caps, Cob, Cop, Cub, Dig, Hep, Hydr, Jacar, Kali-i, Kali-s, Merc-c, Merc, Nat-m, Nat-s, Ol-sant, Puls, Sab, Sep, Sil, Sulph, Thuj, Tussil, Zing.*
Painless — *Cann-i*
Profuse — *Arg-m, Cann-i.*
— **usually profuse, inflammation very high** — *Petrosel*
Profuse - puslike after 2 months — *Cub*
Profuse and scalding urine — *Cub*
Profuse -- yellowish white — *Sep*
Purulent — *Agn, Bar-c, Cann-s, Caps, Chel, Con, Cop, Nat-m, Phos, Ph-ac.*
Purulent -- yellow mucus or greenish — *Kali-s*
— **of pus** -- *Chel, Sil.*
Glutinous — *Cub*
— **of pus with inflammation** — *Sabina*
Puslike bloody — *Sil*
Variable as to quantity — *Cup-m*
Scanty — *Colch*
Scanty : thick — *Rhus-t*
Slight shreddy — *Sil*
Syphilitis in — *Aur-m, Cinnb, Merc, Merc-c.*
Thick — *Calc-s, Cann-s,*
Thick greenish — *Kali-i*
Thick worse at night — *Merc*
— **of thick pus** — *Clem, Cub.*
— **thick after six weeks** — *Cub*
— **at first thin, then thick** - *Mer-c*
Watery — *Cann-s, Fl-ac, Mez, Millef, Nat-m, Sep, Sulph. Thuj.*
Watery mucous — *Cann-s, Fl-ac, Mez, Nat-m, Thuj.*
Whitest — *Gels*
Yellowish white — *Cann-i*

Yellow — *Agn, Ars-s-f, Calc-s, Canth, Caps, Cop, Hep, Nat-m, Nit-ac, Sars, Thuj.*
Yellow worse at night — *Merc*
Stains shirt light yellow, not profuse — *Tarent*
Thick yellow or yellow green — *Puls*
Yellow after 6 weeks — *Cub*
Yellowish or bloody — *Nit-ac.*
Drugs : after abuse of copaiva and cubeba, thin discharge, with burning on urination and frequent urging to stool — *Nux-v*
Dry — *Canth*
Eruptions : following suppressed gonorrhoea — *Clem*
Fever : Febrile disturbance during inflammatory stage — *Acon, Cop, Gels.*
First stage — *Acon, Cann-s, Colch, Cop, Ferr-p, Gels.*
Gleet — *Abies-c, Agar, Agn, Alum, Alumn, Aur-m,. Arg-n, Bar-c, Bar-m, Benz-ac, Bov, Bry, Calad, Calc, Calc-p, Calc-s, Cann-i, Cann-s, Canth, Carb-s, Carb-v, Caps, Chimaph, Cinnb, Cedr, Cinch-b, Clem, Cub, Cupr, Dory, Dulc, Erig, Ering, Ferr, Ferr-p, Fl-ac, Gamb, Graph, Hep, Hydras, Kali-bi, Kali-i, Kali-s, Lyc, Med, Merc, Merc-c, Mez, Mur-ac, Millef, Naph, Nat-m, Nat-s, Nit-ac, Nux-v, Ol-sant, Petr, Pet-rosel, Ph-ac, Phos, Phyt, Plb, Pop-tr, Puls, Pip-m, Sabal, Sabina, Sang, Selen, Sencio, Sep, Sil, Stilling, Sulph, Tell, Tereb, Thuja, Zinc-mur, Zinc.*
— **bad cases** — *Nit-ac*
— **burning** — *Bry*
Chronic — *Agar, Agn, Chim-umb, Ferr.*
— **discharge clear** — *Nat-m*
Chronic with mucopulent discharge — *Cop*
— **with debility** — *Hydros*
— **discharge copious** — *Cub*
— **white painless discharge, more towards morning** — *Mez.*
— **discharge pale** — *Cub*
— **discharge scanty** — *Phos*
— **discharge slimy** — *Cub*
— **discharge causing soiled linen to become stiff** — *Cub*
— **discharge stringy or jelly-like, profuse** — *Kali-bi*
— **discharge thick** — *Hydras*
— **discharge thin, day and night, with formication over body** — *Ced*

— **with eczema latent or visible** — *Kali-m*
— **in fat, lymphatic persons** — *Calc*
— **with disposition to glandular swellings** — *Kali-m*
— **green** — *Bry, Nat-m.*
Yellowish green — *Merc*
— **light headed** — *Cann-i*
— **much heat, little pain** — *Gels*
— **with impotence** — *Agnus*
Intensely itching — *Nat-m*
— **a drop of viscid fluid glues meatus** — *Tell*
— **with sticking together of meatus** — *Camph*
Meatus stuck together in morning — *Sep*
— **worse in morning** — *Aur-m, Aur-n, Ph-ac, Phos, Sep,*
— **at night, staining linen yellow** — *Fl-ac, Sep.*
— **during night, a drop or so staining linen yellowish** — *Sep.*
— **in orchitis after mismanaged gonorrhoea** — *Clem*
Painless — *Agar, Alum, Arg-m, Bar-c, Cann-s, Cop, Ferr, Hep, Hydr, Kali-i, Med, Merc, Mez, Nat-m, Nat-s, Petr, Psor, Puls, Sang, Sep, Sulph, Thuj.*
Prostatic — *Selen*
Protracted — *Caps*
Purulent — *Bar-c, Merc*
Secondary — *Iris*
With want of sexual desire — *Agnus*
Sexual organs debilitated from seminal emissions — *Sep*
Watery — *Mur-ac*
-- **a few drop of white, in morning** — *Ph-ac*
-- **of ten years duration** — *Sulph*
Twelve years duration — *Psor*
for twenty years — *Med*
Yellowish — *Sep*
Yellowish, before urination — *Bar-c*
Last stage — *Nat-m, Sep.*
From leucorrhoea — *Cop*
-- **acrid, or from menstrual discharge** — *Nat-m*
Maltreated — *Brom*
Rheumatism — *Acon, Arg-n, Calc-i, Canth, Clem, Cop, Fl-ac, Gels, Iod, Kali-i, Jacar, Merc, Pr-rub, Merc, Nux-v, Ol-sant, Par, Petrol, Phyt, Puls, Sabina, Sep, Sil, Sulph, Sul-i, Thiosin, Thuj.*
Second stage — *Cal-s, Caps, Kali-m, Sulph.*

— **in first part, when discharge is moderate, much urinary irritation** — *Cop*

— **thick yellow discharge** — *Hydras*

Secondary — *Agnus, Cup-m, Ferr-s, Gels, Hydrocot, Iris, Selen, Tell.*

-- **greenish discharge** — *Kob*

Sequelac — *Agar, Benz-ac.*

Delirium — *Camph, Coca, Kali-s, Merc, Zinc.*

-- **pain in hypogastric region** — *Camph*

-- **impotence** — *Thuja*

Urethra, Chronic itching — *Nit-ac*

-- **after orchitis, hydrocele with sexual weakness** — *Phos*

Prostatitis chronic — *Sulph*

Pulse, weak, rapid — *Camph*

-- **loss of sexual feeling, abuse of Copaiva** — *Lyc*

Spermatic cord swollen — *Cinch*

Strangury from stricture — *Camph*

Stricture — *Cic, Indig, Nit-ac, Thuj*

Testicles, contusive pain — *Arg-m*

Testicles enlargement — *Ham*

Testicles induration of — *Rhod*

Testicles inflamed — *Merc*

Testicles pain in left — *Merc*

Testicles shocks of severe drawing pain into abdomen and down legs to feet — *Merc*

Testicles swelling — *Rhod*

Testicles swollen, especially epididymis — *Cinch*

Testicles swollen hard — *Rhod*

Testicles left swollen, hard, painless — *Brom*

Testicles right, swollen as large as a hen's egg — *Merc*

Testicles tearing in left — *Cinch*

Ulcers in scrotum — *Aur-m*

Suppression of urine with restlessness — *Camph*

-- **difficult urination with sensation of heat and pain, also after coitus** — *Mar-v*

Stool — **frequent urging** — *Nux-v*

Subacute — **especially when injections have been used and prostate is involved** — *Thuja*

Suppressed — *Agnus, Aur, Benz-ac, Brom, Calc, Canth, Chel, Clem, Coca, Crot-h, Daph, Jacca, Kalm, Med, Merc, Mez, Nat-s, Nit-ac, Nat-m, Puls, Sars, Staph, Sulph, Thuj, Verat, Zinc.*

Condylomata — *Thuj*
Conjunctivitis with granulations — *Psor*
— **after Copaiva** — *Benz-ac*
-- **eruptions** — *Clem*
-- **inflammation of eyes** — *Puls*
-- **eyes sensitive to light** — *Psor*
-- **with fever rheumatism, orchitis** — *Gels*
-- **gouty and rheumatic pains** — *Daph*
-- **impotence** — *Thuj*
-- **lameness** — *Psor*
-- **orchitis** — *Kali-m*
Orchitis first right then, left — *Spong*
Photophobia — *Psor*
Prostatitis — *Nit-ac, Thuj.*
Rheumatism — *Con, Psor.*
Articular rheumatism — *Thuj*
Sycosis — *Thuj*
For 15 years — *Hydracot*
Testicles aching — *Nat-m*
Testicles drawing — *Clem*
Testicles hypertrophied — *Bar-m*
Testicles indurated — *Agnus*
Testicles left enlarged, hard, inflamed tender — *Clem*
Testicles left indurated — *Kali-m*
Testicles left inflamed, pain pressing — *Puls*
Testicles pain — *Ant-t*
Testicles right swollen — *Chel*
-- **with swelling of testicles** — *Nux-v*
Swelling of left testicle and epididymis — *Puls*
Testicles swollen — *Mez, Nux-v, Puls.*
Syphilitic — *Eucal.*
-- **with chancroids or chancre** — *Merc*
-- **complicated with** — *Cinnb*
Warts — *Thuj*
— **after abuse of mercury, 4 white pedunculated, dry on mucous — surface of prepuce** — *Lyc*
— **on a sycotic basis** — *Cinnb*
— **complicated with chancre** — *Ph-ac*
— **dry** — *Staph*
— **dry pediculated painless** — *Lyc*
— **Pediculated** — *Staph*
— **Pointy on corona after, chancre** — *Kali-m*

— **Cockscomb — like excrescences of spong — easily bleeding** — *Sulph*

— **In women** — *Aur-m, Corn-s, Cop, Fer, Nit-ac, Plat, Puls, Sep, Thuj.*

Chronic, discharge very acrid — *Petr*

Chronic with ovarian pain — *Plat*

Cutting between during micturition — *Cann-s*

-- **discharge profuse green, with burning and warmth in vagina, particularly during urination** — *Cop*

Painful — *Lact-v*

Painless, discharge, thick, milky, mucous with burning stinging, swelling of labia and cutting pain at mouth of uterus —*Puls*

Leucorrhoea — gonorrhoeal — *Aur-m, Cann-s, Cop, Nit-ac, Plat, Puls, Sep, Thuj.*

-- **from leucorrhoea** — *Cop*

-- **acrid or from menstrual discharge** — *Nat-m*

Gonorrhoea after agg — *Agn, Arg, Caust, Clem, Colch, Cop, Guaiac, Ham, Hydras, Iod, Kali-bi, Kali-i, Kalm, Med, Merc, Mez., Nat-s, Nit-ac, Nux-v, Petr, Ph-ac, Phyt, Podo, Rhod, Sabad, Sabin, Sars, Selen, Sep, Spong, Staph, Sulph, Tereb, Thuj.*

Suppressed from agg — *Acon, Agn, Ant-t, Benz-ac, Clem, Kali-i, Med, Merc, Nit-ac, Nat-s, Puls, Sars, Thuj, X-ray.*

Eyes : in blenorrhoea — *Puls, Thuj.*

-- **granular conjunctivitis** — *Psor*

-- **iritis** — *Cinch*

-- **ophthalmia** — *Acon, Ant-t, Coral, Cub, Eucal, Merc, Nit-ac, Puls, Sil, Spig, Thuj.*

Concomitants : gonorrhoea suppressed — *Acon, Merc, Nit-ac, Puls, Sulph, Thuj.*

Opthalmia — *Acon, Apis, Arg-n, Bell, Ipec, Merc-c.*

Inflammation gonorrhoeal — *Ant-t, Chin, Cor-v, Cub, Med, Merc, Nit-ac, Puls, Spig, Sulph, Thuj.*

Prostate gland : Gonorrhoea after — *Caps, Cub, Merc, Par, Thuj.*

Bladder : Catarrh — gonorrhoea from suppressed — *Benz-ac, Cub, Med, Puls, Sil, Thuj.*

-- **incontinence of urine after repeated attacks** — *Nux-v.*

neck involved sudden urging to urinate — *Petrosel*

more at night — *Merc, Petrosel.*

Genitalia — Conditions gonorrhoea after or suppressed — *Clem, Merc, Mez, Phyt, Puls, Sele, Staph, Sulph, Thuj.*

Impotency : gonorrhoea after — *Agn, Cob, Cub, Hydr, Med, Sulph, Thuj.*

Penis : Gonorrhoea of — *Merc*

Penis -- feeling of heaviness in glans — *Ph-ac*

With phimosis — *Canth, Merc.*

Tearing in left side of prepuce — *Cinch*

Sensibility to contact — *Caps*

Testes : Inflammation — gonorrhoea from suppressed — *Agn, Ant-t, Arg-n, Aur, Bar-m, Bell, Brom, Canth, Chel, Clem, Con, Ham, Kali-chl, Kali-s, Med, Merc, Mez, Nat-c, Nat-m, Nit-ac, Puls, Rhod, Rhus-t, Sel, Spong.*

Testicles : orchitis — *Gels, Ham.*

-- with orchitis and nocturnal pains — *Con*

Contractive pain after — *Cinch*

Cramp-like pain — *Cinch*

-- especially epididymis swelling — *Cinch*

-- tearing in left — *Cinch*

-- orchitis epididymitis — *Aur-m, Clem, Gels, Ham, Puls, Rhod, Spong.*

Glans : gonorrhoea of — *Alum,Cam, Canth, Caust, Chin, Cimb, Lach, Lyc, Merc, Mez, Nat-c, Nat-m, Nit-ac, Petr, Srp. Staph, Sulph, Thuj.*

Scrotum : Swelling gonorrhoea with chronic — *Brom*

Urethra — Biting before, during and after urination — *Cap*

-- bleeding — *Arg-n*

Catarrh — *Hydras*

-- contracted with suppressed gonorrhoea — *Puls.*

Cutting after urination — *Nat-m*

-- burning as in first stage — *Cochl*

-- burning worse at night — *Merc*

Burning during urination — *Chel, Gels.*

Burning shooting pain and increased gonorrhoea with — *Agr-n, Cann-s.*

Patches of induration — *Merc-i-r*

Inflamed with pain, when urinating — *Dory*

Inflamed with pulsating pain throughout — *Cap*

Itching — *Merc-c, Nat-m, Petr, Petros.*

Itching following gonorrhoea — *Nit-ac*

Itching at mouth as at commencement — *Sulph*

Burning in meatus during urination — *Med*

Meatus-conditions-gonorrhoea-after — *Hep, Merc, Sab, Sulph, Thuj.*
Meatus inflamed with tingling — *Cann-i*
Meatus mild ulceration with — *Merc-c*
Pain fever, scanty discharge — *Gels*
Pains terrible — *Ars-s-f*
Feeling as if something remained after urination — *Med*
Scalding during urination — *Cub*
Soreness during urination — *Med*
Stinging — *Merc-c, Mez.*
Stinging coition during gonorrhoea with — *Merc, Mez.*
Swollen - *Thuj*
Throbbing — *Merc-c*
Tickling at orifice with pulsating throughout penis — *Cop*
Tittilating — *Mez*
Sore to touch — *Mez.*
Urinary irritation — *Cop*
Urethritis — *Aur, Cann-s, Cop, Cub, Petrosel.*
Chronic after gonorrhoea 8 years ago — *Mar-v*
Chronic with secretion — *Kali-i*
Chronic with stricture — *Petr*
With acrid discharge — *Sulph*
  -- feels inflamed — *Cann-s*
  -- as if first stages of gonorrhoea — *Cochl*
Urination : Bloody — *Mez*
Itching after — *Cop*
Relieves — *Tereb*
Scalding — *Thuj*
Sudden urging and strangury — *Petrosel*
Conditions of urination-gonorrhoea after — *Can, Canth, Puls,*
Extremities : Knee inflammation suppressed gonorrhoea — *Med, Sil.*
Pain rheumatic — gonorrhoea after suppressed — *Clem, Con, Cop, Crot-h, Daph, Kalm, Lyc, Med, Phyt, Puls, Sars, Sep, Sulph, Thuj.*
Pain : ankle : suppressed gonorrhoea after — *Med, Thuj.*
Swelling knee gonorrhoea after — *Clem, Med.*

CHAPTER 19

Tinea Or Ringworm

It is a group name for a highly contagious, segmented mycelial fungus. It is the commonest, single fungus group of infections found in tropical countries. There are three distinct genera in this group (distinguished by cultural characteristics).

Epidermophyton : It affects only the human skin. There is only one important species E. floccosum.

Trichophyton : It is more virulent than the others. It affects the hair, the glabrous skin, as well as the nails. It includes both the human and animal species. The important species are : T. rubrum, T. Mentagrophyte, T. violaceum, T. verrucosum and T. schoenleini.

Microsporon : Septa on mycelia are very close producing small segments which look like spores but are not so in reality; therefore the name is a misnomer. It affects mainly the hair, and less commonly the glabrous skin. The important species are : M. audounii (human variety) and M. canis and lanosum (animal varieties).

Despite the above classification, it is practical to discuss fungus diseases according to the site of affection.

TINEA CAPITIS

It is rather uncommon in India and the other Asiatic countries except in Kashmir. The causative fungi are the different species of microsporon and trichophyton. Infection takes place from both affected human beings and animals. It is more frequent in boys than girls, because boys have shorter hair, visit barbers more often and play about with each other's caps. The occipital and temporal regions are the sites of choice.

Clinical features : There are three varieties.

The scaly variety is the commonest; it is caused by microsporon. The salient features are : a circular patch or patches of partial alopecia with thin greyish scales; broken lustreless stumps of hair, with may be, a greyish film around them; a greenish fluorescence seen under Wood's light and a positive scraping for fungus. The fungus grows in the stratum corneum of the epidermis, entering the hair follicles through their mouths. Penetrating the cuticle and cortex of the hair, it grows inside the hair as well. Consequently the hair weakens and breaks, producing alopecia, which is usually partial, and broken stumps can be seen. A microscopic examination will show the irregular broken end of the hair, the disturbed hair structure and the mosaic pattern of the mycelia of fungus, both inside the hair structure and also in the scales. It is not just a coincidence that tinea capitis (particularly the scaly variety caused by microsporon) does not affect individuals after puberty. There is a scientific explanation for it, namely, there is an alteration in the function of sebaceous glands at puberty. Specific fatty acids like undecylenic, propionic acid, etc. (Rothman) are produced. These have definite fungicidal properties, with the result that fungi, particularly microsporon, cannot get a hold on the scalp.

The kerion variety is caused more often by trichophyton than by the microsporon of cats and dogs. Kerion is produced either by penetration of the mycelia into the dermis or virulent strains and/or due to sensitivity to the fungus. In the beginning, there are small boil-like lesions with little oozing and no pus. Later red, painless, boggy swellings are produced. These, likewise, have no pus. These lesions are irregularly distributed on the scalp along with the areas of partial alopecia. A greyish sheath is visible on the hair when the latter is pulled out of the kerion; this pulling out of the hair is easy because the hair is only loosely attached. It should be distinguished from folliculitis decalvans and pyoderma.

The black-dot variety is caused by a species of trichophyton (endothrix) in which the mycelia of the fungus grow inside the hair; the hair breaks off flush with the surface of the skin, thereby producing the appearance of black dots. The alopecia may look almost complete, but the black dots can always be detected at the periphery of the lesion. Wood's lamp examination may not show any fluorescence in the black-dot variety of tinea capitis.

Differential diagnosis : In tinea capitis the differential diagnosis is made from other causes of patchy alopecia such as syphilis and alopecia areata. The features of ringworm of the scalp are typical; Wood's lamp and microscopic examinations will help further to establish the diagnosis.

Syphilitic alopecia has an irregular, moth-eaten appearance. Usually affecting the occipital and temporal regions it is accompanied by other features of secondary syphilis. Alopecia areata is characterized by well-defined patches of complete alopecia, absence of dull, broken hair and greyish scales, and the presence of "exclamation mark" hair.

TINEA BARBAE

There are two clinical varieties :

Tinea circinata is characterized by a patch or patches of scaling or vesiculopustules with inflammation most marked at the periphery and accompanied by itching (described in detail under the heading of "Tinea Corporis").

The kerion type as affects the scalp. This variety is common amongst farm workers; it is caused by the trichophyton species, and is conveyed by infected cattle.

Tinea barbae should be distinguished from sycosis barbae, actinomycosis and other granulomas. If the clinical features described above are remembered, the diagnosis is not difficult; it can be confirmed by a microscopic examination. In sycosis barbae there is chronic congestion of the skin of the beard region with superficial, follicular pustules. Actinomycosis produces a hard, indurated, lumpy swelling below the angle of the jaw, chronic suppuration, sinuses and sulphur granules.

TINEA CORPORIS

In practice, this is a very common fungus affection. It is caused by trichophyton in the majority of cases; infrequently, microsporon and epidermophyton have been known to cause it. The latter two produce a milder reaction.

Clinical features: They are typical. Marked itching is a characteristic symptom. There may be one or more lesions which are more or less circular, sharply demarcated from the surrounding skin; their sizes vary, say from that of a one rupee piece to the palm of the hand (or bigger). Confluent patches produce figurate areas. The affected area or areas show vesicles, pustules or scaling; these vary from case to case depending upon the virulence of the fungus and sensitivity of the individual. Inflammation in the form of vesicles and pustules is most marked at the periphery of the lesion. There is a tendency to clearing at the centre; if the central clearing is complete, ringed lesions are formed due to centrifugal spread. The exposed parts of the skin particularly the non-hairy (glabrous) skin, are the sites of choice. The author has often seen tinea corporis develop from tinea cruris; under such circumstances, bit areas of the trunk are affected. The disease is usually chronic, and the course extends over months to years.

Eczematization and lichenification may become the complicating features of chronic cases. Ringworm infection can almost always be confirmed by scraping the active periphery of the lesion, by the demonstration of mycelia under the microscope and by culture. The sources of infection are infected human beings or animals, particularly cattle. Infection is conveyed by direct contact, less frequently, by fomites like clothing.

Differential diagnosis is from nummular eczema (no active inflammatory borders, bilaterally symmetrical patches, usually on limbs, in winter), psoriasis (silvery scales, candle grease sign, distribution), erythematous rashes and lupus.

Prognosis: It has improved and tinea has become curable, if the source of infection is eliminated completely, and the right treatment is given persistently. Half-hearted treatment is demoralizing and results in chronicity. The superficial varieties of this disease do not leave any atrophy or scarring.

Tinea Cruris (Dhobi's Itch)

It is most prevalent in the summer months. It is commonly caused by the epidermophyton and trichophyton from infected toes or nails; fungus may also be conveyed by infected lavatory seats (most commonly in public lavatories) and by laundry clothes. Infection can also be transmitted during sexual intercourse.

Affection occurs on the inner sides of the upper part of the thighs, spreading to adjoining parts of the scrotum, penis, vulva, perineum and later to the buttocks and trunk. Intense itching is the characteristic symptom. It starts as small circinate lesions. Typically, it is seen as well-defined patch or patches of scaling, vesicles and pustules with inflammation most marked at the periphery of the lesions.

Differential diagnosis: It is made from intertrigo, infective eczema and flexural psoriasis. The first two always start at the inguinal cleft which is usually cracked. Inflammation is more marked towards the centre than the periphery. Moreover, the demonstration of fungus clinches the diagnosis of tinea cruris. Flexural psoriasis has no real resemblance to tinea cruris, except that it occurs on the same site; lesions of psoriasis are present on other areas of the body as well.

Prognosis: It is good if the treatment is persisted with the newer fungicidal agents and the predisposing causes are corrected.

TINEA OF FEET AND HANDS

It is very common in tropical and sub-tropical countries; more common in the summer and the monsoon than in the winter. Men are more frequently affected than women. The incidence is directly related to the spread of civilization (Western). Heavy, closed and ill-fitting shoes worn for long hours predispose the individual to infection. The fungus is conveyed from one individual to another through bath mats tubs and swimming pools. Europeans are very sensitive to it; they pick up the infection quickly and suffer from it more severely than the native population. The fungus grows in the stratum corneum of the epidermis in warm and moist areas; for this reason the fourth interdigital spaces of the feet are selectively affected. Here it is seen as a sodden, white membrane covering a red, glazed, fissured skin. Vesicles may be seen at the periphery. This is the chronic interdigital form. There are no symptoms except slight itching. From the fourth interdigital space, the disease may spread to the sole, to the adjoining toes and even to the dorsum of the feet. Lesions may appear as isolated vesiculo-pustules, or bullae, or as patches of erythema and oedema with a scattering of vesicle and pustules; the vesicles may develop into ulcers. Oozing is slight. It is accompanied by intense itching and burning. Secondary infection results in pain, lymphangitis and regional lymphadenitis. This variety has the appearance of an eczematoid or pompholyx eruption. Auto-sensitization produces an identical eruption (which resembles dyshidrosis from which it must be differentiated) on the palms of hands, and may be, the other parts of the body as well.

In the chronic hyperkeratotic variety, well-defined patches of hyperkeratotic, powdery scaling on erythematous-thickened bases are seen on the soles and sides of the feet and the palms of the hands. This condition is asymptomatic except for an annoying roughness. It must be differentiated from other causes of hyperkeratosis like syphilis, psoriasis, menopausal keratoderma, eczema, congenital keratodema, arsenic drug eruption etc. The fungus is rather difficult to demonstrate in this variety. The interdigital variety of tinea of the feet is the most common variety round in practice. A search must be made for this chronic focus in patients presenting dyshidrosis; keratoderma, tinea cruris and tinea unguium.

Diagnosis : If the characteristics described above are borne in mind the diagnosis of tinea of the hands and the feet is not difficult. It should always be confirmed by a microscopic demonstration of the fungus.

Prognosis : The outlook as to complete cure is fair if the disease is treated by an expert and the patient is co-operative.

TINEA UNGUIUM

Synonym : Onychomycosis.

Ringworm of the nails is caused by a species of trichophyton and microsporon. Saprophytes like scopularia and aspergillus have also been incriminated. In contrast to monilial infection tinea affects first the free edges of the nails. One or more nails may be involved but only rarely, all of them. The history usually reveals that the infection has been present for years. Tinea unguium is characterized by opaque, brittle and deformed nail or nails and hyperkeratotic debris under the free edges. There is no pain or itching. The condition is very rarely bilateral and symmetrical. The diagnosis is confirmed by the demonstration of fungus in the hyperkeratotic debris and nail cuttings. The differential diagnosis is arrived at from conditions like psoriasis, moniliasis, eczema, syphilis and dystrophy of the nails.

According to Bendek and Sagher, there is a strong feeling that primary tinea unguium is a rare condition and what we usually take for tinea unguium is pompholyx of the nail due to an internal septic focus, metabolic upset, a run-down condition or emotional stress causing dystrophy of the nail, which acts as suitable debris for the growth of fungus, which according to them is a secondary contaminant.

Prognosis : Because of primary pompholyx, and because the fungus grows inside the hard nail plate which cannot be penetrated by fungicidal agents, the outlook is poor. It has, however, improved.

Homoeopathic Approach

It will be one of the most common complaints in the homoeopathic practice, the patient may visit the homoeopath with various presentations :

(a) Circular discoloured patches.
(b) Itching.
(c) Disfigured nails.

Sometimes the patient may be asymptomatic as in the case when nails are affected. In such asymptomatic cases the constitutional remedy should be considered.

Much depends on personal hygiene and care of skin of the patient. The following advice will be beneficial if it is passed to the patient while starting the homoeopathic treatment :

(a) To keep the linen and the garments clean and to discourage wearing each other's garments. This is especially true amongst children who frequently wear each other's cap while playing games.

(b) The affected part should be washed daily and twice during summer season with soap, preferably calendula and hot water.

(c) To soothe the irritated skin, locally, an ointment prepared by mixing olive oil and calendula external in 1 : 1 proportion should be applied.

(d) It is essential while treating the patient's infection, especially tinea corporis to remove the source of infection either from infected human beings or animals.

(e) In cases of tinea cruris, the underclothing must be sterilized properly and avoid the use of public lavatories.

(f) In cases of tinea on the feet, the patient is advised to wear open type shoes and sandals and to dry the feet properly after bathing; after removing the shoes they should be exposed to mild sun and fresh air.

It is very essential on the part of the homoeopath not to permit the patient to use any local or antifungal agent as this only suppresses the lesion and permits the disease to enter deep into the system affecting the vital organs. Also prolonged use of antifungal agents brings resistance, as a result the infection spreads throughout the body.

DRUGS

Kindly refer to the Chapter on Therapeutics of Eczema and Herpes.

Agar, Ant-c, Ant-t, Ars-iod, Bar-c, Brom, Calc-c, Clac-iod, Chrysar, Dulc, Graph, Jugl-r, Kali-c, Kali-s, Lappa, Lyc, Med, Mez, Nat-ars, Oleand, Phos, Psor, Rhus-t, Semperv-t, Sop, Sulph-ac, Sulph, Tellur, Tub, Ustil, Vinca, Viola-tr.

THE HOMOEOPATHIC HERITAGE
November 1987 - Page No. 667
Tinea Capitis

Lady aged 55, had an eruption involving the greater part of the scalp and ears, extending over the forehead. The scabs are large and thick, and of a yellowish-greenish colour; the hair is matted, from which pus exudes; the forehead is fiery red; the parts involved itch, and are very painful. The patient is irritable, and although there is no general disturbance of the health, yet she says she does not feel well. When quite young she had an attack of tinea capitis, which was treated 'scientifically'. On the break of this suppressed tinea she was under old school treatment, but this time it would be suppressed, and all the applications had only the effect of making her more ill. She received one does of *Mezereum* 1M. On reporting at the expiration of a week I found a decided change in the character of the eruption; the redness on the forehead had disappeared to a great extent. She said she felt better as to her general health than she had for a long time previously. She had for the week three discharges daily of bright red blood from the rectum; these discharges were profuse, no pain, or no especial weakness was noticed. She received but this one dose of the remedy, she steadily improved, and the eruption gradually disappeared and as she states she feels as well as she did when she was a young girl.

The thickness and the colour of the scabs called my attention to *Mezereum*. Lycopodium has moist scabs; Rhus eruptions destroy the hair, eating it off in the progress

MOLLUSCUM CONTAGIOSUM TREATED WITH DULCAMARA

AFTER

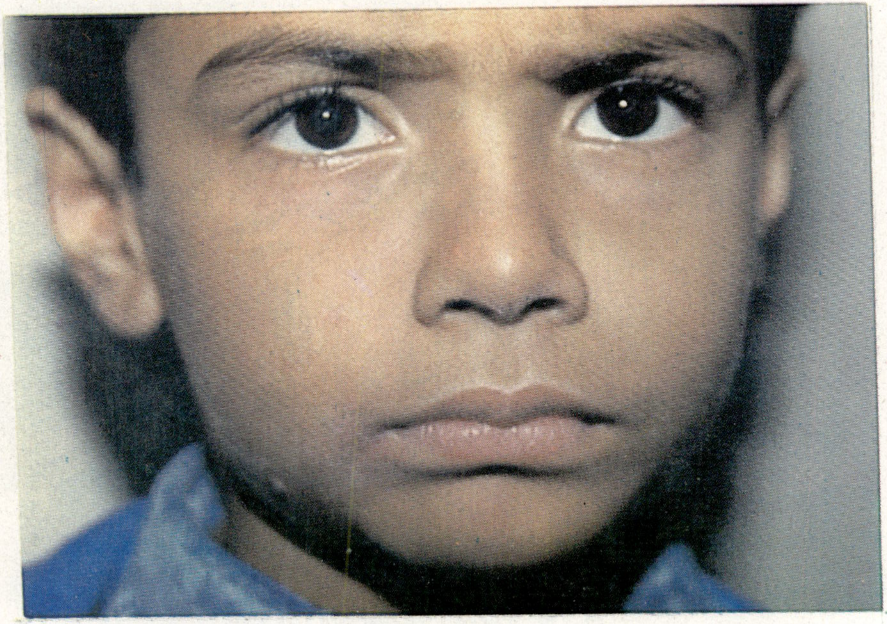

MOLLUSCUM CONTAGIOSUM
TREATED WITH DULCAMARA

BEFORE

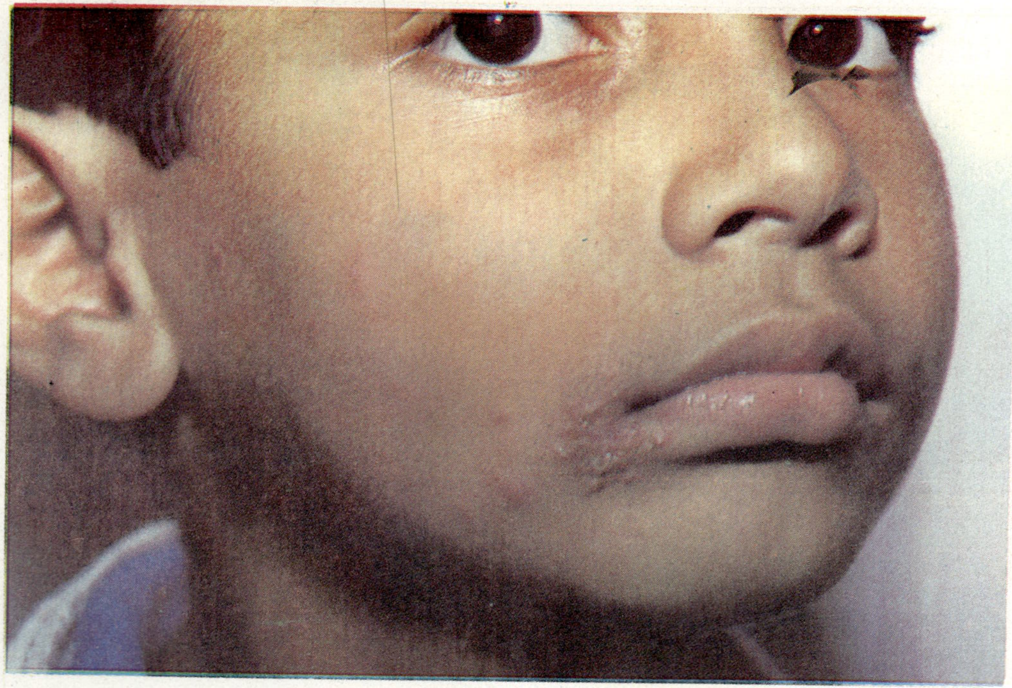

of the eruption, there is a crusty eruption under Staphysagria, but we have a peculiar symptom of Staphysagria wanting; when scratching the itching changes its place, but the part becomes more humid.

Molluscum Contagiosum

It is more common in the summer than in the winter though you come across cases throughout the year. The trunk, neck and face are the usual sites of affection. Infection geared up at gymnasiums, swimming pools, playgrounds, etc. It is contagious; school children are selectively affected.

Features.: The lesions are usually multiple. They are thus multiple, pearly or flesh-coloured, smooth, shiny, papules. The size of a papule varies from that of a pin-head to a split pea. A molluscum contagiosum is a vesicle, but is solid and firm. The top may be flat more commonly umbilicated. When squeezed, cheesy material is ejected. There is usually no pain except when the infection sets in.

Histology Molluscum contagiosum is seen as acanthotic with a well-developed basal cell layer. The prickle cells become round and show eosinophilic masses (inclusion bodies with nuclei pushed to the periphery. The process is more and more marked as the epidermal cells reach the surface. There is slight round cell infiltration in the upper side.

Diagnosis : Molluscum contagiosum is not difficult to diagnose if the above features are remembered. Vesicles, bullae lymphangiomas and warts can all be easily excluded.

Homoeopathic Approach

(1) Refer — Warts.

(2) It should be remembered that lesions disappear spontaneously in many cases; hence claims for cure should be thoroughly scrutinised.

(3) It is a highly contagious disease hence patients should avoid public places like swimming pools, play-grounds, gymnasia, etc.

(4) Local application of salicylic acid, podophyllin, should be avoided at any cost.

Molluscum contagiosum being a viral infection, it indicates the presence of tubercular miasm, hence drugs like *Bacillinum, Tuberculinum* should be used intercurrently. The secondary lesion resembles chicken-pox, hence the use of variolinum, DNA in obstinate and chronic cases.

DRUGS

(1) *Calc-carb, Dulc, Nat-mur, Sil, Sulph*, etc. For detail therapeutics refer the Therapeutics of Warts.

Bacterial Folliculitis

Clinical Presentation

The small 1 to 2 mm pustules of bacterial folliculitis are white in colour and are surrounded by a narrow erythema. Those that are not pierced by a hair are shaped; those that are pierced by a hair are acuminate (pointed). Only a few pustules are present at any one time and there is relatively little tendency for clustering. Fever and lymphadenopathy are not seen. The diagnosis of bacterial folliculitis is usually made on a clinical basis but it can be confirmed by gram stain and bacterial culture, if necessary.

Course and Prognosis

Untreated individual pustules resolve spontaneously in about a week but often as quickly as one heals one or more new pustules appear elsewhere on the body. This spread develops as the result of external inoculation via the finger nails. Hematogenous spread does not occur. On rare occasions bacterial folliculitis leads to deeper infection such as cellulitis or furunculosis.

Pathogenesis

Bacterial folliculitis usually represents infection of the upper hair follicle with Staphylococcus aureus. Streptococci are also occasionally found, but they rarely if ever are the inciting organism. A few cases of Pseudomonas folliculitis have been reported. These occurred during the use of contaminated hot tubs. Minor skin trauma of various sorts usually precedes the development of bacterial folliculitis.

FUNGAL FOLLICULITIS

Clinical Presentation

The dermatophyte fungi Microsporum canis, Trichophyton rubrum, T. mentagrophytes and T. verrucosum may cause a perifollicular abscess which is clinically characterized by the presence of a follicular pustule. All of these organisms except T. rubrum cause sharply marginated,markedly inflammatory plaques upon which the pustules are situated. These pustule studded plaques are rather easily recognized as the zoophilic, inflammatory forms of tinea capitis, tinea barbae and tinea corporis.

Perifollicular pustules due to T. rubrum infection are somewhat harder to recognize. They occur in two settings. First, women with tinea pedis may, in the course of shaving their legs, implant T. rubrum into traumatized follicles. This results in the appearance of scattered but grouped pustules on the lower legs. Second, the erroneous use of topical steroids on plaques of ordinary tinea corporis results in the development of grouped follicular pustules even while the erythema which ordinarily accompanies such lesions is minimized by the anti-inflammatory effect of the steroids. Such lesions are most often seen on the face and dorsal surface of the hands, where they are misdiagnosed at first as being of bacterial origin. Their fungal etiology is often not suspected until they fail to respond to antibacterial treatment.

Course and Prognosis

Folliculitis due to T. rubrum continues its chronic low grade course indefinitely unless treated. Slow peripheral extention occurs even while the central area heals. Fungal folliculitis due to the other, zoophilic organisms eventually resolves spontaneously.

Pathogenesis

Fungal folliculitis is caused by the dermatophyte organisms listed in the paragraph on clinical presentation. Implantation is usually preceded by minor trauma to the skin.

Homoeopathic Approach

Kindly refer the homoeopathic approach of furunculosis. Also for the therapeutics, the reader is requested to refer chapter on Furunculosis.

CHAPTER **20**

Lichen Planus

It is a fairly common, irritating disorder of the skin and mucous, membranes, characterized by purplish or violaceous, polyhedral, flat topped, itchy papules, occurring mostly on the flexor surfaces and in the mouth. The name lichen is derived from the resemblance it has to the purplish lichens that grow on trees in the hills.

It is worldwide in distribution. Its incidence is low. It usually affects young and middle-aged people. The disease is non-infectious.

Etiology : Its cause is unknown. A virus and psychogenic stresses have been blamed. In tropical countries, a lichen planus-like eruption is often brought about by chloroquine and insect bites (lichen planus tropicalis).

Pathology : It is characteristic and, in a typical lesion, it consists of hyperkeratosis, a patchy increase in the stratum granulosum, acanthosis, shortening of the inter-papillary processes, basal cell degeneration, and a well-defined band of round-cell infiltration in the upper corium.

Clinical features : Typically, lichen planus consists of polyhedral, firm, purplish or violaceous papules with shiny, flat tops; very thin, firmly attached scales may be evident on the surface of the papules through a magnifying lens. These are best demonstrated after applying oil to the lesion. The papule is about the size of a split pea (sometimes smaller). The papules may become confluent to form plaques. If the papules enlarge with central clearing, rings are formed (lichen planus annularis). Each ring has a clear, pigmented centre with a reddish or purplish lichenoid periphery. Itching is constant, being more so in dark-skinned people living in tropical climates. Itching produces lichen planus papules along the line of scratching—Koebner's phenomenon — similar to one seen in psoriasis

The rash is bilateral and symmetrical. It is distributed along the fronts of wrists, the flexor surfaces of the forearms, the abdomen, the legs, the genitalia and the back. In about half the number of cases affected, lesions also occur in the mouth, buccal mucosa, less commonly on the lips, tongue and genitalia, as dead white spots, streaks and plaques, or like palms of the hands and the soles of the feet. The mucous membrane lesions are usually asymptomatic, but sometimes cause a little burning and irritation.

It is usually a chronic disease lasting for several months or years. New lesions appear in crops and then disappear spontaneously, resulting in a pigmented skin which takes long to return to normal. The general health of the patient is not affected. The disease may recur. Nails are affected only in a minority of cases. The first change is seen near the cuticle and gradually it extends forwards with the growth of the nail. This results in a nail with rough surface and marked longitudinal striations. If the thinning is severe, the cuticle may grow forward as a pannus. Rarely there may be permanent shedding of the nail.

Variations of Lichen Planus

Annular Lichen Planus : Here ringed lesions with central clearing and raised firm periphery are typically seen. Lichenoid eruption following an insect bite commonly produces this type of lesion on the exposed parts of the body, particularly the face. The number of lesions vary from 1 to 4 or more.

Acute Generalized Lichen Planus : The onset is sudden, the course short, and the rash is generalized. In the early stages, the eruption may not be typical, but characteristic lesions soon become visible. It may merge into chronic lichen planus.

Lichen Planus Verrucosus: It occurs as hyperkeratotic, verrucous, violaceous nodules and patches on the legs. It may occur as such, but is usually accompanied by typical lesions on the legs, wrists, forearms, etc. Itching is severe.

Linear or Herpes-Zoster like Lichen Planus: The linear form, common in children, is seen on the extremities or the face. The lesions rarely occur along the segmental distribution of nerves; when they do, the condition may be confused with herpes-zoster or naevus unius lateralis.

Lichen Plano-Pilaris.: It is usually seen as acuminate, follicular papules with horny spines, accompanied by flat, lichenoid lesions on the chest, back and upper arms.

Bullous Form (Lichen pemphigoides): is rare. Bullous lesions on lichenoid bases are the main features. Course is chronic. Healing is with atrophy.

Diagnosis: The diagnosis of lichen planus is based upon :

1. Demonstration of typical lesions -- polyhedral, form, violaceous (may be difficult to detect in dark skinned people), flat-topped papules with Wickham's stria and very thin adherent scales.
2. Distribution on the flexors, genitalia and mouth.
3. Pruritus.
4. A chronic course.
5. A typical histology.

Differential diagnosis: It is made mainly from other lichenoid eruptions, and, less so, from psoriasis, eczema, warts, naevi, pityriasis rubra pilaris. The mucous lesions of lichen planus must be differentiated from the lesions of leukoplakia, the mucous patches of syphilis and aphthous stomatitis. On the scalp it must be distinguished from discoid lupus erythematosus, pseudo pelade, favus,etc.

Other Lichenoid Eruptions

Lichen Spinulosus : It is characterized by pin-head sized, follicular, flesh coloured papules with horny spines. The papules are grouped in patches. Children are commonly affected. The sites of affection are the abdomen, buttocks and legs. The condition is asymptomatic, and clears up with a good nourishing diet containing plenty of animal fats, extra vitamins, tonics and the local application of animal fats or cod liver oil.

Lichen Syphiliticus : The salient features are : Follicular papules with induration; slight itching; lymphadenopathy; mucous patches; and a history of exposure. The V.D.R.L. is positive.

Lichen Simplex Chronicus : Lichenification or neurodermatitis is another term used for this kind of lichenoid eruption.

Lichenoid Drug Eruptions : These occur commonly in the tropics and in dark skinned people. An idiosyncracy to certain drugs, e.g., Arsphenamine, gold, chloroquine, mepacrine, hydroxychloroquine, quinine, and certain phenothiazine derivatives, para-amino-salicyclic acid, thiazide diuretics and aminophenazole (Dapatazole) may result in lichenoid eruption which may stimulate lichen planus. Contact with chemicals used in the processing of coloured photographic films may, in sensitized individuals, produce similar eruptions.

Lichen Nitidus : It consists of discrete, pink or flesh-coloured, asymptomatic papules, grouped in patches. The typical sites are the genitalia, inner sides of thighs, lower abdomen and at times wrists. It is a benign disease.

Lichen Striatus : An uncommon form occurring in children. It usually affects upper limbs and occasionally the legs. Lesions consist of flesh-coloured or darker lichenoid papules arranged in a linear fashion, usually unilateral and along the long axis of a limb. Streak may be only a few centimetres in length or extend along the entered suggesting a linear naevus. Histopathology is non-specific. No active treatment is necessary as the eruption has a tendency to disappear spontaneously. Sometimes occlusive corticosteroid dressings are definitely beneficial in aborting the disease.

Lichen Myxoedematosus : A very rare but definite entity, practically independent of thyroid pathology. Lesions consist of discrete, localized papular, annular or discoid, lichenoid plaques. This is associated with infiltration and at times lymphoedema. Itching is only minimal. General health is not affected. Basal metabolic rate, erythrocyte sedimentation rate and other tests for metabolic defect are normal except that blood lipids may show slight change. Thyroid extract may benefit an occasional patient.

Prognosis : Lichen planus is a chronic disease lasting for years. The disease occurs usually once in a lifetime; more than one attack may be seen. On involution, there is pigmentation which takes a long time to disappear. There is usually no constitutional disturbance.

Homoeopathic Approach

Lichen planus should be considered as a constitutional disorder and not merely a local disease. The disease is characterised by relapses and remissions and the course of the illness is chronic. Hence case should be taken to treat the disease at its earliest so that we can give relief to the patient from the pruritus which is one of the most annoying symptoms of the disease.

Psychogenic stress is known to induce the relapse in many individuals; hence while taking the history of the patient it is important to discuss the mental state in great detail. At no cost corticosteroid should be advised to the patient, if he is already on corticosteroid then it should be tapered off at the earliest. Soothing lotion preferably calendula mother tincture in 1:10 dilution should be advised to the patient. The following points should be considered while taking the history :

(i) Psychosomatic aspects of the patient.

(ii) Pruritus should be enquired into in detail with its modalities and concomittant.

(iii) Lichen Planus is known to have many variants hence sound knowledge of its manifestations should be known to the treating physician.

Psychotherapy in obstinate cases can be given along with homoeopathic drugs.

Certain variants of lichen planus e.g. lichen striatus are known to disappear spontaneously. Hence one should be aware of the natural course of the disease.

Drugs given below are found useful in cases of lichen planus. The reader is advised to refer therapeutics of eczema and psoriasis for its characteristic symptoms.

Agar, Alum, Am-m, Anac, Ant-c, Ananth, Apis, Ars, Ars-iod, Bell Bov, Bry, Castan, Calad, Chin-ars, Dulc, Lod, Jugi-c, Kali-ars, Kali-iod, Kreos, Led, Lyc, Merc, Merc-s, Nabul-s, Nat-c, Plant, Phyt, Rumex, Sars, Sep, Steph, Sul, Sul-iod,

Sycosis

It simply means chronic folliculitis due to staphylococci affecting the hairy regions of the body. In order of frequency, the beard region, neck scalp, legs, arms and pubic region are most often involved. Characteristically, this condition is seen as small, superficial, follicular pustules; some rupture to discharge beads of pus, the rest dry up to form crusts. Folliculitis develops rapidly. involving more and more follicles. Soon the infection becomes chronic; the skin looks congested, swollen and infiltrated. Usually no pain is present; itching and burning are the only symptoms. The eruption looks unsightly and is annoying. In the beard region (Sycosis barbae), the chin and upper lip are most affected; the eruption later spreads to other parts. There is no oozing and weeping at any stage; this feature helps in differentiating the disease from follicular infective eczema in which the whole of the beard region is rapidly involved and oozing is a dominant feature.

Sycosis Nuchae.: On the back of the neck, sycosis has a tendency to produce small. Keloidal papules and nodules (Acne keloides nuchae) which are chronic and relapsing. It starts as discrete, follicular papules, other develop into firm nodules or plaques of thick, scar-like tissue by coalescence. The hair appear twisted and tangled. It is accompanied by marked itching and occasionally pain.

Sycosisi Lupoides is a rare, chronic and progressive folliculitis of the beard region and scalp. It is seen as a small, smooth, atrophic patch of alopecia, surrounded at the periphery by small follicular papules. It is presumably caused by staphylococcus or virus. The prognosis is bad. X-ray therapy, local hydrocortisone injections and broad-spectrum antibiotics (systematically or locally) are worth trying.

Folliculitis decalvans is comparatively an acute and severe skin disease involving the scalp. Furunculosis, abscesses and cicatricial alopecia are the important clinical features.

Etiology : The most common causative organism of sycosis is staphylococcus aureus; less commonly, other staphylococci. Discharges from the nose, throat and teeth are the source of these organisms. They may enter the skin through slight injuries or abrasions caused by shaving. Use of unhygienic shaving kit, blunt razors, fine shaving by stretching the skin and shaving against the grain of hair tend to cause sycosis. Folliculitis has a tendency to occur amongst people working in dusty and dirty environments, e.g. miners, building workers and sweepers. Workers handling or coming in contact with oil tend to develop oil acne which must be distinguished from primary sycosis. Predisposing causes are many. Seborrhoeic diathesis is a common feature. Sedentary habits, under-nutrition or obesity, diabetes, unhygienic living, neurotic temperament and emotional strain are the common predisposing factors.

Differential Diagnosis : Tinea barbae can be distinguished from this condition by the presence of deep-seated, indurated, boggy swellings, and microscopic examination for fungus. Secondary eczematization and follicular infective eczema, on the other hand, can be distinguished by the features described above. Impetigo has special features like interfollicular epidermal involvement, tense bullae and stuck-on honey-coloured crusts etc. In etiological diagnosis, seborrhoeic diathesis and or acute seborrhoeic dermatitis must be seriously considered.

Prognosis : The course of sycosis is chronic; it is marked by exacerbations and remissions. The disease can continue for years. The prognosis is good if proper treatment is given and the patient co-operates. Only a very small percentage of cases are intractable.

Homoeopathic Approach of Sycosis Barbae

Cases of chronic folliculitis come in plenty to a homoeopath, as the course is chronic and frequently the disease recurs with conventional treatment. I would like to stress the following points for the same :

(1) Trying to eliminate the septic focus from the nose, throat and teeth, as these outlets are the frequent roots of infection. The person should be shifted from the dusty environment and one should take due precaution in general health of individual with correct homoeopathic medicines and exercises.

(2) Avoiding trauma to the affected part viz. by shaving in one direction; by keeping away strong soap and irritating oils like mustard oil, by using sharp razor blades to prevent repeated shaving by keeping the hair short and by refraining from fine shaving which would necessitate stretching of the skin.

(3) Under no circumstances X-ray therapy or Staphylococcin vaccine should be permitted as it suppresses the expression of disease thereby making the disease more chronic.

(4) For annoying itching and burning sensation, locally a mixture consisting of calendula external with water in 1:1 ratio.

(5) Folliculitis is a disease which is characterized by remissions and relapses and hence all due care should be taken whilst evaluating the condition.

SYCOSIS BARBAE

Ant-Tart : There is presence of eruption around the mouth. Thick pustular eruption like pocks which leave bluish-red marks on healing, leaving ugly blue, red scars. The most characteristic symptom is that the individual pustules is as large as pea and is distended with pus. Profuse salivation with thick white pasty tongue is one of the important concomitants.

Cal-Carb : The skin of the face is rough and dry covered by humid scabby eruptions in the form of clusters with burning pain. There is scanty discharge of thin pus. The face appears pale, puffy and pasty with swelling of lower lip. Lips are full of cracks and they bleed easily. The submaxillary glands are swollen.

Cicuta-V : Eruptions are present on the face, are confluent, purulent and of a deep red colour. There is formation of burning scab with yellowish serum on the upper lip, cheeks and chin. Also thick honey scurf is present on chin, upper lip and lower portion of cheek. The eruption is accompanied with swelling of submaxillary gland and insatiable appetite.

Graphites : Eruptions that affect the skin around the nose, mouth and lips. They are full of cracks which ooze glutinous discharge which forms into thick crust. There is presence of itching and burning sensation along with stinging pains. The itching is worse at night and by warmth of bed. The other concomitant symptoms are constipation, tendency to obesity and disposition to catch cold.

Kali-Bi : The eruptions of Kali-bi resemble those of small-pox. There is presence of vesiculopustular eruptions with burning pains and tendency for ulceration. The discharges from the eruptions are yellow, sticky, acrid and offensive. There is presence of itching which is worse from heat, worse in hot weather and worse on undressing. It is specially indicated for persons who are fleshy, fat, light complexioned, who are subjected to catarrh and to syphilitic history.

Lithium-Carb : There is excessive dryness of skin with presence of scabby, tettery eruptions on

hands, head and cheeks which are preceded by red raw skin.
There is a presence of dull stitching pain in the eruption which ultimately ends in itching. Barber's itch is more prominent on the right side of the face. Uric acid diathesis and rheumatic complaints are associated concomitants.

Lycopodium : Eruptions that affect the face, behind the ears, corners of the mouth, in patches, characterized by loss of hair with oozing of watery or yellowish fluid. Tendency to form cracks and ulceration in the eruption which later on heals. Offensive perspiration, right sided affection and 4-8 p.m. aggravation are important concomittants.

M.I.R. : There is presence of vesicular papular eruption on the face, especially on the cheek. The eruptions are full of small fissures and cracks. Presence of sycosis barbae in patients with syphilitic background.

Rhus-Tox : Corners of the mouth, lips are surrounded by erythematous vesicular eruptions with oozing of watery, yellowish fluid. There is formation of painful yellow crust. Itching is worse by scratching, worse by warmth (Rhus-v. is better by hot application).

Staphysagria : The eruption are characterized by thick scabs which itch violently. There is presence of biting and itching sensation, as of vermin, which changes place on scratching. The skin symptoms alternate with joint pain.

Sul-Iod : In obstinate cases of barber's itch, this is an extremely important medicine, where the papular eruption on the face is prone to suppuration. There is presence of itching which is worse in a warm room and by warm application. The discharges are acrid, which produce burning sensation wherever it comes in contact with the skin. Lymphnodes surrounding the eruption are enlarged and swollen.

Thuja : The eruption typically affects the beard and whiskers. There is presence of foul pustules, with sunken apices. The eruptions itch or burn violently whenever the patient applies cold water. Greasy skin, presence of warts sweetish odour of the perspiration are few of the important concomittants.

CHAPTER 21

Pemphigus Vulgaris

Diagnostic Hallmarks

1. Distribution : Oral mucous membranes and upper trunk.
2. Large, shallow erosions which heal very slowly.
3. Biopsy : acantholytic intraepidermal bulla.
4. Immunofluorescent studies : IgG in a network around epidermal cells.

Clinical Presentation

The bullae of pemphigus vulgaris arise from normal appearing skin; there is no surrounding inflammation. The blisters are also extraordinarily fragile. For that reason intact bullae are found only during the first day or two of their existence. Thereafter the blister roof is broken leaving a bright red, shallow erosion which requires weeks or months to heal. The initial lesions are usually found on the upper trunk and back but, since new lesions develop faster than old ones heal, there is gradual extension elsewhere with special predilection for face, groin and axillae. The prominence of these crusted erosions often obscures the fact that the patient has, in fact, a bullous disease.

Oral mucous membrane lesions are practically always present and they frequently precede the cutaneous lesions by weeks to months. These oral lesions begin as blisters but they too quickly break down to form shallow erosions. The oral erosions of pemphigus are particularly likely to occur in the posterior mouth. The accompanying discomfort interferes with chewing and swallowing. The resultant malnutrition contributes to the extreme debility which develops in untreated patients.

A suspected clinical diagnosis must be confirmed by biopsy. Light microscopy reveals a characteristic intraepidermal vesicle with loss of epidermal cell cohesion (acantholysis). Direct immunofluorescent studies carried out on perilesional skin demonstrate a pathognomonic pattern of IgG deposition in a network-like pattern surrounding the epidermal cells. Complement is also sometimes present. More than 90% of patients will also have circulating auto-antibodies. These antibodies can be demonstrated on indirect immunofluorescent studies where they are noted to fix to antigens which lie on the cytoplasmic membrane of epithelial cells. The titer of these antibodies reflects in a general, although not highly accurate manner the severity of the disease. To a limited degree the antibody titer can also be used to monitor the response of the disease to therapy.

Atypical Presentation : Pemphigus foliaceus is an uncommon form of pemphigus in which the intraepidermal clefting occurs high in the epidermis rather than just above the basal layer. Patients with pemphigus foliaceus develop erosions which are more superficial than those found in pemphigus vulgaris. Oral involvement is less often present and patients do not become as debilitated. Some patients with pemphigus foliaceus have a high frequency of facial erythema and may, in addition, have a variety of lupus-like laboratory findings. The combination of these findings is known as the Senear-Usher syndrome. A form of pemphigus found in Brazil (fogo selvagem) has epidemiologic features which suggest an infectious etiology.

Course and Prognosis

Pemphigus begins most commonly in mid to late adult life. It is a chronic disease which, left untreated, inevitably leads to severe debility and death. With vigorous, early treatment the mortality rate is approximately 15%. Other autoimmune diseases are found with unexpected frequency in patients with pemphigus and a small but significant number of patients have thymomas and a variety of other internal malignancies.

Pathogenesis

Pemphigus is considered to be an autoimmune disease. IgG antibody and sometimes complement are deposited at the site of epidermal cell damage; these same antibodies are regularly found in the circulation. Moreover, cause an epidermal lesion identical with that found in the original disease. The antigens responsible for this autoimmune reaction are unknown but they appear to be located on the exterior surface of certain epithelial cells. Further evidence of an autoimmune etiology includes the frequent association of pemphigus with other autoimmune diseases and the occasional presence of a thymoma. Genetic factors are probably also important. Pemphigus occurs much more frequently than can be explained by chance. As is perhaps apparent from the discussion above, the pathogenesis of pemphigus shares many remarkable similarities with that of lupus erythematosus.

Pemphigoid

Diagnostic Hallmarks

1. Distribution : starts on the extremities but becomes generalized.
2. Tense, tough blisters mostly arising from normal skin.
3. Individual lesions heal well spontaneously.
4. Immunofluorescent studies : IgG and C_3 in a linear pattern at the dermal epidermal junction.

Clinical Presentation

Patients with pemphigoid characteristically develop the disease after the age of 60. Crops of large bullae, 2 to 5 cm in diameter, appear first on the extremities but within a short period of time commence appearing on the trunk as well. Occasional lesions are seen on the scalp, palms, soles and oral mucous membranes.

In most instances the bullae arise from normal appearing skin but a few may occur against an erythematous background. When lesions of this latter type predominate, distinction from bullous erythema multiforme a subepidermal location. For this reason the roofs are not easily broken and the bullae stay intact for many days. In fact blisters outnumber erosions whereas the reverse is true in pemphigus.

The bullae are usually filled with clear fluid but occasionally some are tinged with blood. Old lesions heal as rapidly as new lesions appear. Thus progression of the disease with its accompanying disability is not as prominent as it is in patients with pemphigus. Some patients are completely asymptomatic but itching often is present and occasionally it is very severe.

A clinical diagnosis must be confirmed by biopsy. Light microcopy reveals a subepidermal blister with a perilesional inflammatory infiltrate containing an increased number of eosinophils. Biopsies of perilesional skin for direct immunofluorescence reveal a band of immunoglobulin and complement at the dermal-epidermal junction. The immuno-globulin which is deposited is usually IgG but in a small percentage of cases, .IgA is found instead. Approximately 70% of patients will also have circulating auto-antibodies directed at the basement membrane zone. These can be demonstrated with indirect immunofluorescent studies.

Pemphigoid Variants : Cicatricial pemphigoid is a rare disease in which erosive disease of mucosal surfaces (particularly the eyes and the mouth) is followed by scarring. Cutaneous bullae are not prominent but when they occur they too may heal with scarring.

Localized pemphigoid is similar to conventional pemphigoid except that the lesions remain restricted to a single segment of the body. This variant most commonly occurs on the lower legs of older women.

Course and Prognosis

Pemphigoid is a chronic disease which persists indefinitely. New lesions develop as rapidly as old lesions heal such that 10 to 20% of the skin surface is continually involved. Debility due to the disease itself is not great but it is additive with that due to advanced age and intercurrent disease. Death due to superimposed infection occurs in 5 to 10% of patients.

Pathogenesis

Pemphigoid is an autoimmune disease directed toward one or more antigens at the dermal-epidermal junction. Immunoglobulin and complement are always found at the basement membrane zone and 70% of patients also have circulating antibodies which fix to the dermal-epidermal junction of certain epithelial tissues. Unfortunately, and unlike the situation in pemphigus, injection of these antibodies into an appropriate substrate does not result in the formation of blisters.

Genetic factors are also less impressive than they are in pemphigus. There are no racial or national groups which seem particularly predisposed to the disease and HLA typing has failed to reveal patterns which consistently differ from those of the normal population.

A considerable number of patients with pemphigoid appear to have an associated systemic malignancy. However, these patients are of advanced age and when matched against similarly aged control groups the incidence of tumours does not seem to be statistically increased.

Homoeopathic Approach

Pemphigus is one of the important causes of vesiculobullous eruption. It is important on the part of the homoeopath to recognize pemphigus because of the serious prognosis it is associated with. Whenever a homoeopath is confronted with a bullous eruption, answer to the following questions must be sought :

(a) Is the eruption localized, regional or generalised?
(b) Has it symmetrical or asymmetrical distribution?
(c) Is it groove or discrete, polymorphus or monomorphus?
(d) Are the mucous membranes involved?
(e) Do the bullae occur as such; or on erythematous bases?
(f) Are they tense or flaccid, with serous or purulent content?
(g) What are the shapes and sizes of bullae?
(h) Any Niklosky's sign?
(i) Are there accompanying signs like itching or pain?
(j) Any accompanying scaling or crusting?
(k) What kind of a surface does one see when the roof of the bullae is removed?
(l) How is the general health of the individual and are there any toxic symptoms?

Since the cause of Pemphigus on most occasions is autoimmune, hence the need of constitution remedy to treat the condition. It is essential to take the help of a dermatologist for reviewing the case of pemphigus when treated homoeopathically. If the patient does not improve with homoeopathic treatment, one can take help of corticosteroids temporarily and then revert back to homoeopathy once the patient is in remission stage.

Good nursing is by far the most essential part of management. Locally the bullae must not be ruptured and a linen dipped in the mixture of calendula external and water in the ratio of 1 : 4 should be applied to prevent secondary infection. The patient must be protected from cold. The diet must be nutritious. When blisters are present in the mouth, the patient has difficulty in mastication and swallowing. When this is the case, he should be given bland fluids or semi-solid diet. Whenever the skin around the eye is involved, the eye should be cleaned with very dilute solution of euphrasia, preferably 1 : 30. The use of antibiotics should not be permitted because of their serious side effects; instead patient should be recommended a good vitamin supplement, as these patients suffer from vitamin deficiency.

Drugs

Anacardium : There is great burning of skin with scarlet redness over the whole body. The body is covered with blisters from the size of a pin-head to a pea. There is presence of intense itching with mental irritability. It is worse in the evening and by application of hot water.

Antipyrine : There is presence of erythema with intense itching. Bullae appear and disappear quite soon. Pemphigus affects the mucous membrane of the oral cavity which is characterized by burning of the mouth and gums; ulcerations of lips and tongue, with oedema and puffiness of face.

Arsenic Alb : There is intense itching, burning and swelling due to bullous eruptions which have a tendency to either suppurate or turn gangrenous. The burning and itching sensation is worse by application of cold and scratching. The patient is extremely restless and develops early prostration in the sickness. Patient feels better with warm application. There is aggravation of all the complaints.

Alum-T : The appearance of skin is scarlet red with raw bloody surface everywhere. The discharges that ooze out from the bullae are very acrid and produce inflammation and destruction of surrounding tissues. It also has special affinity for mucous membrane of the oral cavity where it produces mucosal lesion of pemphigus. There is sore raw and burning feeling in the oral cavity. Corners of the mouth are sore and cracked. The throat is swollen, burns and is extremely raw. The patient is hot and gets worse in a warm room.

Bufo : There is presence of itching and burning sensation in bullae which is better by bathing in cold water. The bullae tend to suppurate easily. Bullae which open and leave a raw surface, exuding an ichorous fluid. There is presence of bullae on palms and soles. There is marked lymphangitis of the surrounding part.

Caltha : There is presence of bullae which are surrounded by a ring and they itch greatly; on the 3rd day they are transformed into crusts. There is much itching. Face is swollen, especially around the eyes. Bullae have tendency to suppurate easily.

Cantharis : There is presence of bullous eruptions showing excessive tendency to turn gangrenous. There is presence of burning sensation which is relieved by cold application. There is ulcerative pain in the lesion whenever it is touched. There is generalised oversensitiveness. accompanied by excessive weakness. Urinary troubles can be important concomittants.

Causticum : There is presence of large bullae on the chest and back with sensation of soreness. The patient feels better in a warm room and warm weather. There is a sensation of burning, itching and rawness. Progressive weakness accompanying the pemphigus. Warts, long standing worries and local paralysis are important concomittants.

Carb-Oxy : The whole skin is covered with large and small vesicles of pemphigus. The most important concomittant associated with pemphigus are sleepiness and coldness on the surface, especially hands are icy cold.

Copaiva : Here the mucous membrane is first affected then the skin. There is presence of excessive foetid discharge. Presence of pemphigus in people having past history of gonorrhoea.

Crotalus-H : Pemphigus with low typhoid like or septic condition. The contained fluid assumes a dark, bloody character, threatening gangrene. The eruptions are surrounded by purplish mottled skin and oedema. Pemphigus may alternate with internal affections like diarrhoea.

Dulc : Pemphigus chiefly affects skin of face, genitalia and hands. A thick brown yellowish discharge oozes out which later on turns into crust. There is presence of pruritus which is worse in cold wet weather. Glands surrounding the pemphigus get enlarged and suppurate. The eruptions are known to aggravate during menstruation.

Jug-c : Eruptions that start in the axilla and then spread to the back and chest. There is

PEMPHIGUS TREATED WITH SEPIA & GRAPHITES

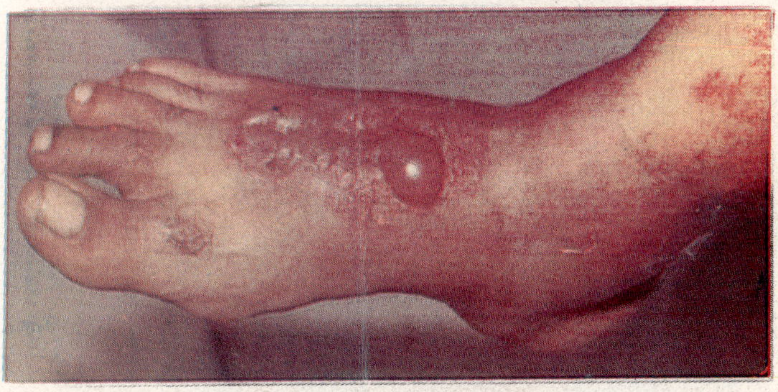

BEFORE

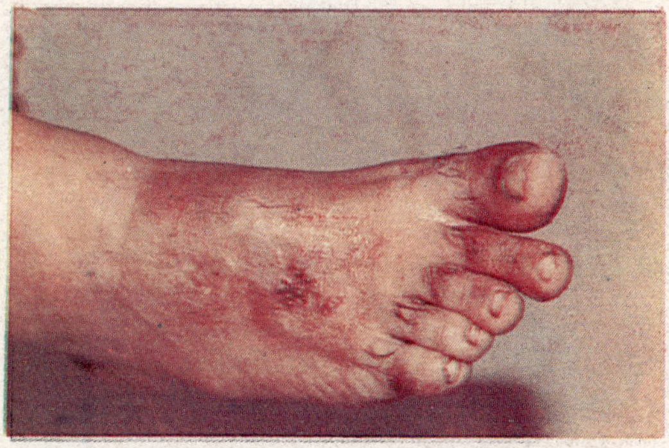

AFTER

MELANOSIS -- AFTER INSECT BITE --TREATED WITH VESPA

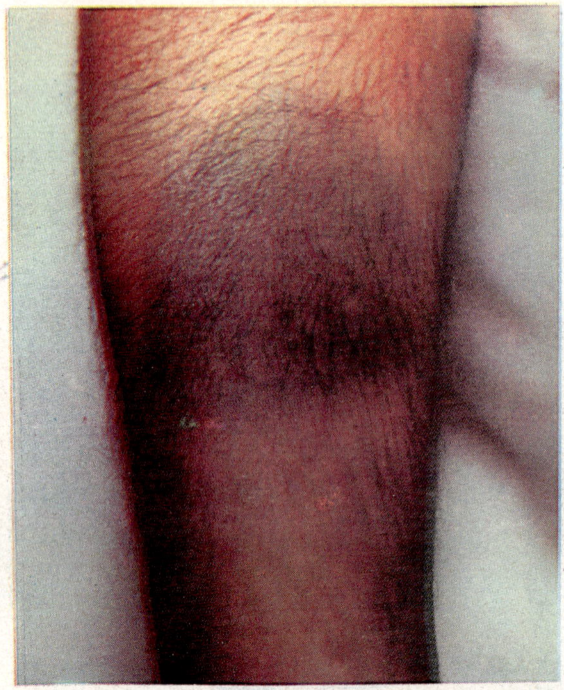

presence of itching and burning which is better by scratching. Gastro-intestinal concomittants are usually associated with pemphigus.

Lachesis : The eruptions are bluish black, the fluid within the vesicles is haemorrhagic and individual bulla is surrounded by purplish blue discoloration. The eruption has tendency to develop gangrenous condition which later on turns into gangrenous ulcers. There is presence of severe prostration, inflammatory fever, quick intermittent pulse, fainting, nausea, spasmodic and bilious vomiting, convulsions and cold sweat.

Mancinella : There is presence of very large blisters which, when ripe, turns into heavy brown crusts. The serum that oozes out from bullae is extremely sticky. Depressed mental state and pain in the thumb are important concomittants.

Merc-cor : There is burning and redness of skin with formation of bullae. The eruptions gradually lead to ulceration with swelling of the gland. A past history of gonorrhoea or bloody dysentery are important concomittants.

Ran-B : There are constantly repeating eruptions or blisters, secreting an offensive gluey matter, forming crust and healing from the centre. The acrid discharge makes the surrounding part sore. There is presence of burning and itching sensation which is aggravated by slightest touch. The skin is sensitive to cold air.

Ran-Scleratus : Large isolated blisters which burst and form an ulcer, discharging acrid, ichor making the surrounding part sore. There is boring and gnawing pain within the vesicle.

Rhus-Tox : Confluent blisters, containing a milky or watery fluid with peeling of skin. The skin appears red and swollen. The bullous eruption suppurates very easily. There is sensation of burning and itching which is worse by scratching and better by local application of heat. Overall, the patient is worse in the night and wet weather and better in dry weather.

Scrop Nodosa : Pemphigus eruptions, especially in and around the ears. The bullous eruptions turn gangrenous.

Thuja : Bullous eruptions are present, especially on the covered parts of the body. Discharge from the bullae is extremely offensive. There is presence of itching and burning which is worse in the evening, night and after scratching. Patient feels better by touch.

CHAPTER **22**

Hair Loss (Alopecias)

Hair loss is separable into two major categories : that which occurs with associated scalp disease and that which occurs in the absence of scalp disease. In separating these two categories one must ignore the presence of mild, non-inflammatory dandruff since this condition is almost universal in prevalence and is rarely if ever associated with significant hair loss.

Alopecia with scalp disease

Tinea Capitis : Sharply localized patches of alopecia are an integral part of tinea capitis. This hair loss is characterized by the fact that the hair are broken off at, or close to, the surface of the skin. This results in the presence of fine stubble which if too short to palpate is sometimes visible as a series of black dots within the patch of alopecia. The patches of alopecia in tinea capitis are also characterized by their sharp margination and their confinement precisely to the area of scalp disease. The associated scalp disease consists of a sharply marginated scaling plaque with varying degrees of inflammation. Infection with *M. audouinii* and *T. Tonsurans* may be relatively non-inflammatory whereas those due to *M. canis* and *T. mentagrophytes* may be bright red and edematous. Such kerion formation may be accompanied by pustulation around some of the follicles. Only the *Microsporum* infections fluoresce under

Wood's lamp illumination. Confirmation of a suspected instance of tinea capitis depends on performance of KOH preparations and fungal cultures. Treatment of tinea capitis is almost always accompanied by complete regrowth of hair.

Lupus Erythematosus : Localized patterns of hair loss regularly develop when lesions of discoid lupus erythematosus occur in the scalp. Here too the hair loss is very sharply localized. However, since the centre of such lesions is hypopigmented and scarred, it may appear at first glance as if scalp disease is not present. In such cases careful examination of the margins will reveal the annular, active erythematosus border which is distinctive of the disease. The scalp lesions of discoid lupus erythematosus rarely occur alone; the presence of typical facial lesions helps to suggest the correct diagnosis. Hair loss also occurs in systemic lupus erythematous but it is more diffuse and is often unassociated with scalp disease.

Diseases Associated with Hair Loss

- Alopecia with scalp disease
  - Localized loss
    - Tinea capitis
    - Discoid lupus erythematosus
  - Diffuse loss
    - Seborrheic dermatitis
- Alopecia without scalp disease
  - Localised loss
    - Alopecia areata
    - Secondary syphilis
  - Diffuse loss
    - Telogen effluvium
    - Male and female pattern loss
    - Hypothyroidism

Seborrheic Dermatitis : Many patients with inflammatory dandruff (seborrheic dermatitis) complain of diffuse hair loss. Such loss is probably real although it is seldom visible to the examiner. When present it occurs from all portions of the scalp and thus lacks the patchiness found in tinea capitis and discoid lupus erythematosus. The underlying scalp disease is that of a mild inflammatory, scaling process. The amount of scale varies with the frequency and vigor with which the patient shampoos. Seborrheic dermatitis of the scalp severe enough to result in hair loss is generally accompanied by seborrheic dermatitis of the retroauricular and nasal folds. Alopecia associated with seborrheic dermatitis may be continuous but it is not progressive. For this reason visible baldness should not be ascribed to seborrheic dermatitis. Hair regrowth occurs when seborrheic dermatitis is adequately treated.

Alopecia without Scalp Disease

Alopecia Areata: Alopecia areata is a disease in which there are sharply localized, circular patches of sudden hair loss unaccompanied by any visible evidence of scalp disease. Typical lesions are 2 to 3 cm in diameter. Often only a single lesion is present but careful examination may reveal two or three additional lesions in other areas of the scalp. In less typical cases, multiple, larger patches of hair loss are present and in very rare instances total hair loss (alopecia totalis) occurs. Alopecia areata typically affects the scalp but the process can involve the eyebrows, eyelashes, beard area, axillae and pubis. The disease can occur at any age but it is most commonly found in late childhood and the early teen years.

The course and prognosis in alopecia areata are highly variable. Patients destined to undergo complete remission generally develop only a few small patches. These grow quickly to a maximum size of 2 to 3 cm and then remain stable in appearance for 6 to 12 months. Thereafter new hair, which are often initially white in colour, begin to regrow. By 18 months the process is completely healed. Patients with larger or more numerous patches of alopecia have a poorer prognosis. Individual patches of alopecia may expand centrifugally for many months before undergoing stabilization. An estimate of the likelihood of continued expansion can be obtained by gently tugging on the hair at the edge of the bald spot. Several hairs will be removed with each tug in cases where expansion is actively evolving; no loose hairs will be found in cases which have reached stabilization. A few patients with numerous large patches of alopecia eventually obtain complete regrowth. Most go through years of dynamic equilibrium in which new patches develop as quickly as old patches regrow. A very unfortunate few patients go on to total alopecia; The outlook for total regrowth in these individuals is extremely poor. Patients with alopecia areata who have obtained complete remission have about 25% chance of developing one or more subsequent episodes later in life.

The cause of alopecia areata is unknown. Genetic factors are probably important since approximately 30% of patients have a positive family history of the same disease. There is also considerable evidence pointing toward an autoimmune etiology. Patients with the more severe forms of alopecia areata are rather likely to have autoantibodies directed against thyroid cells, parietal cells, adrenal cortex cells or intracellular proteins. Vitiligo, another autoimmune disease, is seen with increased frequency in patients with alopecia areata. Finally, recent immunofluorescent studies, which are as yet inconclusive, have shown the occasional deposition of immunoglobulins at the site of affected follicles. Emotional factors probably also play a role although it is often difficult to decide whether those present are a cause or a result of the disease.

There are difficult decisions to be made regarding the treatment of alopecia areata. The lesions which respond best to therapy are the small, unobtrusive lesions which also are the most likely to resolve spontaneously. The larger, more objectionable lesions are extraordinarily resistant both to spontaneous regression and to therapy.

Secondary Syphilis : Patients with secondary syphilis of many months' duration often develop a peculiar pattern of patchy, "moth eaten" alopecia. The large number of patches, their smaller size and their indistinct margins help to separate this condition from that of alopecia areata. The hair loss is transient; regrowth occurs following adequate homoeopathic therapy.

Telogen Effluvium : Telogen effluvium is a diffuse type of alopecia which occurs when numerous but scattered hair follicles simultaneously change from the growing (anagen) phase to the resting (telogen) phase of the hair growth cycle. This may be contrasted to the situation in alopecia areata where a similar switch to telogen phase occurs in a tightly localized area.

Patients who seek medical attention for diffuse hair loss of telogen effluvium type seldom have alopecia visible to the examiner.

However, proof of increased hair loss is easily obtained by gently tugging at random tufts of hair. One or more telogen hairs will be removed with each tug in patients with telogen effluvium. Only an occasional loose hair will be found in individuals with normal hair growth. Alternately, the magnitude of the hair loss can be determined by asking the patient to save and count individual hairs found on the pillow, in the hairbrush and in the basin or bathtub. Most individuals with telogen effluvium will report the loss of approximately 400 hairs per day, a number approximately 4 to 5 times that expected from individuals with normal hair growth.

Telogen effluvium is seen more commonly in women than in men. Moreover, telogen effluvium is frequently found in the postpartum state and following the discontinuation of oral contraceptive pills. These observations suggest that hormonal factors play a role in pathogenesis. However, the process is also seen following physiologic stress (high fever, myocardial infarction, cerebral vascular accidents) and in association with psychologic stress suggesting that other, unknown factors may also be important.

Patients with telogen effluvium rarely if ever progress to clinically significant baldness. Most instances of telogen effluvium resolve spontaneously over 6 to 12 months period. No effective treatment is recognized.

Male and Female Pattern Baldness : Both men and women may develop a distinctively patterned type of hair loss as according to age. In men the loss is most noticeable at the vertex and in the bitemporal regions of the scalp. In women the loss is usually restricted to the vertex. In both sexes some overall diffuse loss may also occur. Pattern loss may be seen as early as the third decade in men but is rarely apparent prior to the sixth decade in women.

Genetic factors are important in the pathogenèsis of pattern loss. Both the degree of loss and the age at which it starts seem to occur in familial patterns. Hormonal factors are likewise important since men castrated at a young age do not develop pattern loss, regardless of genetic factors, until and unless supplemental testosterone is administered. The hormonal aspect of pattern loss in women is much less clear although the delay in onset until cessation of reproductivity suggests the possibility that estrogens are protective.

In a general sort of way there is a correlation between the age at which onset begins and the severity of eventual loss. However, the hair loss, regardless of how early it begins, is not linear with time. Individuals may go through short periods of intense loss followed by longer plateau periods of relative stability.

Hypothyroidism.: Diffuse hair loss unassociated with scalp disease is occasionally seen in women with moderate to severe hypothyroidism. The mechanism through which this occurs is unknown but it seems unlikely that it is directly related to serum levels of thyroid hormone since replacement, while preventing further loss, fails to reverse the process.

Homoeopathic Approach of Hair Falling

Whenever patient presents with either alopecia or hairfall always examine the scalp to rule out any atrophy or scarring of the scalp skin. Scarring of the scalp is seen as a shining surface, diminution or absence of hair core, loss of skin elasticity and wrinkling, it feels like thickened scar tissue when palpated. Atrophy is seen as wrinkling, thinning and loss of elasticity. It is important to remember that in cicatricial cases, hair never grows back, while in non-cicatricial cases, they do, if the cause can be controlled and treated. Treatment consists of finding the cause and its elimination, reassurance and improvement of general health with good nourishing diet, vitamins and minerals. In debilitated individuals, Alfa-Alfa mother tincture can be given. A quiet relaxing holiday is very beneficial.

Local treatment consists of :

(a) Avoid repeated and too frequent combing and shampooing.

(b) Avoid excessive use of oil and oily preparation, especially in seborrhoeic individuals.

(c) Light massage of the scalp with any of the following preparations :

Take equal parts of Sepia, Arnica and Jaborandi mother tincture, mix it in 300 ml. of pure coconut oil. Shake vigorously and gently massage the scalp twice a day, when there is hair falling in active phase and once a day when hair falling has become stationary and regrowth is desired.

Drugs

Acid-Fluor : Large patches entirely denuded of hair. The new hair that grows is dry and lustreless and breaks off easily. The patient must comb the hair often because it mats at the end. Itching of the head with falling of the hair. Falling of the hair because of syphilis.

Aloe : The hairs come out in lumps, leaving bare patches; eyelashes also fall out with frequent frontal headache.

Am-Mur : Large accumulation of bran - like scales, with falling of the hair, which has a deadened and lustreless appearance with great itching of the scalp.

Ant-Crud : Losing hair from nervous headache.

Ars-Alb : Touching the hair is painful, bald patches at or near the forehead. The scalp is covered with dry scabs and scales, looking rough and dirty, extending sometime even to forehead, face and ears.

Aur-Met : Syphilitic alopecia.

Anantherum : Falling of hair from beard and eyebrows.

Bar-C : Baldness, especially of the crown. In young people the scalp is very sensitive to touch.

Borax : Hair is rough and horny, cannot be combed smooth. Hair tangled at the tip, and stick together.

Calc-c	:	Hair falls out especially when combing. Dryness of hair, great sensitiveness of scalp, with yellowish or white scales on scalp. There is sensation of coldness of outer head.
Cantharis	:	Hair fall out when combing, especially during confinement and lactation. There is presence of enormous dandruff with scales on the scalp.
Carb-Veg	:	Falling out of hair, after severe disease or abuse of mercury, with great sensitiveness of scalp to pressure. Hair fall out more from the back of head, after severe illness or parturition.
China	:	Hair sweats much and falls out.
Graph	:	Falling of beard and eyebrows.
Helleborus	:	Losing hairs from the eyebrows or pudenda.
Hepar-S	:	Hair fall out here and there with bald spots.
Hypericum	:	Alopecia from headaches caused by concussion of brain.
Kali-C	:	Alopecia after fever, dry hair repeatedly falling off with dandruff.
Lycopodium	:	Hair become grey early. Hair fall off after abdominal disease, after parturition with burning, scalding and itching of the scalp, especially on getting warm from exercise during the day.
Mancinella	:	Losing hair after severe acute diseases.
Merc	:	Hair fall out mostly on sides and temples without any headaches.

Nat-Mur	:	Hair fall out if touched mostly on forepart of the head, temples and beard. Scalp is very sensitive. Face is shiny as if greasy.
Nit-ac	:	Profuse falling of hair, especially of vertex with eruption. It may be due to syphilis, nervous headaches debility or emaciation. The scalp is sensitive.
Petroleum	:	There is much itching of the scalp with severe dandruff and falling of hair.
Phos-Ac	:	Gnawing grief changes hair of the young.
Phos	:	Round patches of scalp, completely deprived of hair, falling off of the hair in large bundles on the forehead and on the sides above the ears, the roots of the hair seems to be dry, the denuded scalp looks clear, white and smooth. There is presence of copious dandruff.
Plumbrm Met	:	Great dryness of hair. It falls off even from beard.
Sarsaparilla	:	Mercuro-syphilitic affections of the head with sensitiveness of scalp with falling off of hair.
Selenium	:	Hair fall off when combing; also hair fall from eyebrows, whiskers and genitals. There is tingling and itching sensation on the scalp which feels tense and contracted.
Sepia	:	Losing hair after chronic headache.
Silicea.	:	Premature baldness. Itching of the scalp before menses.
Sphingurus	:	Falling of hair, especially from beard and whiskers.
Staphy	:	Hair falls off mostly from occiput and

around the ears, with humid foetid eruption or dandruff on the scalp.

Sulphur : The hair is very unruly — sandy, hard and lustreless, growing in all directions. The scalp is sore to touch. There is violent itching of the scalp which is worse by getting warm in bed.

Thuja : White scaly dandruff with dry hair.

Vinca Minor : Hair falls out in single spots and white hair grows there. The skin of the scalp oozes moisture with matting of hair. There is irresistable desire to scratch.

Wiesbaden : By the use of this remedy, the hair will grow rapidly and darker.

HAIR

Hair baldness (falling out) — *All-s, Sat, Anac, Apis, Fluor-ac.*
— **especially on crown** — *Bar-c*
— **premature** — *Sil*
— **in young people** — *Bar-c, Sil.*

Hair bristling (brushing, electric, on end, grasped, pulled, rises) — *Acet-ac, Ver.*
Hair, brittle — in brain disease of children — *Kali-c*

Hair brushing (bristling, combing, roots), painful : *Carb-s*
— **will not remain brushed** — *Med*

Hair, disposition to change colour (gray) — *Kali-iod.*

Hair does not bear combing (brushing, roots, touch) — *Asar*

Hair crawling — *Ver*

Hair, crisp — *Kali ars, Med.*

Hair cutting, complaints from — *Bell, Glon, Phos.*

Hair, dishevelled — *Ver*

Hair dry, (brittle, lustreless, rough) — *Aloe, Alum, Badiag, Hippo, Kali-ars, Med, Psor, Sul, Thuj,*
— in brain diseases of children — *Kali-c*
— in cholera — *Calc*
— in marasmus — *Calc*

Hair, electrical (bristling) — *Med*

Hair, as if standing on end — *Acon, Arn, Carbo-v, Chel, Mur-ac.*

Hair, falling out — *Amb, Bar-c, Calc-p, Canth, Carbo-a, Chel, Form, Kali-iod, Kali-s, Kreos, Magn-c, Merc, Sil, Sul,*
— on vertex — *Nitr-ac, Zinc.*

Hair, frowsy — *Bor*

Hair, feeling as if grasped roughly (pulled) — *Cinch.*

Hair, turns grey prematurely (white) — *Camph, Lyc.*

Hair, greasy — *Phos-ac*

Hair, growth, slow, short — *Thuja*

Hair, heaviness and heat of it distract her affection oi brain — *Glon*

Hair, lank and long — *Sul*

Hair, lustreless (dry) — *Hippoz, Med, Psor.*

Hair, luxuriant (growth on parts not otherwise covered by hair) — *Thuj*

Hair, moist (Plica, sticky) — *Hyper*

Hair, oily (Greasy) — *Bry, Merc, Pho-ac.*

Hair, picked at continually — *Lach*

Hair, plica polonica (Sticky) — *Ant-t, Fluor-ac, Jacea, Lyc, Sars, Ver, Vinca.*

Hair, pulls - *Ars, Bell, Cupr, Dig, Lil-t, Med, Tarn, Tub, Xanth,*

Hair, as if pulled (bristling on end, grasped)— *Acon, Aeth, Arg-n, Kali-n, Lach, Mag-c, Mag-m, Phos, Selen,*

Hair, rises (bristling) — *Acon, Bar-c, Cham, Canth, Chel, Glon, Laur, Meny, Mur-ac, Sul-iod, Ver-a, Zinc.*

Hair, roots (brushing, combing, touch) : destroyed by eruption (tinea) — *Ars*
— **painful** — *Coloc*
— **painful, when combed as from ulceration** — *Chel*
— **painful, especially to touch** — *Cinnab*

Hair, rough (dry) — *Bor*

Hair, splits — *Bor, Thuja.*

Hair, sticks together (plica), must comb it continually — *Psor.*

Hair, tangles easily — *Bor, Psor.*

Hair, constant attempt to tear in children — *Bell.*

Hair, thin (falling out) — *Thuj.*

Hair, touch (brushing, combing, roots), painful — *Apis.*

Hair, snowy white on deadened parts (grey) — *Ars-h.*

CHAPTER 23

Nail Diseases

Nail Dystrophy

Damage to the nails as a result of trauma or disease results in nail dystrophy. This is defined as the presence of a misshapen or partially destroyed nail plate. Soft, yellow keratin often accumulates between the dystrophic nail plate and nail bed, resulting in elevation of the former. Various common causes of nail dystrophy are discussed below.

Trauma: Trauma to the tips of the digits occasionally results in the formation of a subungial haematoma. The severe pain which accompanies this problem can be relieved by piercing the nail plate with a heated needle or paper clip. Large subungual hematomas result in sloughing of the nail plate weeks to months later. Permanent scarring sometimes accompanies trauma. The nail plate thicken often in an unevenly grooved or ridged pattern. A small amount of soft keratin may accumulate between the nail plate and nail bed. Nails scarred in this manner seem particularly predisposed to the subsequent development of onychomycosis. Unfortunately, surgical removal of the nail plate is simply followed by regrowth of an equally dystrophic nail. Cosmetic improvement can be obtained if one cements a false nail on top of the dystrophic nail plate.

Onychomycosis : Fungal infection is an extremely common cause of toe-nail dystrophy. The great toe-nail seems particularly prone to infection; involvement of the other toe-nails is less common. Infection of the finger-nails occurs only in nails previously traumatized or when nail involvement is part of tinea manum. Interestingly tinea manum never involves more than one hand. The likelihood of onychomycosis increases with age; children are rarely if ever involved. Nails in men are somewhat more frequently involved than are those in women.

The first sign of onychomycosis is generally the development of a small area of onycholysis (separation of the nail plate from the nail bed) at the distal tip of the nail. Shortly thereafter a buildup of soft yellow keratin occurs in the space created by the onycholysis. Eventually the entire nail plate is lifted and the end result if partially destroyed, heaped up, and mishaped, yellow nail. The entire process is asymptomatic unless a thickened toe-nail begins to press against the top of the shoe.

Most onychomycosis is due to infection with *Trichophyton rubrum* but in a few cases *Epidermophyton floccosum* and *Trichophyton mentagrophytes* may be recovered. Treatment is the same regardless of which organism causes the disease.

Psoriasis : Nail dystrophy occurs in a considerable proportion of patients with psoriasis. Most often nail changes follow the development of cutaneous lesions but, on rare occasions, they may precede any other clinical evidence of the disease. Several types of nail dystrophy are recognized. The specific clinical appearance depends on whether the pathology occurs in the nail matrix or the nail bed. In either case the psoriatic lesions responsible for these changes are hidden within the matrix or bed and are not visualized as clinical lesions.

Onycholysis occurs as the result of nail bed involvement. In early lesions the normally smooth, curvilinear distal junction of the nail plate with the nail bed becomes irregular. In more advanced disease, soft, yellow keratin accumulates between the nail plate and nail bed in a manner clinically indistinguishable from that which occurs in onychomycosis. The earliest reflection of nail matrix disease is the development of stippling or pitting on the surface of the nail plate. This type of pitting occurs only in patients with alopecia, areata and psoriasis. More advanced involvement of the nail matrix in concert with nail bed disease leads to the development of grossly mis-shapen nails. These more serious nail dystrophies are often accompanied by inflammatory, arthritic changes in the distal interphalangeal joint.

Arteriosclerotic Changes of the Toe-nails : A decrease of blood flow to the small vessels of the toes regularly results in the development of nail dystrophy. The nail changes found in these circumstances are clinically identical with those seen in onychomycosis; the two diseases can be correctly identified only when KOH preparations and fungal cultures are carried out. Arteriosclerotic dystrophy is seen only in the toe-nails; finger-nails are not affected.

Beau's Grooves : Beau's grooves are 1 mm wide depressions in the nail plate which extends horizontally from one lateral nail groove to the other. All nails are simultaneously affected. The groove occurs as the result of decreased nails construction during an episode of significant physiologic stress. Beau's grooves most commonly develop following dramatic illnesses such as myocardial infraction and periods of high fever. Similar grooving also develops after isolated periods of high fever. Similar grooving also develops after isolated periods of severe malnutrition. These grooves develop as the nail plate is forming in the nail matrix. Because of the slowness with which the nail plate grows, the groove first becomes visible at the posterior nail fold several weeks after the original insult. The groove then remains in the nail plate, slowly moving distally during the several months it takes for the nail plate to renew itself completely.

Clubbing : Clubbing of the distal fingers is identified by the following three criteria : (1) flattening of the groove, or angle, formed by the junction of the proximal nail plate and the paronychial fold; (2) rounding of the nail plate such that the distal edge begins to curve around the distal tip of the digit; and (3) widening or thickening of the digit from the distal interphalangeal joint to the tip. Clubbing is most commonly seen with chronic pulmonary or cardiopulmonary disease but also occurs with some tumours, especially those of the lung parenchyma. A somewhat similar, but not identical, process occurs in the thyroid acropachy of Grave's disease.

Nail Splitting : Splitting of the nail plate can occur in either of two forms : cracks which are oriented parallel to the length of the finger or through separation of the nail plate layers such that "flakes" of nail chip off the distal edge. Some instances of splitting occur as the result of scar formation within the nail matrix but most are idiopathic. Splitting generally worsens with aging. Cosmetic improvement can be obtained by applying multiple layers of clear finger-nail polish such that the cracks, fissures and flakes are cemented together. False finger-nails can also be cemented over the underlying dystrophic nail.

Warts : Periungual warts often distort the nail plate. In most instances the dystrophy is not permanent and the nail plate returns to normal following therapeutic or spontaneous resolution of the warts. Permanent nail dystrophy occasionally occurs when warts have been present for long periods of time or when they have been aggressively treated with destructive modalities such as electrosurgery.

Nail Colour Changes

White Banding :Horizontal white banding or opacification (Terry's nails, half and half nails, Muercke's lines) occurs in a variety of settings. Clear cut distinction among the various types of white nail banding is not usually possible. In most instances these changes are seen in the presence of hypoalbuminemia accompanying chronic hepatic or renal disease.

Brown Banding : Brown banding occurs in either of two directions : a vertical band running from the posterior nail fold to the distal tip of the nail or a horizontal band running from one lateral nail fold to the other. The former occurs as the normal finding in black patients and can be seen secondary to the presence of a nevus or melanoma in the nail matrix of white patients. Because of the risk of melanoma such lesions, when newly acquired, should be biopsied. The other, horizontal bands of pigment, may be found in Addison's disease and following systemic administration of various cancer chemotherapeutic agents.

Splinter Haemorrhages : Splinter hemorrhages occur as thin dark red lines 1 to 3 mm in length. They represent small haemorrhages at the junction of the nail plate and the nail bed. These hemorrhages are carried outward to the distal tip of the finger as the nail grows. The presence of these hemorrhages is believed by some to be a helpful diagnostic sign of bacterial endocarditis and trichinosis but their frequent occurrence in totally healthy individuals makes their significance doubtful in most clinical settings.

Onycholysis

If you look at the distal tip of your finger-nail you will notice that the free edge where it overhangs the nail bed is white. This opacification occurs because of the second air-nail interface which is present on the underside of the nail. In situations where the nail plate is separated from the nail bed, a similar white opacification occurs. This separation is known as onycholysis. Bacterial organisms sometimes colonize this blind pocket. These organisms add colour : *Pseudomonas species* results in a green colour and *Proteus species* results in a brown or black colour. Onycholysis is a non-inflammatory, asymptomatic condition.

Onycholysis is most commonly caused by infection with *Candida species*, especially *C. albicans*. These *Candida* infections occur with particular frequency in individuals such as dish-washers, bartenders, waitresses and dentists who are regularly involved in wet work. Onycholysis due to candida infection is often, but not always, accompanied by paronychial swelling and inflammation. Onycholysis also occurs in psoriasis and is somewhat less often seen with trauma, hyperthyroidism and as a result of photochemical separation in patients taking tetracycline.

The diagnosis of onycholysis due to candidiasis is generally made on a clinical basis. KOH preparations are not very productive but positive cultures can usually be obtained from pieces clipped from the overlying nail.

Paronychial Inflammation

Candida Paronychia : Infection with *Candida* species (usually *C. albicans*) is the most common cause of paronychial inflammation and swelling of the fingers. It occurs with considerable frequency in people such as dish-washers, bartenders and waitresses who are regularly involved in wet-work. *Candida* paronychia is characterized by : (1) lack of pain, (2) lack of warmth,

(3) absence or paucity of pus, and (4) chronicity. Onycholysis frequently accompanies candidal paronychia. The diagnosis is usually made on a clinical basis. KOH preparations are difficult to carry out and often there is even insufficient material for culture.

Bacterial Paronychia : Bacterial paronychia is an acute, painful process. It is usually preceded by an episode of trauma such as the tearing of a hang-nail. It presents with all the classical signs of a bacterial process : redness, warmth, swelling and tenderness. Gentle pressure on the swollen tissue often results in the expression of a drop of pus which can then be picked up on an applicator for culture. From a practical standpoint, however, culture is not usually necessary.

Herpetic Whitlow : Herpetic whitlow is the name given to paronychial infection with *Herpesvirus hominis* type I or type II. Like bacterial paronychia, this infection occurs acutely and is associated with redness, swelling, warmth, exquisite tenderness and regional lymphadenophathy. It is regularly confused with bacterial paronychia but careful examination will reveal the presence of multiple, grouped, minute vesicles. The disease is an occupational hazard for individuals such as nurses, dentists and dental assistants who are routinely involved in mouth care. Herpetic whitlow runs its course in approximately 10 days. There is no specific therapy.

Ingrown Toe-nails : Ingrown toe-nail is the most common cause of paronichial inflammation of the great toe. It develops when the sharp edge of the great toe-nail pierces the surrounding fold of a paronychial tissue. Ingrown toe-nail is likely to occur when one or more of the following are present : (1) nail is curved to a greater degree than normal (2) the toe-nail is clipped back too far allowing tissue to roll up over it; (3) athletic endeavours which require sudden stops ("toe jamming") are carried out; and (4) ill-fitting shoes are worn such that the toe of the shoe presses against the nail and surrounding tissue. Bacterial infection regularly develops in the paronychial tissue traumatized by the presence of an ingrown nail.

Therapy of an acute ingrown nail requires that the nail corners be lifted free of the surrounding; inflamed paronychial tissue. This is easily (although uncomfortably) carried out by the application of mosquito forceps to the nail plate. With the plate lifted a small pledget of cotton can be wedged under the nail. This programme leads to gratifying improvement within a week at which time surgical correction, if necessary, can be carried out. Such surgery generally requires permanent removal of a portion of the nail plate and nail matrix.

Homoeopathic Approach

It is said in medicine that nail changes can be the tell-tale signs of patients occupation, a systemic disease of vascular and neurogenic disorders, of the patients nutritional state and dermatological affections.

General Remarks

(1) First of all identify the clinical manifestations in the nail, then try to catch whether it is starting proximally or free end.

(2) It is important to establish this fact besides making sure whether all the nails on hands and feet are involved or there is unilateral affection or only single nail is affected. Single nail involvement is usually due to some local cause; unilateral involvement is usually due to neurological or circulatory cause, while bilateral symmetrical involvement is usually due to the systemic cause or generalized dermatosis.

(3) Try to sort out the exact cause of it by history and a complete physical examination — dermatological, systemic, nutritional, etc.

(4) Local causes in the form of trauma, manicuring and dermatosis are very important; hence they must be considered before systemic cause is presumed.

(5) A simple olive oil massage helps to bring back the shine and lustre of the nails.

In treatment, emphasis should be made on prescribing constitutional deep-acting remedy. Local treatment is rather unsatisfactory. General health of the patient must be improved by nourishing diet, supplementary vitamins, etc. The overall outlook is rather gloomy in most affection, unless the primary cause can be corrected. Even then, enough time should be allowed for the new nail to grow.

Drugs

Alumina	:	Panaritium with brittle nails, lancinating pains and tendency to ulceration of the finger-tips; gnawing beneath the finger-nails, with crawling along the arm as far as the clavicle; nails brittle or thick, spots on nails.
Anthracinum	:	Violent burning pain in panaritium; absorption of pus into the blood; gangrenous destruction; cerebral symptoms.
Antimonium Crud	:	Deficient growth of nails; split nails, growing cracked and thick (split hoof in horses); thick, horny, callosities of skin.
Apis Mel	:	Burning, stinging, throbbing panaritium, which is hard and has a white, sickly bleached out appearance, characteristic of the bee sting; very sensitive to touch; the finger swells rapidly, with tense glossy-red surface, extending up to forearm.
Arnica	:	Ulceration around the roots of nails, with painful soreness of the ends of the fingers.
Asafoetida	:	Whitlow, with violent nightly pains and threatening necrosis of phalanx.
Berberis	:	Pain under finger-nails, with coldness of feet, extending up ankles and swelling of some of the finger-joints.
Bryonia	:	Tight, compressed feeling with pressing-out sensation, as if the finger needed more room, dark, congested part; chilly feelings at times, but dry heat and burning tearing, shooting pains more prominent; at first cold applications pleasant, later moist hot poultices more agreeable; dry mouth without thirst or great thirst; bitter taste; dry stool; dry skin; pulse fast; frequent and strong.

Bufo : Bluish black swelling around nail, followed by suppuration; *pains run in streaks up the arm to axilla* : after slight confusion, tearing pain, with redness along whole arm, following lymphatic vessels into armpit, causing painful glandula swellings.

Dioscorea : *Disposition to Felons* : frequent sharp pains in bones of fingers, one finger at a time, sensation as of a brier in the middle finger of each hand with throbbing, darting, stinging pain next to the bone and very tender to pressure; nails brittle; jumping; darting pains in corns.

Fluoric Acid : Felon, particularly *Bone felons*, with offensive discharge; > from cold applications; phalanges swollen far above their natural size, on dorsum of finger an opening discharges ichorous pus; panaritium, also simple onychia with ulceration; sharp sticking pain at root of right thumb-nail. Nails grow more rapidly, crumpled or longitudinal ridges in them; soreness between toes; soreness of all the corns. It promotes expulsion of necrotic bones.

Graphites : Ingrowing toe-nail; sides and roots of the finger and toe-nails become sore, ulcerate and swell, they are exceedingly painful, violently burning and throbbing, then suppuration and proud flesh. Given at the beginning it absorbs the ailment in a few hours, hypertrophy of nails.

Hepar Sulph : Superficial erysipelatous onychia around the root of the nail; Before suppuration Hep. After it — Lach; thumb livid, violent throbbing, cutting, burning pain, lymphatics inflamed, lump in axilla; patient sensitive to touch and cold; subject to it every winter; decided yellow colour of the skin;

pulse can be plainly felt, and the patient cannot bear the weight or pressure of a poultice though > by warmth generally.

Hypericum : Panaritium; injuries of parts rich in sentient nerves, particularly fingers and toes and matrices of nails; pains severe and of long duration; mechanical injuries by splinters or needless under nails; squeezing or hammering of toes and fingers.

Lachesis : Maltreated cases of some standing, when gangrene is threatening or has already set in, emitting an intolerable odour (Ars); pricking in the ends of fingers.

Ledum : Consequent to injuries, but only in first stage, as by pulling off abruptly a hang-nail, during sewing; nightly itching of feet.

Lycopodium : Inflammation extending over whole hand; dark-red swelling; belching, bloated abdomen, emptiness in stomach, with yawning.

Mercurius : Inflammation in the cellular tissue beneath the cutis, in the sinews, their fasciae, and their phalangeal joints; pains not violent, more throbbing than shooting; patient extremely sensitive to heat and cold.

Natrum Sulph : Living in damp dwellings or workshops, pale appearance, lassitude and dull headache in the morning, chilly and feverish in the evening. A blister on the unguilar phalanx, followed by deep-red swelling; festering at root of nail; great pains, more bearable outdoors than in the room.

Nux-Vomica : Suppuration in palmar surface of finger or thumb with throbbing or burning pain < by warmth and by letting the hand down, in the evening after sundown; more comfortable in bed.

Rhus-Tox : Slow local development, frequent remission; dark-red erysipelatous, with little blisters or oedema; pain running up the armpit.

Sepia : Itching with throbbing, shooting and burning at intervals or alternately; part dark-red and pus visible.

Silicea : Affection of periosteum; moderate redness or heat, deep-seated inflammation, violent shooting pain deep in the finger, worse in the warm bed, sleepless at night, pain being unbearable, with great restlessness, irritability even unto convulsive jerks; opening with a surrounding wall of proud flesh, pus malignant, discoloured; it promotes expulsion of necrotic bones; ingrowing toe-nail; tearing pains as if the bones would be actually torn out, preventing all sleep, *Frequent crops of boils*; chronic foetid foot-sweats, slightest draught unbearable.

Sulphur : Hang-nails; complementary to Apis in panaritium.

Thuja : Finger-nails distorted, crumbling, soft, discoloured (Graph., Nitr-ac., Sil.), toe-nails brittle and distorted; ingrowing toe-nails.

NAILS

Nails, affected in general : *Alum, Am-m, Ant-t, Ars, Aur, Bar-c, Bell, Bor, Bov, Calc-c, caust, Chel, Chin, Coch, Colch, Con, Dig, Dro, Grap, Hell, Hep-s, Iod, Kali-c, Lach, Lyc, Mag-s, Mar, Merc, Mosch, Mur-ac, Nat-m, Nit-ac, Nux-v, Par, Petr, Pho-ac, Plat, Puls, Ran-b, Rhus-t, Rut, Sabad, Scil, Sec-c, Sep, Sil, Sul-ac, Thuj*

Around — *Calc-p*

Black — *Crot-h, Grap.*

Blue - *Aur, Chel , Chin , Coch , Dig, Dros, Ip, Lyc, Manc, Nat-m, Nux-v,Petr, Plb, Sil, Ver-v,*

Brittle - *Ālum Ars, Calc-c, Calc-fi,* **Graph**, *Lept, Merc, Nat-m , Sabad, Sep, Sil, Spi, Thuj.*

Burning as of — *Caust, Con, Elap, Nit-ac, Sars, Vinc.*

Burrowing — *Caust*

Crumbling — *Merc, Sil, Thuj.*

Crawling under — *Lach*

Deformed, thickened, etc —*Alum, ant-c, Ars, Calc-fl, Caust, Ferr, Grap, Merc, Sabad, Sep, Sil, Sul, Thuj.*

Discoloured —*Ant-c, Ars. Caust. Ferr, Graph, Mur-ac, Nit-ac, Sil, Sul. Thuj.*

Exfoliating —*Ferr, Graph, Merc.*

Falling off —*Ant-c, Ars, Bor, Canth, Chloral, Croc, Form, Graph, Hell, Merc, Scil, Sec-c, Sil, Sul, Thuj, Ust.*

Sensation — *Ap, Pyro.*

Growing slowly — *Ant-c, Sil.*

Hang-nails — *Calc-c, Lyc, Merc, Nat-m,' Rhus-t, Sang, Stan, Sul.*

Horny growths under —*Ant-c, Graph.*

Ingrown —*Coloc, Graph, Kali-c, Mar, Sil, Sul, Sul-io.*

Needles under as if — *Led*

Numb and tingle -- *Colch*

Pain under — *Carb-v, Caust, Flu-ac, Graph, Hep, Kali-c, Merc, Sil.*

Painful _ *Am-m, Ant-t, Bell, Caust, Graph, Hep, Kali-c, Mag-s, Mar, Merc, Nat-m,, Nit-ac, Nux-v, Par, Puls, Ran-b, Rhus-t, Sabad, Scil, Sep, Sil, Sul.*

Panaritium — *Anthx, Ap, Ars, Flu-ac, Hep, Lach, Merc, Nat-s, Rhus-t, Sil.*

Prickling — *Colch*

Ribbled; ridged, furrowed — *Ars, Sabad*

Sensitive — *Calc-c, Con, Hep-s, Mag-s, Merc, Nat-m, Nux-v, Petr, Pho-ac, Scil, Sep, Sil, Sul, Thuj.*

Sore, smarting pain, etc. —*Alum, Ant-c, Calc-c, Caust, Graph, Hep-s, merc., Mez, Mag-s, Nat-m, Nux-v, Puls, Sep, Sul.*

Soft —*Thuj*

Splinters under, as of — *Calc-p, Coc-c, Colch, Flu-ac, Hep-s, Nat-m, Nit-ac, Petr, Plat, Ran-b, Sil, Sul.*

Splitting cracked — *Ant-c, Ars, Flu-ac, Nat-m, Rut, Sabad, Scil, Sil.*

Spotted —*Alum, Ars, Nit-ac, Sep, Sil, Spig, Sul, Thuj*

Suppuration — *See Ulcerative pain.*

Thick —*See deformed above.*

Throbbing under — *Sul.*
Tingling in — *Colch.*

Ulcerated, Onychia — *Alum, Am-m, Ant-c, Ars, Aur, Bar-c, Graph, Bell, Bor, Bov, Calc-c, Calc-fl, Caust, Chin, Cist, Con, Graph, Hep-s, Lach, Lyc, Mar, Merc, Mur-ac, nat-m, Nat-s, Nit-ac, Petr, Pho-ac, Plat, Puls, Ran-b, Rhus-t, Rut, Sabad, Scil, Sec-c, Sep, Sil, Sul, Sul-ac, Sil-ic, Sul-io, Thuj*

Ulcerative pain —*Am-m, Bell, Berb, Calc-p, Caust, Chin, Graph, Hep-s, Kali-c, Mag-s, Merc, Mosch, Mur-ac, Nat-m, Nux-v, Puls, Ran-b, Rhus-t, Rut, Sep, Sil, Sul, Sul-ac, Thuj*

Yellow —*Amb, Ant-c, Ars, Aur, Bell, Bry, Calc-c, Canth, Carb-v, Caust, Cham, Chel, Chin, Con, Ferr, Hep-s, Ign, Lyc, Merc, Nit-ac, Nux-v, Op, Plb, Puls, Sep, Sil, Spig, Sul.*

HOMOEOPATHY AND COMPARATIVE MEDICINE
February 1957
Page No. 37 - Case No.1.

A Case of Whitlow Cured
(by Mr. K.P. Balakrishna Rai)

Patient — My wife aged 23 years.

On December 20, 1955, my wife complained that there was slight swelling with inflammation and burning on the phalanx around the nails of her right hand. I did not give her any medicine as I thought the complaint will get cured spontaneously. On December 24, all the symptoms aggravated, the part was red and swollen with signs of impending suppuration. She could not touch anything and the pain was intolerable with nightly aggravation. She applied some cooling Ayurvedic remedies, which gave her no relief and she wanted me to have it operated by a doctor. The portion of 'Silicea' among the lectures of the Grace Medical Mission now came to my mind. On the 25th morning, I gave her six doses of *Silicea* 12x, a dose of two pills to be taken every hour. After taking the 6 doses there was much relief. She had undisturbed sleep that night. Next day she was able to use her fingers without feeling any pain or discomfort. As there was improvement, I increased the interval between the doses and gave only three doses that day. On the third day, I observed that the pus had all been absorbed and the finger looked normal. This confirmed my belief in the curative principles of Homoeopathy and many cases of whitlow and similar affections of other patients were since treated by me with *Belladonna*, *Hepar* and *Silicea* and no surgical intervention was called for in any of them. Thank God that a layman like me could render such medical aid.

CHAPTER **24**

Pruritus

Introduction

The Hindustani equivalent for pruritus is '*kharash*' or '*khujli*'. It is a symptom and scratch marks are its sign. The amount of advertisements this symptom has inspired and the number of panaceas it has brought forth, indicates what a common and annoying condition it must be. Pruritus interferes with activity and sleep; so it becomes a social problem. The intensity of itching excited by a stimulus varies with the sensitivity of the skin and the mind, from person to person. Tramps, for instance, hardly feel mosquito bites; people with morbid minds, on the other hand, may start scratching at a mere suggestion. The skin and the nervous system are closely related because of their common origin in the embryo; for this reason, mental stress cannot only start itching, but also complicate several skin disorders, particularly pruritus.

The exact mode in which pruritus is produced still remains obscure, but it is believed that pruritus is produced by the activation of the nerve endings of pain, which are present in the papillary layer of the corium, due to summation of subthreshold stimuli. In comparison, intermittent stimulation results in tickling and threshold stimuli produce pain. There are no known special nerve endings concerned specifically with itching. The itch sensation terminates centrally in the thalamus; that is why comatose patients itch and people scratch in dreams.

Pathophysiology of pruritus still eludes satisfactory explanation and understanding. Histamine and certain proteoses (and enzymes) whether introduced from outside or liberated as a consequence of antigen-antibody reaction evoke pruritus. Threshold of pruritus is lowered in thin skinned individuals under emotional stress and loneliness. People prone to sense of heat at more prone to pruritus.

Results of Itching

Local — Scratch marks. Broken hair.
Excoriations. Polished nails.
May be secondary pyoderma, eczematization and even ulceration.
Lichenification.
Pigmentation and even depigmentation.

General — Interference with physical and social activities.
Irritability.
Insomnia.
Exhaustion and wasting.

Causes of Pruritus

(a) **Physical and Physiological**

1. Rough clothing, wool next to skin, tight clothes.
2. Heat, cold, dryness, humidity. Hot and cold baths also produce itching.
3. An unclean body, dirt and dust accumulated in the absence of frequent bathing.
4. Hot, spicy food and alcohol causing cutaneous flushing.

(b) **Itching Dermatoses** (itching caused by a skin disease of Infection)

1. Animal, parasites — scabies, pediculoses, insect bites, fleas, bugs, mites, mosquitoes, etc.

2. Ringworm.
3. Dermatitis and eczema.
4. Urticaria, angioneurotic oedema.
5. Lichen planus.
6. Neurodermatitis — localized and disseminated.
7. Prurigo simplex, nodularis, atopic.
8. Psoriasis patients itch in tropical climate.
9. Mycosis fungoides and reticuloses.
10. Erythrodermas.
11. Prickly heat.
12. Dermatitis herpetiformis.
13. Local stasis, Schamberg's disease.

(c) Local Irritation by discharges, etc.

(d) Systemic Disorders producing itching, but perhaps no skin lesions.

1. Hepatic diseases.
2. Renal diseases.
3. Diabetes, myxoedema.
4. Drugs — Morphia, Cocaine, Barbiturates.
5. Animal parasites — intestinal worms, trichiniasis, onchocerciasis.
6. Anaemia and leukaemias.
7. Senility.
8. Pregnancy and oral contraceptives.
9. Internal malignancy.

(e) Psychogenic

1. Neurasthenia.
2. Neurodermatitis.
3. Agarophobia.
4. Prurigo.

General Discussion

Syphilides hardly ever itch except when present in moist areas or when they are scrofulosorum in type. Besides the above list of causes of pruritus, regarding which information can be obtained in the respective chapters dealing with them, there are some special varieties of pruritus — pruritus ani, pruritus vulvae and pruritus scrotum. Before proceeding to the method of tackling a case of pruritus, lay emphasis on the following :

1. One should look for evidence of dermatoses, insect bites etc. The majority of cases of itching fit in the group of itching dermatoses. The patient must be completely unclothed, examined fully in natural or fluorescent light; the clothes should also be scrutinized for lice and other parasites. The distribution of pruritus and the nature of the lesions decide the exact etiological diagnosis.

2. Physical factors like heat, cold, clothing, diet, etc. should not be forgotten. Even if a physical factor is not the primary cause, common experience has shown that in almost all patients pruritus is aggravated by exposure to the sun, change of temperature, movement of air, by cold or hot bath and peripheral vascular dilatation resulting from the intake of alcohol and hot spicy food.

3. When pruritus is present without skin lesions, a complete systemic examination including rectal and vaginal examination should be undertaken along with an examination of the urine for sugar, albumin, etc. Stool test; haemogram; blood sugar, cholesterol, urea, uric acid, liver function tests, X-ray of the chest and bones; psychiatric and emotional assessment.

4. Any drug habit or association must be brought out in the history.

5. Only in the absence of the above factors and in the presence of definite evidence of psychogenic involvement, must be a diagnosis of psychogenic pruritus be accepted. It must be borne in mind that any pruritus can become worse or exaggerated due to secondary mental involvement establishing a vicious circle.

General Treatment

It consists of :

1. Eliminating the cause.

2. Removing the exciting factors. The patient must be properly clothed; avoid sudden changes of temperature;

indulge in luke-warm baths; take simple bland food and avoid excess of tea, coffee and alcohol. The bowels must be kept open.

3. Reassurance.

Senile Pruritus

Strictly speaking, the term implies generalized itching in elderly people, usually after the age of 50 to 60, with senile, atrophic dry skin; itching is precipitated by rough or wollen clothing, sudden changes in temperature, baths, etc. The other known causes of pruritus and itching dermatoses are absent. Though itching becomes generalized sooner or later, to begin with it may be confined to the trunk or the lower extremities. The course is usually progressive and the outlook is rather poor. The treatment consists of :

1. Massage with olive oil calendula mixture in 1:6 ratio.
2. Protection from the physical exciting causes.

Summer Pruritus

It is a fairly common complaint during the summer months in the hotter parts of tropical countries. In northern India, it is seen in between the months of April and August, but it occurs in its worst form during the monsoon. Dry heat frequently causes pruritus, but the other more common causes of summer pruritus are; profuse perspiration which results in clothes sticking to the body; dusty environment; uncleanliness; heat spots and prickly heat. It is more common in people who are overweight and overclothed for the climate. The treatment should be emphasis on correcting the responsible causes, improving the general health of the patient, encouraging him to use thin clothing, to live and work in cool hygienic environments. Airconditioning, if possible is very helpful. A talcum dusting powder massage is also beneficial. For an extreme case, holiday at a cool hill station is the answer.

Winter Pruritus

It implies itching in the cold winter months in certain individuals; the itching disappears with the onset of the warm weather; other known causes of pruritus are absent. Itching occurs mostly on the trunk, thighs and arms on undressing. Exposure to cold weather is the precipitating cause, though dry skin, a run-down condition, the use of strong alkaline soaps, a very cold or very hot bath and woollen clothes tend to cause pruritus. The treatment consists in correcting the exciting and predisposing causes, in bathing properly, clothing the body suitably and improving the general health. The palliataive treatment is the same as discussed above.

Pruritus Ani

It may occur as such, or be associated with pruritus vulvae and scrotum. It is a fairly common complaint seen as simple pruritus with a sodden anal skin, but sooner or later sequelae of pruritus like excoriations, pyoderma, lichenification and eczematization develop to complicate matters. Pruritus ani is more common in males than females. It is common in Asiatic countries because of heat and perspiration causing maceration, frequent gastro-intestinal disorders, hot spicy food and the high incidence of intestinal worms, etc.

Etiology. The common cause of pruritus ani are :

(a) Local causes (Inside the anus) : Threadworms.
Fissure-in-ano.
Haemorrhoids, polypi and fistula. Moist anus due to improper drying.
Chronic constipation or diarrhoea.
Hot spicy or sensitising foods.

(b) Skin Diseases : Tinea, monilial infection, intertrigo.
Condylomata lata and acuminatum.
Seborrhoeic dermatitis.
Psoriasis; eczema.
Pediculoses.
Lichen sclerosus atrophicus.
Contact dermatitis to toilet paper, enemas.

(c) Systemic : Use of antibiotics and other drugs.

			Diabetes. Achlorhydria. Reticuloses. Senility.
(d)	Spread of Pruritus from Vulval Region	:	Also from the scrotopenile region in conditions like diabetes, leucorrhoea, pelvic tumours.
(e)	Psychogenic Pruritus	:	Neurodermatitis.

Diagnosis : In pruritus the diagnosis is mainly etiological; hence before any treatment is instituted the patient must be subjected to a thorough examination and investigation to establish the cause. Firstly, cutaneous diseases and the possibility of pruritus having spread from neighbouring areas must be ruled out. If both these groups of causes are absent, the gastro-intestinal tract must be completely investigated by history taking, repeated stool examinations, a rectal swab, a protoscopic examination, etc. Only when no etiological factor is identified may primary psychogenic causes be considered as producing the neurodermitis.

Treatment consists of :

1. Reassurance.

2. Eradication of causes. In early and mild cases, this alone is enough. The diet should be simple, light and wholesome. All indigestible foodstuffs — chillies, condiments, curries and alcohol must be with-held. Anal region should be lubricated with oil at bath time.

3. The affected part must be kept clean, cool and dry. Underwears should be cotton and loose.

Pruritus Vulvae

It is a common and often very distressing form of localized pruritus occurring by itself or in association with pruritus ani or itching of the groins and adjacent parts of the thighs. Itching may either be confined to the vulval skin or include the vaginal walls and urethral orifice. Simple pruritus soon gets complicated by excoriations, lichenification, eczematization and pyoderma. It is common in married women, 30 to 35 years of age. Occasionally, it comes across in children and adolescents.

Etiology

(a) Cutaneous diseases of the vulval region.
Scabies, pediculoses.
Tinea.
Contact dermatits due to contraceptives, douches, pessaries, medicated sanitary pads, toilet paper and local medicaments.
Lichen planus.
Psoriasis.
Herpes progenitalis.
Intertrigo, infective eczema, seborrhoeic dermatitis.
Condylomata lata and acuminatum.
Lichen sclerosus et atrophicus, leukoplakia.
Senile vulvitis and kraurosis vulvae.
Filariasis — elephantiasis, and schistosomiasis.
Lymphogranuloma venereum causing esthiomene.
Fox Fordyce's disease.

(b) Local causes in the vaginal and urinary tract.
Vaginal discharge — monilial or trichomonas infection.
Cystitis, vaginitis and cervicitis.
Acid urine and also urinary incontinence.
Urethral stones.
Pregnancy and pelvic congestion.

(c) Spread from neighbouring areas.
Anus — thread worms and pruritus ani (other causes).
Thighs — tinea, intertrigo, etc.

(d) Systemic.
Diabetes.
Drug eruptions, especially antibiotics.
Achlorhydria.
Senility.
Liver disease.
Malignancy.
Reticuloses.

(e) Psychogenic.
Neurodermatitis due to sexual frustration, perversion sex, guilt or fear of venereal disease.

Diagnosis : Since the diagnosis is mainly etiological, emphasis should be laid on eliciting the cause before prescribing any treatment. A complete examination should be made of the skin of the vulval region for cutaneous disease, and also of the urogenital tract, the anus, and the neighbouring regions. Routine investigations include examination of urine for sugar and acidity; of stools for ova and vaginal discharge for infective flora. Though mental and emotional factors are responsible for a great deal of chronic pruritus vulvae (both primarily and secondarily), physical organic causes must first be exluded. The help of a psychoanalyst and a social worker may prove useful in tracking down the psychogenic causes.

Prognosis : Pruritus vulvae can be most distressing; in a small percentage of cases, it becomes an obstinate complaint.

Treatment : The basic principles of treatment are almost the same as those applied in general pruritus and pruritus ani. They consist of :

1. Reassurance, particularly about the absence of cancer, or other contagious diseases.

2. Keeping the affected part clean, dry and lubricated.

Pruritus Scrotum and Penis
It is fairly common complaint in young or middle aged persons in tropical countries. According to the author's experience, pruritus of the male genital organs is more common than pruritus vulvae in India. The reasons for this may be that : (1) Shy Indian women do not come forward for consultation as men do. (2) Nutritional deficiencies affect the scrotum causing itching.

Itching may be mild, moderate, or very severe and distressing. The skin becomes thickened, rugose, excoriated and lichenified.

There may be a secondary complication of pyoderma; and itching from the scrotum of anus may also spread to the perineum.

The common causes are :

1. **Pruritus on the penis** :
   (a) Glycosuria.
   (b) Herpes progenitalis.
   (c) Pediculoses, scabies.
   (d) Contact dermatitis due to contraceptives, pessaries, etc.
   (e) Irritation by vaginal discharges.
   (f) Prostatic affections.
   (g) Neurodermatitis.
   (h) Spread of itching from neighbouring areas, other cutaneous diseases, etc.

2. Pruritus on the scrotum :
   (a) Scabies, pediculoses.
   (b) Contact dermatitis due to contraceptives, irritation by vaginal discharges, etc.
   (c) Excessive sweating.
   (d) Intertrigo starts at the junction of the penis with the scrotum.
   (e) Chaffing by underwear, loin cloth or suspendory bandage.
   (f) Tinea cruris.
   (g) Nutritional deficiency.
   (h) Use of broad spectrum antibiotics.
   (i) Neurodermatitis.
   (j) Spread of itching from neighbouring areas and other cutaneous diseases including sebaceous cysts.

Treatment is similar to that employed in pruritus vulvae and ani.

Pruritus in Pregnancy

Besides, the usual causes of pruritus, there is a small group of dermatoses characterized by pruritic papules and urticarial plagues that occur predominantly, if not exclusively during pregnancies, clearing up on delivery and recurrence with subsequent pregnancies. These conditions now number nine, and of these, four stand out as distinct entities either because their mechanism of production is now elucidated (herpes gestationis, pruritus gravidarum, auto-immune progesterone dermatitis of pregnancy) or because of unique clinical and laboratory findings (impetigo herpetiformis).

Drugs

Aethusa	:	Pimples on vulva, itching when patient becomes warm.
Aloe	:	Itching and burning in anus, preventing sleep; itching of prepuce; itching, especially of legs.
Alumina	:	Itching of orifice of urethra; pruritus vaginae; itching in eye-lids, anus, scrotum and shoulders. *Rough Skin all over the body.*
Alumina	:	Intolerable itching of whole body, especially when getting warm and in bed, scratches till the skin bleeds, which is then painful; itching piles, with burning excoriation and great sensitiveness; itching, throbbing and stitches in vagina.
Ambra	:	Voluptuous itching on scrotum; severe itching on pudenda, must rub parts, swelling of labia; *Pruritus vulva during pregnancy.*
Ammonium Carb	:	Violent itching of skin, after scratching burning blisters appear; itching and stinging of skin keep him awake; though lessened by scratching; itching and burning at anus; itching at genitals.
Antimonium Crud	:	Itching of skin, feels sore if scratched; itching of penis, of tip of glans; biting, itching, as from salt on left side of scrotum.
Antimonium Tart	:	Violent itching of pudena, pustules on external genitals.
Argentum Met	:	Intolerable itching, as from crawling, on head and body, unchanged by scratching,

even motion of skin is almost unbearable; pruritus scroti.

Argentum Nit : Itching smarting mostly of thighs and axillae, when warm in bed; skin brown, tense and hard.

Arsenicum : Itching with burning or an eruption emitting watery fluid like sweat and attended with much constitutional weakness; chronic cases; senile pruritus in broken-down constitutions, < from cold applications, > from warmth; itching of genital organs.

Caladium : Pruritus vulvae during pregnancy and after miscarriage; *pruritus vaginae induces onanism*, with mucous discharge and pimples around parts; violent itching on external genitals compelled her to scratch in spite of punishment, reduced her in mind and body; violent itching eruption on scrotum, < at night, dry and scaly, violent corrosive itching, burning, must touch parts, but cannot scratch there, no swelling, but much heat, in face frequent sensation as if a fly were crawling there, > from cold water.

Calcarea Carb : Itching and stitches in internal or external vulva < towards evening or after going to bed; severe itching on various parts of body in bed; violent irritation about chest, back, neck and shoulders, in calves of legs, followed by a reddish rash; < at night.

Cantharis : Pruritus vulvae, especially from masturbation, itching intense; pruritus, with strong sexual desire, *during climaxis*; itching changing place, as from fleas.

Causticum : Itching over whole body at various parts, on tip and wings of nose, face, scrotum, back, arms, palms, dorsum of feet, preventing sleep; itching of orifice of urethra, scrotum and skin of penis.

Chelidonium : Itching of skin; crawling and itching in rectum and on perineum; sticking and itching in anus; itching and creeping in scrotum and glans.

Coffea : Voluptuous itching, would like to scratch, but parts are too sensitive, the least itching of skin prevents sleep.

Collinsonia : Prutitus vulvae, *accompanied by Haemorrhoids*, obstinate constipation during dysmenorrhoea or in pregnancy, < when lying down, parts swollen and bulging; itching intolerable, making her almost delirious, > by bathing in cold water.

Conium : Violent itching of pudenda and even within vagina, day and night, < just after menstruation; erratic itching of all parts of body, as from fleas.

Croton Tig : Frequent corrosive itching on glans and scrotum, < while walking; intense itching of female genitals, < at night, > by very gentle scratching; eruptions on body itch very much, cannot bear severe scratching but a mere rub suffices to allay the itching.

Cuprum Acet and Ars : Skin sensitive to contact with clothing;itching, especially of arms and legs, < undressing at night and in bed, with slight relief only from scratching of coarse rubbing; sleep disturbed and unrefreshing; pruritus ani; scrotum constantly moist and damp.

Dolichos Pruriens : Intolerable itching all over body *in pregnant women*, < at night preventing sleep, and from scratching, no perceptible eruption on skin, constipation jaundice; *itching without erup-*

		tion, first on feet every winter higher up, after 7 years reaches him upto abdomen.
Euphorbium	:	Itching of mons veneris; burning itching in different parts of body which induces scratching.
Ferrum Met	:	Pruritus recti, he cannot sleep at night on account of the itching; the worms creep at night out of the anus.
Fluoric Acid	:	Pruritus ani; itching within and around anus, on perineum.
Graphites	:	Pruritus ani; with moisture and tendency to form little vesicles; itching in vulva, < *just before menses* (Con., *After menses*), especially for persons inclined to obesity; continual itching, < at night, nothing visible upon skin before scratching, which causes nodules and long welts.
Hamamelis	:	Itching at anus, which feels sore, as if raw; pruritus of female parts; soreness and smarting on small spots, not very sensitive to touch.
Helonias	:	Excessive pruritus vulvae, which is puffed, hot red and itching terribly; labia swollen and covered with a curdy, white deposit, like aphthae; leucorrhoea of a bad odor, easily changing to flow of blood.
Hepar-Sulph	:	Itching of penis and at fraenum preputii; smarting itching of vulva, little pimples around ulcer, with leucorrhoea; burning itching of body, with white vesicles after scratching; unhealthy skin, slight injuries suppurate.
Hydrastis	:	Pruritus vulvae, with profuse leuccorrhoea and sexual excitement.

Ignatia : Itching of skin of a fine pricking character resembling flea-bites, and changing from one place to another; itching better from gentle scratching; when getting heated in the open air.

Iodum : Papules that are very apt to run together or around which the skin in brownish and covered with scales; irresistible nocturnal itching, compelling one to scratch and thus causing insomnia, cachectic appearance, emaciation and dyspepsia.

Kali carb : Furious itching in region of mons veneris; burning itching herpes, moist after scratching (Kali brom).

Kreosotum : Itching towards evening so violent as to drive one almost wild; soreness and smarting between labia and vulva, offensive discharges.

Lachesis : Itching at anus, < after sleep; burning itching of whole body with yellow or purplish blisters.

Lac Caninum : Slight excoriation and itching of the external labia, feels at times as if caused by something alive in it, crawling about and itching terribly; same sensation on shoulders and neck, occasionally on hands, < towards evening and when warm.

Ledum : Violent itching on *dorsum of ankles and feet*, especially at night, < after scratching; itching rash on wrist-joint, all of them much > in warmth of bed.

Lilium Tig : *Pruritus most marked after menses* (Con); voluptuous itching in vagina with fullness in parts; stinging in left ovarian region.

Lycopodium : *Diurnal itching* (Natr. m), biting itching when becoming warm during the day; itching eruption at anus, painful to touch; itching of inner surface of prepuce.

Magnesia Mur : Itching on genitals and scrotum, extending to anus, formication over whole body, < while sitting, > by exercise and motion.

Mercurius : Moist, itch-like eruption on hand, with rhagades, < at night; when warm in bed, zoster with itching and tendency to suppurate.

Mezereum : Inveterate cases with unbearable nocturnal itching burning, especially in parts where there is very little fat deposited, < evening and from warmth; general coldness and twitching of the subcutaneous muscles; burning sensation changes place after scratching.

Muriatic Acid : Itching of scrotum, not relieved by scratching; organs weak, penis relaxed.

Natrum Mur : Diurnal itching (Lyc.); itching, soreness and moisture between scrotum and thighs, pus-like smegma on glans; itching and crawling sensation at the corona glandis; leucorrhoea causes itching; with yellow complexion; itching of female external parts, with falling off of the hair; itching of skin, but no rash (Dol) after violent exercise.

Natrum Sulph : *Itching while undressing* between scrotum and right thigh, small scabs, itching > by scratching, also on forehead, scalp, neck, chest, sycosis.

Nitric Acid : History of syphilis or psora, skin around anus dry and cracked, with tendency to bleed from scratching; and fissure; *falling off of the hair from genitals*; itching, swelling and burning of vulva and vagina; itching of shins, bleeding when scratched, small scabs form; skin dark, dirty.

Oleanaer : *Itching of skin when undressing* (Natr-sulph); after stool itching and burning in rectum and anus; skin sensitive all over, the mere friction of the clothing makes it sore, raw and painful.

Opium (Morphine) : Redness and itching of skin, very troublesome all over, fine pricking, rarely sensitive to touch.

Petroleum : *Itching humid herps on scrotum* between scrotum and thighs, on perinaeum, soreness and moisture on female genitals, with violent itching; itching herpes, followed by ulcers.

Platina : *Furious itching inside of uterus*, pruritus vulvae voluptuous tingling, with anxiety and palpitation of heart (Coff.), sensation of soreness, tingling, smarting, itching, burning, with inclination to scratch on different parts of body.

Psorinum : *Pruritus from amenorrhoea, with phthsis*, during pregnancy, pimples, itching violently, about nipples, oozing a fluid; itching between fingers; heat and itching of soles; body itches intolerably, < in bed and from warmth; scratches until it bleeds, which relieves.

Pulsatilla : Itching and burning on inner and upper side of prepuce; itching, < at night from pastry or pork, from delayed menses > from cold water, pruritus senilis.

Rhododendron : Itching and sweat on scrotum, soreness between scrotum and thighs.

Rumex : Itching < by cold, > by warmth; more formication than burning, chiefly when undressing, > by every exposure to cold air.

Silicea : Prurigo formicans, during night itching sensation as if ants were crawling over the skin; itching humid spots on genitals, mostly on scrotum; sweat on scrotum; itching at pudendum; itching of soles, driving to despair.

Staphisagria : *Pruritus genitalium in newly married people*, with frequent urging to urinate; voluptuous itching of scrotum; stinging itching vulva.

Sulphur : Voluptuous itching burning, < evenings and in bed; chronic cases with itching, burning, stinging at anus, < after scratching.

Tarentula Hisp : Intense pruritus of vulva and vagina. < nights, with dryness and heat of the parts.

Teucrium (Marum ver.) : Cannot sleep on account of the intense itching of the anus, causing him to toss and roll at night.

Zincum : Crawling in skin of whole body, < only by rubbing, frequent violent itching as from fleabites, especially on back and abdomen, < at night, excessive itching during menses, inducing masturbation, with fidgets of feet and lower extremities (Canth., masturbation); itching in bends of joints; sudden itching, here and there, in bed at night, goes off by contact.

SCABIES

It is a contagious diesease caused by a parasitic mite called Sarcoptes Scabiei. The disease is contacted by intimate contact with infected individuals, or through infected bed linen or clothing.

The parasite, Sarcoptes scabiei, is a mite with four pairs of legs unlike bugs, lice and fleas, which have only three pairs of legs. The female is 400 to 800 m in size, and grey in colour. This parasite is just visible to the naked eye. The male is smaller than the female, and has a very brief span of life; it dies shortly after copulation. The impregnated female acarus, having burrowed her way into the horny layer of the epidermis, lives there for about two months. In these burrows, she lays eggs which develop into larvae. They pierce the roots of the burrows, find shelter in the pores of the skin, and develop into adult mites. The life-cycle of the acarus, from the ovum to the adult stage is from 13 to 21 days.

Clinical Features

1. **Nocturnal Pruritus** — Intense itching which is worse at night. The young acri piece of the burrows in the warmth of the bed and try to reach the pores. Usually there is no itching in the first four to six weeks of contacting the infection, because the itching is due to the development of sensitization to some of the products (saliva-scabin) of the mite, and about this much time is required for it. In case of reinfection, itching starts early.

2. History of exposure or multiple cases in the family.

3. Burrows are a very important feature of the disease. They represent the path traversed by the parasite in the horny layer of the skin. They are tortuous. Their lengths vary from a quarter of an inch to one inch. They are flesh coloured, with dark dots here and there. If the roof is lifted with a fine needle, the mite can be demonstrated. The common sites of burrows are : The fingers, the inter-digital webs, the palms, the wrists, the points of elbows, the anterior axillary folds, around the nipples, the abdomen, the buttocks, the genitalia, the legs and the feet. The neck and the face are not involved, except in children. By scratching and secondary infection the burrows are deformed or mutilated and hence, are often difficult to demonstrate. For this reason, they are not absolutely essential for diagnosis.

4. Fine, pin-head sized, follicular papules. Besides, papulo-pustules on erythematous bases (Studs) are commonly

seen. They are helpful in diagnosis. Scabetic dermatitis and dyshidrosis-like eruption, following an attack of scabies have been reported by the author. Occasional individual dermal nodules may develop due to deeper penetration by the acarus or a severe dermal reaction to the toxins of the acarus.

5. Excoriations and scratch marks.

Complications

(a) Impetiginization.
(b) Eczematization.
(c) Secondary lymphadenitis.

If untreated, the disease may last for months. Ultimately natural desensitization may develop.

Homoeopathic Approach

Scabies is one of the common cutaneous disorder caused by animal organism in developing countries. Since it is an infectious disease, it is essential to know the mode and root of infection. These organism produce infection in three different forms :

(1) **Trauma** : In the process of burrowing to the skin in search of food, sucking blood or laying eggs. Most of the anthropodes fall into this group.

(2) **Secondary infection** : The traumata may become secondarily infected with ordinary pyogenic infection giving rise to different types of pyodermas.

(3) **Transmission of specific infectious disease** : From the public point of view this feature deserves the utmost attention, and hence the eradication of causative animal vectors should form an important part of therapy.

Always consider scabies homoeopathically as external manifestation of internal psora, haphazard or irrational treatment leads to further separation of psora which ultimately leads to involvement of vital organs, like lung, heart, etc.

The most commonest complaint that the patient presents to us is pruritus, hence the above modality should be thoroughly scrutinized.

Often scabies get secondarily infected in such a case, one has to observe properly the discharge, the appearance presence of crust, etc.

Preventive measures : Personal hygiene and daily bath, separate clothes, bed linen and towels should be advised. Use of medicated soap containing calendula and oil of lavender.

Dr. Hering finds for the itch a successful practice of sleeping with the twigs of populus balsamifera in the bed. Balsam of Peru, if genuine, stirred in water and the clearer portion is used as bath is next best.

I have personally varified the advise of Dr. Hering by even applying Balsam Peru mother tinture locally on the lesion about 3 times a day. It is extremely soothing to the skin at the same time prevent secondary infection.

The following remedies are indicated :

Ars-Alb : The eruption appears on the bends of knees. The eruptions could be dry as well as full of small pustules.
There is presence of burning and itching which is worse at night, application of cold water > by local application of warmth. The scabies has tendency to alternate with bronchial asthma.

Anthrakokali : Eruption with itching appearing during the night and disappearing during the day time; also the eruption decreases during full moon. The eruptions are present, especially of scrotum, hands, tibia and dorsum of feet. Intense thirst in an important concomittant.

Carbo-Veg : The eruptions are dry almost over the whole body, especially worse on extremities. There is presence of itching which is worse after undressing at night. Scabies can occur after abuse of mercurial salts. Concomittant symptoms like dyspepsia, belching, passing flatus should help the physician to select drug. Once infection takes place, there is presence of acrid, bloody, foul discharge. The pus smells like asafoetida. There is presence of excessive burning in the lesion which is worse by local application of heat as well as cold.

Causticum : It is an extremely important drug when scabies are suppressed by local application of Mercury and Sulphur. There is excessive itching of whole body at night, also when secondarily infected there is presence of humid vesicles oozing corroding pus. The other concomittant symptoms are yellowish looking skin, warts, involuntary urination when coughing, sneezing or walking. The patient on the whole is extremely sensitive to cold air.

Croton-Tig : The eruptions are present on genitals, vertex, temples, extremities, etc. There is violent itching and burning in the lesions and skin becomes sore if scratched as a result the patient is better by gentle rubbing. Gradually the eruption becomes pustular which burst and form crust.

Hepar-Sulph : The eruptions that resemble scabies are present on folds of skin, hands and feet. The eruptions are pustular and crusty, oozing a foul, old cheese like discharge. The skin is extremely sensitive to cold air. The itching is worse at night and better by warm application. Presence of scabies in an individual where eruptions are suppressed by Mercury.

Lycopodium : Eruptions on the scalp, extremities, genitals and abdomen. The eruptions are yellowish brown, moist, purulent. Itching and burning sensation is worse by warmth and better by cold application, especially itching while burning is better by local application of heat. GIT concomittants like weak digestion, craving for sweets, flatulence should help one to prescribe the drug.

Merc-Sol : Eruption that typically affects bends of elbow, genitals, extremities, etc. The appearance of skin is dirty, yellow, rough and dry. Secondary infection sets in early and there is presence of pustules which liberate bloody corroding tenecious, sticky, offensive pus. There is presence of violent voluptuous itching over whole body, principally in evening or at night. It is worse by heat of bed and sometimes attended by burning after scratching.
Itching is so severe that patient develops insomnia. There is general tendency to free perspiration but patient does not get relieved.

Psorinum : This nosode should be used in those cases of scabies where one has a repeated history of scabies in the past or scabies are suppressed with the help of conventional medicine resulting into internal affection e.g., asthma, migraine, heart trouble, etc. The eruptions are present on bends of elbow. The scabies appear in every winter and disappear in summer. There is presence of violent itching, worse by warmth of bed or by scratching.

Rhus-V : Vesicular eruption resembles erysipelas. The appearance of skin is dark red. There is presence of itching which is relieved by hot water.

Sepia : The eruption is predisposed to crack and ulcerate as soon as it appears. There is presence of itching and burning sensation which is worse in the evening, open air. Better in warm room; scabies come periodically every spring. It is also useful in those cases of scabies after previous used of Sulphur.

Sulphur : It is one of the supreme remedy in homoeopathy which is used for recurrent maltreated, obstinate, suppressed cases of scabies, as a result of irrational homoeopathic treatment or when mercurial or sulphur ointment are used to suppress the lesion. There is presence of voluptuous tingling and itching in the bends of joints in between fingers, as soon as he gets warm in bed, also it is worse when undressing. Itching is accompanied by burning and soreness, especially after scratching. The skin appears rough and scaly with formation of little vesicles and pustules.

CHAPTER 25

Diseases Of The Sweat Glands

Common Disorders of the Sweat Apparatus

Functional	Hyperhidrosis, anhidrosis, bromhidrosis, Chromhidrosis, Dyshidrosis.
Infections	Periporitis, Abscesses, Hidradenitis, Suppurativa.
Inflammatory and sweat retention	Milaria, Fox-Fordyce's disease, Dyshidrosis, Exfoliativa.
Tumours	Cystic-hydrocystoma. Naevoid-Syringoma. Malignant tumours.

Hyperhidrosis

It may be generalized or localized, physiological or pathological, transient or permanent. Besides being uncomfortable, hyperhidrosis may interfere with social and occupational activities. Furthermore, exaggerated sweating, predisposes to maceration of the skin, growth of fungus (dermatophytes, monilia and microsporon furfur), miliaria, intertrigo, secondary dermatitis, contact eczema and keratoderma.

The causes of hyperhidrosis are :

Generalized

1. Physiological — Exertion, emotional embarassment.
   High atmospheric temperature combined with humidity.
   Alcohol, tea, spicy food (Gustatory). Drugs like pilocarpine.

2. Pathological — Fevers like malaria.
   Shock-cold, clammy sweats.
   Endocrine-thyrotoxicosis, acromegaly.
   Debility and wasting disease (diabetes tuberculosis).

Localized

The common sites are : the palms and the soles, the axillae, the groins and the forehead. The causes are : heredity, autonomic imbalance, emotional stresses, neurasthenia, local deformity e.g. flat feet.

Palmar and plantar hyperhidrosis can be distressing. It may be complicated by bromhidrosis (on the feet, due to bacterial decomposition), keratoderma (the palms and the soles), ringworm (feet), contact dermatitis (particularly on the feet due to the sweat dissolving the chemicals, from footwear), and dyshidrosis (the palms and the soles). In the flexures, particularly the axillae, the groins and the ano-genital region, hyperhidrosis tends to cause intertrigo, contact dermatitis (in the axillae from clothing), dermatitis (scrotum) and monilial infection (groins and inframammary regions).

Prognosis : It is uncertain. There is remote possibility of spontaneous resolution; otherwise the outlook is poor. Condition persists until the cause is removed.

Treatment : It consists of :

1. Improving the general, physical and mental health of the patient; also of cutting down hot spicy food, tea, alcohol and tobacco. Living in the cool, fresh air, in loose thin clothing which allows evaporation of sweat, should be encouraged. Constant emotional stresses, strains and excitement must be avoided and physical exertion reduced.

2. The cause or causes must be removed. For instance, in localized hyperhidrosis of the feet, deformities like flat-footedness should be corrected; if there is obesity, the weight should be reduced.

3. Symptomatic treatment. It is important in the localized type of hyperhidrosis.

Bromhidrosis

Foul-smelling sweat is usually confined to the feet, and less often, to the axillae and the genitalia. It usually results from hyperhidrosis and bacterial decomposition of sweat. It may also be produced by the intake of valerian, asofoetida, onions and garlic in food and, occasionally, in diseases like gout and diabetes. The treatment is similar to that employed for localized hyperhidrosis, namely sterilization of clothing and socks by boiling, of shoes by formalin, frequent changes of clothes and footwear and the wearing of open chappals.

Anhidrosis

Diminished sweating is more common than complete absence of sweating. It is uncomfortable for two reasons — (1) The patient feels a sense of dryness of integument, (2) The patient cannot tolerate heat easily, and there is danger of hyperpyrexia and heat stroke. The common causes are — congenital xeroderma, ichthycosis and atrophy of the skin and congenital ectodermal defects.

Localized anhidrosis is seen in patients after they have been affected by sympathectomy, Horner's syndrome, leprosy and other neurogenic disorders. Destruction of sweat glands in radiodermatitis and scleroderma also produces localized anhidrosis. In atopic dermatitis blocking of sweat ducts may also produce partial or complete anhidrosis. The treatment consists in correcting the causative factors.

Generalized anhidrosis can be treated with warm baths, mild exposures to the sun and pilocarpine injections.

Homoeopathic Approach

The approach consists of improving the general state : mental, physical and hygienic conditions. Also of cutting down hot spicy food, tea, alcohol and tobacco; living in the cool fresh air, in loose thin clothing which allows evaporation of sweat, should be encouraged.

(1) Constant emotional stresses, strain and excitement must be avoided and physical exertion reduced.

(2) The cause or causes must be removed, for instant localised hyperhydrosis of feet, deformities like flat foot should be corrected. If there is obesity, the weight should be reduced.

(3) In cases of hyperhydrosis, one should wear sandals or chappals or open type shoes. Socks should be changed twice a day. Avoid nylon or woollen socks. Wearing of sleevless shirt and blouse should be encouraged in the cases of axillary hyperhydrosis.

Baryta Carb : Foetid foot-sweat toes and soles get sore : checked foot-sweat, followed by lameness, tonsillar angina, etc. sweat increased in presence of strangers; offensive sweat of one (mostly left) side; sweat increased by eating; sweat returning every other eveining; soles feel bruised at night, keep one awake; callosities on soles, which are painful on walking; cramps in soles of feet, < while walking or dancing.

Bryonia : Sweat in short spells, and only on single parts; profuse and easily excited sweat, even when slowly walking in the cold open air; profuse night and morning sweat; sour or oily sweat, night and day; sour sweat at night, preceded by thirst; oppressive drawing in head when the sweat is about to terminate, and succeeded by a muddled condition of the head; vaporous exhalation of the skin from evening till morning.

Calcarea Carb : Sweat during the slightest exercise, even in cold open air. (Sep., sweat after the exercise, when sitting quietly); during first sleep; morning sweat; most profuse on head and chest; clammy night sweats, only on legs; foot-sweat makes feet sore; feet cold and damp.

China : Copious, profuse oily sweat, easily excited during sleep or motion; *exhausting night sweats*, greasy sweat on the side on which he lies; increased thirst during sweat; partial cold sweat on the face or all over body, with thirst; sweats **easily**, especially at night in sleep; hectic fever, with profuse debilitating night sweats.

Hepar Sulph : Cold, clammy, frequently sour or offensive smelling sweat; perspires day and night, without relief, or first cannot sweat at all and then sweats profusely; night or morning sweat with thirst.

Hydrastis : *Offensive sweat on genitals*; excessive sweat of axilla and about genitals; clothing feels uncomfortable about groins.

Jaborandi : *Copious sweating and salivation*; profuse secretion from most of the glandular structures of the body, perspiration starts on fore-head and face and then spreads all over body, most profuse on trunk, profound prostration after sweating; unilateral left sided sweat; profuse night sweats (Pilocarp).

Mercurius : Profuse sweat at night, towards morning with thirst and palpitations; from exertions, even when eating; evening in bed before falling asleep. Sour, offensive, or cold clammy, oily (China), and causing burning of skin; with all pains, *but giving no relief* < by the weakness.

Phosphorus : Sweat mostly on head, hands and feet, or only on forepart of body, with increased urine, *profuse clammy night sweats < during sleep* (Samb, < when awake, no sweat when sleeping), without relief.

Sambucus : *Dry, burning heat during sleep, giving way immediately on waking to profuse sweat*, first on face and then extending over whole body, continuing more or less during waking hours; on going to sleep again the dry heat returns, with cold hands and feet, but still he shuns uncovering; profuse, weakening sweat, day and night, lasts during the apyrexia.

Sepia : Free and sudden perspiration from a nervous shock or from exertion, the sweat, coming out after the exertion is over or the shock passed and when one is sitting quietly (Calc., sweat during exertion). Night-sweat on chest, back and thighs, from above downward to the calves, smelling sour offensive or like elder blossom; profuse morning sweat after awakeing; *offensive foot sweat*, causing cold heels and soreness of toes; every third night sour, offensive sweat, like elder bloosoms; crippled nails.

Silicea : *Nocturnal head sweat keeps the child awake*, profuse sweat of head, the body being dry or nearly so; copious offensive foot sweat, with rawness between toes and itching of soles, driving to despair; periodical sweat; debilitating, sour and offensive night sweats, mostly after midnight.

Stannum : Sweat comes on after he falls asleep, and as soon as he moves he is chilly on back and shoulders; often *sequela of weakening diseases*, sweat smells mouldy, musty, most profuse on neck, especially night and morning; hectic fever, anxious heat, as if sweat would break out.

Thuja : Sweat, either of those parts alone which are covered (Bell, Chin, Spig.) or of those alone which are uncovered, while covered parts are dry and hot; sweat most copious on upper part of body, except head; sweat on perineum; foetid sweat on toes, with redness and swelling of tips; on soles of feet, nails crippled, brittle or soft; *sweat during sleep, but stops as soon as he awakens* : oily, foetid sweat; sweetish odour exhaling from skin, accompanying abdominal or pelvic disorders; suppressed foot sweat.

SWEAT

Sweat : Sweatiness in general : *Acet-ac, Agar, Ag-c, Alum, Ambr, Am-c, Am-m, Anac, Ang, ant-c, Ant-t, Ap, Arg, Arn, Ars, Asar, Aur, Bar-c, Bell, Ben-ac, Bis, Bor, Bov, Bro, Bry, Calad, Calc-c, Calc-p, Camph, Canth, Caps,, Carb-an, Carb-ac, Carb-v, Caust, Cham, Chel, Chin, Cic, Cina, Clem, Coff, Colch, Coloc, Con, Croc, Cupr, Cyc, Dig, Dros, Dul, Euphr, Ferr, Flu-ac, Gels, Glon, Graph, Guai, Hell, Hep-s, Hyos, Ign, Iod, Ip, Jab, Kali-c, Kali-n, Kreos, Lach, Lact-ac, Lau, led, Lith-c, Lyc, Mag-c, Mag-m, Mang, Merc, Mez, Mos, Mur-ac, Nat-c, nat-m, Nit-ac, Nux-m, Nux-v, Op, Par, Petr, Phos, Pho-ac, Plat, Plb, Psor. Puls. Ran-b, Ran-s, Rheum, Rhod, Rhus-t, Rut, Sabad, Sabin, Samb, Sars, Sec-c, Selen, Seneg, Sep, Sil, Spig, Spong, Stan, Staph, Stram, Stro, Sul, Sul-ac, Tarax, Thuj, Val, Ver-a, Vio-o, Vio-t, Zinc.*

Absent (inability to sweat) : *Acon, Alukm, Ambr, Am-c, Ap, Arn, Ars, Bell, Bis, Bry, Calc-c, Can, Cham, Chin, Coff, Colch, Dulc, Eup-p, Graph, Hyos, Iod, Ip, Kali-c, Led, Lyc, Mag-c, Mar, Merc, Merc-c, Nat-c, Nit-ac, Nux-m, Nux-v, Old, Op, Phos, Pho-ac, Plat, Puls, Ran-s, Rhus-t, Sabad, Samb, Scil, Sec-c, Seng, Sep, Sil, Spong, Stap, Sul, Thuj, Verb, Vio-o.*

Biting, smqarting : *Cham, Con, Flu-ac, Ip, Tarax.*

Bloody : *Arn, Ars, Calc-c, Can, Crot-h, Hell, Lach, Lyc, Nux-m, Nux-v, Phos.*

Brownish yellow, staining : *Ars, Bell, Carb-a, Graph, Lach, Mag-c, Sele, Thuj.*

Clammy, Sticky : *Acon, Agar, Aloe, Anac, Ant-t, Arn, Ars, Bry, Calc-c, Camph, Carb-a, Carb-ac, Carb-v, Cham, Chin, Coloc, Dig, Ferr, Flu-ac, Hell, Hep-s, Iod, Jat, Kali-bi, Lach, Lil-t, Lyc, Merc, Mez, Mosch, Nat-m, Nux-v, Ox-ac, Phos, Pho-ac, Plb, Sec-c, Spig, Sul-ac, Tab, Ver-a.*

Cold : *Act-ac, Acon, Agar, Air, Aloe, Amb, Am-c, Anac, Ànt-t, Arn, Ars, Asaf, Aur, Bar-c, Bell, Bry, Bufo, Calc-c, Calc-p, Can, Caps, Carb-v, Chin, Cimi, Cina, Cocl, Coff, Con, Croc, Cupr, Dig, Dulc, Elap, Euphor, Ferr, Fer-p, Gels, Graph, Hell, Hep-s, Hyd-ac, Ign, Ip, Jast, Kali-bi, Kali-p, Lach, Lil-t, Lob, Lyc, mang, Merc, Merc-c, Mur-ac, Naj, Nat-c, Nit-ac, Nux-v, Op, Ox-ac, Petr, Phos, Pho-ac, Plb, Puls, Pyro, Ran-s, Rhe, Rhus-t, Rut, sabad, Sec-c, Sep, Spl, Spong, Stap, Stram, Sul, Sul-ac, Tab, (Icy), Terb, Thu, Ver-a, Ver-v, Vip.*

Easy sweatiness, profuse : *Agar, Amb, Am-c, Amy-n, Am-m, Anac, Ant-t, Ars, Asar, Bell, Bor, Bro, Bry, Bufo, Calc-c, Calc-p, Canth, Carb-a, Carb-v, Caust, Chin, Coloc, Con, Dulc, ferr, Flu-ac, Gels, Graph, Guai, Heo-s, Hyos, Ign, Iod, Ip, Kali-c, Kali-n, Kreos, Lach, Led, Lyc, mag-c, Mag-m, Merc, nat-c, Nat-m, Nat-n, Nit-ac, Nux-v, Op, Petr, Phos, Pho-ac, Psor, Puls, Rhe, Rhod, Rhus-t, Sabad, Sars, Selen, Seng, Sep, Sil, Spig, Spong, Stan, Stp, Stram, Sul, Sul-ac, Thuj, Val, Ver-a, Zinc.*

Fetid (bad smelling) : *Am-c, Am-m, Arn, Ars, Bapt, bar-c, Bell, Bov, Canth, Carb-a, Carb-v, Coloc, Con, Crot-h, Cyc, Dio, Dulc, Euphr, Ferr, Flu-ac, Graph, Euai, Hep-s, Kali-c, Kali-p, Lach, Lac-c, Led, Lyc, Mag-c, Mag-m, Merc, Merc-c, Nit-ac, Nux-v, Petr, Phos, Plb, Psor, Puls, Rghod, Rhus-t, Selen, Sep, Sil, Spig, Staph, Stram, Sul, Thuj, Ver-a, Zinc.*

Flies, attracting : *Bry, Calad, Pul, Sep, Thuj.*

Greasy (oily) : *Agar, Aur, Bry, Bufo, Chin, Flu-ac, Mag-c, Merc, nat-m, Plb, Rhus-t, Selen, Stram, Thuj.*

Hot : *Acon, Amy-n, Anac, Ant-c, Asar, Aur, Bell, Bis, bry, Camph, Canth, Carb-v, Cham, Chin, Coff, Dig, Dros, Hell, Ign, Ip, Kreos, Lach, Led, Lyc, Op, Par, Phos, Pip-n, Sabad, Sep, Sil, Stan, Staph, Stram, Thuj, Ver-a, Vio-t.*

Onions or garlic, odour of : *Artem, Bov, Lach, Lyc, Kali-p, Osm, Phos, Sinap, Tell.*

Sour odour : *Arn, Ars, Asar, Bell, Bry, Bufo, Calc-c, Carb-v, Caust, Cham, Chin, Colch, Ferr, Flu-ac, Graph, Hep-s, Hyos, Ign, Iod, Ip, Kali-c, Lact-ac, Led, Lyc, Mag-c, Merc, Nat-m, Nat-p, Nit-ac, Nux-v, Puls, Rheum, Rhus-t, Sep, Sil, Spig, Staph, Sul, Sul-ac, Thu, Ver-a.*

PARTIAL SWEAT

Partial sweat of single parts, spotted : *Acon, Agar, Ag-c, Ambr, Am-c, Am-m, Anac, Ang, Ant-t Arg, Arn, Ars, Asaf, Asar, Aur, Bar-c, Bell, Bor, Bov, Bry, Calad, Calc-c, Calc-p, Camph, Canth, Caps, Carb-a, Carb-v, Cham, Chel, Chin, Cic, Cina, Clem, Cocl, Coloc, Con, Croc, Cupr, Cyc, Dig, Dros, Dulc, Euphr, Ferr, Graph, Cuai, Hell, Hep-s, Hyos, Ign, Iod, Ip, Kali-c, Kali-n, Kreos, Lau, Led, Lyc, Mag-s, Mag-m, Mang, Merc, Mez, Mosch, Nat-c, Nat-m, Nit-ac, Nux-v, Op, Par, Petr, Phos, Pho-ac, Plat, Plb, Puls, Ran-s, Rheum, Rho, Rhus-t, Ruta, Sabad, Sabin, Samb, Sars, Scill, Sec-c, Sele, Sep, Sil, Spig, Spong, Stann, Staph, Stram, Stro, Sul, Sul-ac, Tarx, Thuj, Val, Ver-a, Vio-t, Zinc.*

Head : *Acon, Ambr, Ant-t, Apis, Bell, Bor, Bov, Bry, Bufo, Calc-c, Cam, Carb-a, Car-v, Caust, Cham, Chin, Cina, Coloc, Carb-v, Dig, Frap, Guai, Ham, Hep, Ip, Kali-c, Lau, Led, Mag-c, Mag-m, Merc, Merc-c, Mez, Mosch, Mur-ac, Nat-m, Nit-ac, Nux-v, Op, Par, Petr, Phos, Pho-ac, Plb, Puls, Rheum, Rhus-t, Ruta, Sanic Sec-c, Sep, Sil, Spig, Sul, Sul-ac, Tarax, Thuja, Val. Ver-a.*

Ears : *Act-sp, Calc-c, Old, Puls, Zinc.*

Nose : *Bell, Cina, Hell, Lau, Mar, Nat-m, Rheum, Ruta, Tub.*

Face : *Acc, Alum, Ambr, Am-m, Ang, Ant-t, Arg, Arn, Ars, Asaf, Bell, Bor, Bry, Calc-c, Camph, Can, Caps, Carb-a, Carb-v, Cham, Chin, Cic, Cina, Cocl, Coff, Con, Croc, Cupr, Dig, Dros, Dulc, Guai, Hell, Hep-s, Hyos, Ign, Ip, Kali-c, Lau, Led, Lyc, Mag-c, Merc, Mosch, Nat-c, Nat-m, Nux-v, Op, Par, Petr, Plat, Plb, Puls, Ran-s, Rheum, Rhus-t, Ruta, Sabad, Samb, Sars, Sep, Sil, Spig, Spong, Stann, Staph, Stram, Sul, Sul-ac, Thuj, Val, Ver-a, Vio-t.*

Forehead : *Am-c, Ang, Calc-c, Cina, Crot-t, Guai, Hell, Led, Merc-c, Mosch, nat-c, Nat-m, Nit-ac, Nux-v, Ol-an, Op, Ran-s, Rheum, Sars, Sec-c, Staph, Sul, Val, Ver-a.*

Upper lip : *Acon, Coff, Kali-bi, Kali-c, Med, Nux-v, Rheum.*

Epigastrium : *Bell, Bor, Kali-n, Nux-v, Sec-c.*

Abdomen : *Ambr, Anac, Arg, Arg-n, Asar, Canth, Cic, Dros, Ip, Merc, Nux-v, Phos, Plb, Rhus-t, Sele, Staph.*

Groins : *Anac, Canth, Selen, Sep, Thuj.*

Genitals : *Ag-c, Alum, Am-c, Ars, Aur, Bar-c, Bell, Calad, Calc-c, Canth, Carb-a, Carb-v, Con, Dio, Flu-ac, Hep-s, Ign, Lyc, Mag-m, Merc, Mez, Pho-ac, Puls, Rhod, Sele, Sep, Sil, Staph, Sul, Thu.*

Female genitals : *Alum, Aur, Bell, Calc-c, Canth, Cic., Con, Dio, Flu-ac, Hep-s, Ign, Merc, Petr, Puls, Sele, Sep, Sil, Sul, Thu.*

External throat and neck : *Alum, Bell, Can, Cham, Clem, Coff, Euphr, Ip, Kali-c, Mang, Nux-v, Rhus-t, Spig, Stann, Sul.*

Nape : *Anac, Ars, Calc-c, Chin, Ferr, Hell, Hyos, Mag-c, Mang, Mosch, Nit-ac, Nux-v, Pho-ac, Pul, Sep, Sil, Spig, Stann, Sul, Tub.*

Chest : *Agar, Anac, Arg, Arn, Asar, Bell, Bov, Bufo, Calc-c, Canth, Chin, Cocl, Dros, Euphr, Grap, Hep-s, Ip, Kali-n, Lyc, Merc, Merc-c, Nat-m, Nit-ac, Phos, Pho-ac, Plb, Puls, Rhus-t, Sabad, Sec-c, Sele, Sep, Sil, Spig.*

In axillae : *Asar, Bov, Bry, Calc-c, Caps, Carb-a, Carb-v, Dulc, Hep-s, Kali-c, Lach, Merc-c, Nat-m, Nit-ac, Petr, Phos, Rhod, Sabad, Scil, Sele, Sep, Sil, Sul, Sul-ac, Tell, Thuj, Ver-a, Zinc.*

On Back : *Acon, Anac, Ars, Bufo, Calc-c, Caust, Chin, Coff, Dulc, Gual, Hep-s, Ip, Lach, Led, Lyc, Mur-ac, Nat-c, Nit-ac, Nux-v, Par, Petr, Phos, Pho-ac, Puls, Rhus-t, Sabin, Sep, Sil, Stann, Stram, Sul.*

Hands : *Acon, Ag-c, Ambr, Am-m, Anac, Ant-t, Ars, Bar-c, Bell, Bry, Bufo, Calc-c, Cam, Canth, Caps, Carb-v, Cham, Chin, Cimi, Cina, Cocl, Coff, Coloc, Con, Dig, Dulc, Ferr, Flu-ac, Hell, Hep-s, Ign, Iod, Ip, Kreos, Lau, Led, Lil-t, Lyc, Merc, Merc-c, Nat-c, Nat-m, Nit-ac, Nux-v, Petr, Phos, Pho-ac, Puls, Rhe, Rhod, Rhus-t, Sars, Sep, Sil, Spig, Sul, Thuj, Ver-a, Zinc.*

Palms : *Acon, Am-m, Amy-n, Anac, Arg-n, Bar-c, Bapt, Bry, Calc-c, Calc-p, Camph, Caps, Cep, Cham, Con, (Cold), Dig, Dulc, Flu-ac, Hell, Ign, Kali-bi, Kali-c, Kreos, Lau, Led, Lyc, Manc, Merc, Nit-ac, Nux-v, Phos, Pip-n, Psor, Rhe, Rhus-t, Spig, Sul.*

Feet : *Acon, Am-c, Ang, Apis, Arn, Ars, Bar-c, Bell, Bry, Calc-c, Camph, Can, Canth, Carb-a, Carb-v, Chel, Cimi, Cocl, Coff, Coloc, Cupr, Cyc, Dros, Euphr, Flu-ac, Graph, Hell, Hep, Iod, Ip, Kali-c, Kre, Lach, Led, Lil-t, Lyc, Mag-m, Mang, Merc, Mez, Mur-ac, Nat-c, Nat-m, Nit-ac, Petr, Pho, Pho-ac, Phyt, Plb, Puls, Ran-b, Rhus-t, Sabad, Scil, Sec-c, Sele, Sep, Sil, Staph, Sul, Thuj, Zinc.*

LIST OF REFERENCE BOOKS

GENERAL TEXT BOOKS

DISEASES OF THE SKIN
by ***Andrews. G.C.***; Philadelphia, W.B. Saunders Co., 1971.

SKIN, OTHER DISEASES
by ***Fox and Farqubar*** : London, Churchill & Co., 1976.

AN INTRODUCTION TO DERMATOLOGY
by ***Percival, G.H.***; Edinburgh & London, E & S. Livingstone Ltd., 1967.

DERMATOLOGY IN GENERAL MEDICINE,
by ***T.B. Fitzpatrick***; **II Edition**. New York. McGraw Hill Book Corporation, 1979.

PRACTICAL DERMATOLOGY, III Edition
by ***I.B. Sneddon***; London, Edward Armold & Co., 1977.

DERMATOLOGY AND INTERNAL MEDICINE

SKIN MANIFESTATIONS OF INTERNAL DISORDERS
by ***Wiener, K***; St. Louis, C.V. Mosby Co., 1947.

DERMATOLOGY CLUES TO INTERNAL DISEASES
by ***Behrman, H.T.***; *New York*, Grune, 1967.

THE CUTANEOUS MANIFESTATIONS OF SYSTEMIC DISEASES
by ***Downing, J.G.***; Springfield, III, Charles C. Thomas, 1974.

ATLASES

ATLAS OF THE COMMON SKIN DISEASES
by ***Semon & Moritz***; Bristol, John Wright & Sons, 1975.

A COLOUR ATLAS OF DERMATOLOGY
by ***G.M. Levene***, London, Wolfe Medical Publications, 1979.

SKIN PATHOLOGY

A GUIDE TO DERMATOHISTOPATHOLOGY
by ***Pinkus. H. & Mehregan, A.H.***;
New York, Appleton Century, 1980.

MYCOLOGY

MEDICAL MYCOLOGY
by ***Dey, N.C.***; Calcutta, 1968.

PSYCHOSOMATIC DERMATOLOGY

EMOTIONAL FACTORS IN SKIN DISEASES
by ***Witikower, E., & Russel, B.***; *New York*, Paul B. Hoeber, 1953.

VENEREAL DISEASES

MODERN DIAGNOSIS AND TREATMENT OF THE MINOR VENEREAL DISEASES CANIZARES
by ***O. Springfield,*** III, Charles C., Thomas, 1973.

ALLERGY

PRACTICE OF ALLERGY
by ***Vaughan. W.T***; St. Louis, C.V. Mosby Co., 1966.

SPECIAL DERMATOSES

HANDBOOK OF TROPICAL DERMATOLOGY
by ***Simons, R. D. G.***, Ph.; *Houston.*

REPERTORY OF THE HOMOEOPATHIC MATERIA MEDICA
by J.T. Kent. A.M., M.D. 4th Indian Edition, 1982.

THE CHRONIC DISEASES — THEIR PECULIAR NATURE AND THEIR HOMOEOPATHIC CURE
by ***Dr. Samuel Hahnemann***, Translated from the second enlarged German Edition of 1935, by ***Prof. Louis H. Tafel***.

THE ENCYCLOPEDIA OF PURE MATERIA MEDICA A Record of the positive effects of Drugs upon the healthy human organism.
Edited by ***Timothy F. Allen***, A.M. M.D.

POCKET MANUAL OF HOMOEOPATHIC MATERIA MEDICA COMPRISING THE CHARACTERISTIC AND GUIDING SYMPTOMS OF ALL REMEDIES (CLINICAL AND PATHOGENETIC)
by ***William Boericke***, M.D. 9th Edn. 1984.
Revised and Enlarged with the addition of a *Repertory* by ***Oscar E. Boericke***, A.B., M.D.

HOMOEOPATHIC THERAPEUTICS
by ***Samuel Lilienthal. M.D.*** 3rd Edition.

A DICTIONARY OF PRACTICAL MATERIA MEDICA
by ***John Henry Clarke. M.D.*** 3rd Edition
by ***R.E. Dudgeon, M.D.***, London, 1955.

MATERIA MEDICA PURA
by ***Samuel Hahnemann***, Translated from the latest German Edn. by ***R.E. Dudgeon***, M.D. 1980.

MATERIA MEDICA OF HOMOEOPATHIC MEDICINES
by ***Dr. S.R. Phatak***. M.B.B.S. 1982.

CONCISE REPERTORY OF HOMOEOPATHIC MEDICINES,
by ***Dr. S.R. Phatak,*** M.B.B.S., 2nd Edn., 1985.

A COMPARISON OF THE CHRONIC MIASMS
(Psora, Pseudo-Psora. Syphilis. Sycosis)
by ***Phylltis Speight.***

BOENNINGHAUSEN'S CHARACTERISTICS AND REPERTORY
Translated, compiled and augmented by ***C.M. Boger,*** M.D.

SYNTHETIC REPERTORY PSYCHIC AND GENERAL SYMPTOMS OF THE HOMOEOPATHIC MATERIA MEDICA,
Dr. Med Horst Barthel, M.D., 3rd Improved Edn.

DISEASE OF THE SKIN INCLUDING THE EXANTHEMATA,
by ***Frederick M. Dearborn,*** A.B., M.D., 2nd Edn., 1974.

REPERTORY OF HERING'S SYMPTOMS OF OUR MATERIA MEDICA,
by ***Calvin B. Knerr,*** M.D.

HANDBOOK OF MATERIA MEDICA AND HOMOEOPATHIC THERAPEUTICS,
by ***Timothy Field Allen.*** A.M., M.D.I.C.D.,
Reprint 1979.

THE GUIDING SYMPTOMS OF OUR MATERIA MEDICA,
by ***C. Hering***, M.D.

MATERIA MEDICA, by ***J.T. Kent.***

INDEX

ACANTHOLYSIS
◘ in pemphigus, 54, 57
Acanthosis
◘ meaning of, 23-4
Acne 42
◘ approach, 354-59; cases, 359-60
◘◘ comedones in, 17
—Conglobata, 34
—Necrotia, 3, 40
◘ Repertory, 362-64
—Rosacea, 29, 37, 41, 49, 64
◘ Course, 353; hallmarks, diagnostic, 353
◘◘ pathogenesis, 353-54
—Simplex cases, 361
—Vulgaris, 29, 31, 41, 42, 49, 65, 75, 76-7
◘ course 351; hallmarks, 349
◘◘ pathogenesis, 351-52
◘ presentation: atypica, 350-51
◘◘ clinical, 349-50
◘ prognosis, 351
Acryocyanosis, 110
◘ and chilblains, 109
Acrosclerosis
◘ and chilblains, 109
Actinomycosis, 33, 37, 41, 52, 62
—madurae, 43
Acute Eczema
◘ see Eczema, Acute
Acute generalized Lichen Planus
◘ see Lichen planus
Acute painful corns
◘ see Corns, acute painful
Acute sunstroke
◘ see Sunstroke, acute
Adamson's fringe
◘ definition, 11
Addison's disease, 28, 49
Adipose tissue, 7, 18
Alcohols
◘ constituent of sebum, 16
Allergic dermatoses
◘ see Dermatoses, allergic
—Purpura
◘ see Purpura
Allergy
◘ cutaneous, 46-8
◘ sense of heat in, 27
◘ tests, 58-60
Alopecia(s), 49
◘ and scalp disease, 513ff
◘ approach, 518ff; meaning, 34
◘◘ Repertory, 522-24
—Areata, 515-16
Anagen, 12, 13
Antiphylactoid purpura
◘ see Purpura
Analplasia
◘ see Mitotic figures
Androgens, 11, 16, 17
Angioma, 25
—brain, 49
Angioneurotic oedema
◘ see Oedema
Angular stomatitis
◘ see Stomatitis
Anhydrosis, 75, 565
Annular Lichen Planus
◘ see Lichen Planus
Anthrax, 31
◘ development, rapid, 43
Anthropathica Psoriasis
◘ see Psoriasis
Antigens, 45, 46, 50
Apocrine Glands
◘ see Glands
Arrector pili muscle, 25
◘ meaning, 13
Arrector Pilorum muscle, 11
Arteriosclerosis, 49
◘ changes of toe-nail, 527
Arthus' phenomenon, 46
Asthma, alternating with:

¤ eczema, case study, 270-73
¤¤ scabies, 73
Atopic dermatitis
¤ see Dermatitis
—Eczema
¤ see Eczema
Atrophy, 24, 31
¤ meaning, 35
Avitaminosis, 37, 48

BACKWARDNESS, ECONOMIC
¤ and contagious diseases
¤¤ see Disease, contagious
Bacterial folliculitis
see Folliculitis
Bacteriological studies
cultures, 51; mears and
stains, 50-1
Baldness
¤ pattern: femals, male, 517-18
Banding
¤ see Nail colour changes
basal cell(s)
¤ see Basal germinal cells
Basal cell epitheliomas
¤ development of, 44
Basal germinal cell(s), 24
¤ function of, 7
Basal lamina, 6-7, 10, 58
Basement membrane
¤ see Basal lamina
Basophil(s), 45, 46, 60
—Degranulation Test (Shelly), 60
Bazin's disease, 43
¤ see Nail Dystrophy
Benign late Syphilis
¤ see Syphilis
Besnier's Prurigo
¤ see Eczema, atopic
Biological tests
¤ see under respective names
Biopsy, 55
¤ technique, 56
Blackhead
¤ see Comedone
Blood flow
¤ and skin temperature, 17
Body heat regulation, 17-8
Boils, 26, 74
¤ Repertory, 413ff
Bowen's disease see Epithelioma(
Bromhidrosis
¤ definition, 565
Bronze diabetes, 48
Bubo
¤ formation, 453-54
¤ in left groin: case, 450-51
Buerger's disease, 43, 49
Bullae, 24, 25
¤ causes, 30
Bullous disease(s), 58
¤ form, 494
Bunion(s)
¤ approach, 94-5; description, 94
¤ Repertory, 95; type, 94-5
Burrow
¤ meaning of, 35
Bursa Lymphocyte cells, 44-5
Bursae lesions
¤ see Lesions

CALLOSITIES
¤ see Calluses
Calluses
¤ see Corns and Calluses
Candida albicans, 22
—Paronychia, 529-30
Carbuncle, 31, 48
Case-taking
¤ and lesions, primary, 28
Catagen, 12, 13
Cells,
¤ axions of, 16
—, dendritic
¤ see Dendritic cells
—epidermal, 24

◘ maturation, 24
—epithelial, 12, 13
—mesenchymal, 20, 21
Chancre
◘ see Syphilis
—, Syphylitic
◘ see Syphylitic Chancre
Chancroid, 42
◘ approach, 433ff; complications,
◘◘ 453-54; development, 44;
◘◘ diagnosis: 454, differential, 454-55;
◘◘ etiology, 452; features: clinical, 452-53, distinguishing, 455;
◘◘ treatment, 455
Chaps
◘ repertory, 101-05
Cheiropompholyx
◘ see Dyshidrosis
Chemical eczema
◘ see Contact Dermatitis
"Chhapaki"
◘ see Urticaria
Chicken pox, 29, 30, 31, 33, 34
◘ course, limited, 43
Chilblains, 40, 43, 69
◘ and: acrosyanosis, acro-sclerosis, crurum, Erythro-cyanosis, 109
◘ cases, 115-16; diagnosis, 109-10; history-taking, 112; repertory, 116-17; symptoms, 112; treatment, 111-15
Chloasma, 28, 41, 49
Chronic diseases
◘ Hahnemannian theory of, 72ff
Chronic eczema
◘ see Eczema, chronic
—Erythroderma
◘ see Erythroderma, chronic
Chronic Pyoderma
◘ see Pyoderma, Chronic
Circinata
◘ examples, 35-6; meaning, 35
Climata
◘ and skin diseases, 2
Clinical dermatoses
◘ see Dermatoses
Clinical lesions
◘ see Lesions, clinical
Clubbing
◘ see Nail dystrophy
Cold
◘ affections, due to, 110-11
◘ stress on, by: Ayurveda, Galen, Hippocrates, 27
—sweating
◘ meaning, 15-6
Comdedones, 17
◘ description, 35-6
Condyloma acuminata (warts)
◘ see Warts
—acuminatum, 24, 42, 44, 75
Condylomata, 75, 78
—lata, 38, 42
—verruca, 75
Congenital ectodermal defects, 22
—Ichthosiform Erythroderma, 228
Constitution
◘ stress on, by : Ayurveda, Galen, Hippocrates, 27
Contact Dermatitis
◘ see Dermatitis
Contact eczema
◘ see Eczema
Contagious diseases
◘ see Diseases, contagious
Corium
◘ and: blood vessels, bullae, cysts, 25; infiltration, 24-5, neoplasms, 25
◘ see also Dermis
Corneum stratum
◘ see Stratum Corneum
—layer
◘ body water content maintained by, 15
Corns
◘ acute, painful: treatment, 88-90
◘ and callosities: repertory, 90-4

¤ and calluses approach, 84-8; cases, 86-8; causation, 84; characteristic, 85; course, 82-3; description, 83-4; differnce between, 83; hallmarks: diagnostic, 82; location, 84; presentation: clinical, 82; prognosis, 82-3; therapy, 83; treatment: previous, 84; review, 85
Corps ronds and grains
¤ see Darier's disease
Cortex
¤ see Hair shaft
Countries, tropical
¤ see Tropical countries
—Western
¤ see Western countries
Crawling sensation (formication), 26, 27, 72
Crurum
¤ and chilblains, 109
Crust
¤ causes, 32-3; description, 32
Cryglobulin test, 61-2
Cushing's disease, 49
Cutaneous allergy
¤ see Allergy, cutaneous
—Cysts
¤ see Cysts, cutaneous
—diseases
¤ see Skin diseaes
—Disorders
¤ and systemic diseaes, 48-9
—lesions, 37, 128-29
¤ and systemic disorders, 48-9
—scars
¤ removal of, 1
—vessels
¤ reaction of, 17
Cuticle, 12, 14
Cutis laxa, 25
—Vera
¤ see Dermis
—Verrucosus, 24
Cysts(s), 25
—cutaneous
¤ causes, meaning, 35
—dermoid, 22, 35
—Pilonida, 22, 35
-Sebaceous, 35
Cystineurea
¤ Cystine in, 16
Cytocrine
¤ secretion of, 5
Cytological examination, 56-7
Cytoplasmic Organelles
¤ see Stratum Corneum

DARIER'S DISEASE, 23, 37
Dark field examination, 51
Dark ground illumination test, 422, 454
Dendrites
¤ Dendritic cells, see Epidermis
Depigmentation, 29
¤ caused by, 81
Dermal leishmaniosis, 29, 34, 40ff
¤ character of, 44
—Vascular plexuses, 17
Dermatitis, 28, 32, 33, 62
¤ causes, 216; definition, 214-15; environment: correction, 241-42; etiology, 215-17; histopathology, 215; immunology, 217-18; prognosis, 240; treatment, 240ff.
—artefacta
¤ see Dermatits autophytica
—Atopic, 40ff, 59, 60, 69
—Autophytica, 238
—Contact, 40ff
¤ allergens, 223
¤ and photodermatitis, 218-19
¤ approach, 242ff; causes, 219ff; diagnosis, 2, 221
—Discoid, 35, 42, 43
—Eczematoid, Infectious, 223-225
—Exfoliative, 32, 36
¤ causes, 227; classification, 228-30

——epidemic (Savill), 229
——(Hebra), 229
——Neonatorum (Ritter), 228
——Primary (Wilson), 228-29
—Herpetiformis, 25, 30, 40, 42, 49, 58
—infantile case, 286
—Infective, 42
—Medicamentosa, 238
—Occupational
¤ agents, causative, 225-26; examples, 246-47
—Perioral
¤ characteristics, 239-40
—Seborrhoeic, 23, 32, 33, 41, 42, 65, 68, 319, 514-15
¤¤ development, 44
—Solar
¤ affections, 118-19; treatment, 119ff
—Varicose, 236-37
¤ treatment, 237
Dermatological diagnosis, 40
—disorders
¤ and sebaceous glands, 17
—terms, 36ff
—practice
¤ laboratory and other aids, 50ff
—treatment, 63ff
Dermatology
¤ and general medicine, 1; case-taking, 38 ff; pattern, 8; practice, 2; scope, 2
Dermatomycosis
¤ diagnosis of, 51-2
Dermatoses, 68
¤ and Western countries, 1
—Man-made prevention, 3
¤ see also Skin diseases
¤ caused by, 81; chemical, 1; diagnosis, 41ff; localized, 40-1
¤ photosensitization
¤¤ classification, 123-4
¤ psychogenic, 1
—allergic, 27, 75
¤ diet in, 64ff
Dermic papule
¤ description, 29
Dermis, 4, 12, 14, 17ff, 23, 24, 72
¤ neoplasms in, 25; structure, 7-8
Dermoid cysts
¤ see Cyst(s)
Desmosomes
¤ see Stratum Malpighis
"Dhapar"
¤ see Urticaria
Dhobi's itch
¤ see Tinea Cruris
Diabetes, 23, 62
¤ bronze, 48
¤ glucose in, 16
Diathesis, skin
¤ see Skin diathesis
Discoid dermatitis
¤ see Dermatitis
—Eczema
¤ see Eczema Discoid, and nummular
Disease(s)
¤ classification: Hahnemannian, 74-80; nosological, 72-3
—contagious
¤ and: backwardness, illiteracy, 1-2; superstitions, 1
—Cutaneous
¤ see Skin diseases
—Entity
—History of, natural, 43-4
—Man-made
¤ percentage, 3
—Skin
¤ see Skin diseases
—Systemic
¤ and cutaneous disorders, 48-9
—tropica, 2
Disorders, cutaneous
¤ see Cutaneous disorders
Disseminated Eczema

¤ see Eczema
Disseminated gonococcal infection
¤ see Infection
Dorpharyngeal infection
¤ see Infection
Drug eruptions
¤ see Eruptions
Drug rash
¤ see Rash
Dryness
¤ stress on, by
¤¤ Ayurveda, Galen, Hippocrates, 27
Dyshidrosis, 43, 49
¤ characteristics, 238-39; diagnosis, etiology, treatment, 239

ECCRINE GLANDS
¤ see Glands
Economic backwardness
¤ see Backwardness, economic
Ectoderm, 19
¤ structure, 20
Eczema, 23, 24, 29, 30, 32, 33, 41, 75
¤ approach, 21, 77ff; cases, 273-74, 275-85, 286-88; definition, 214-15; diagnosis, 2; repertory, 265ff; treatment, 278-83
—acute
¤ diet in, 65-6; treatment, 249
—and Dermatitis
¤ see Dermatitis and Eczema
—and Goitre
¤ case, 284-85
—alternating with:
¤ asthma, case study, 270-73
—Atopic, 64, 232ff
¤ diagnosis, 233-34; etiology, 234; features, clinical, 233; prognosis, 234; stages, 233
—Capitatis
¤ case, 277=78
—Contact, 42, 43, 48
¤ and cosmetics, 70
—Chronic, 33, 37
¤ treatment, 249ff
—discoid, 49
—disseminated
¤ characteristics, 235-36; diet in, 65-6; SOH in, 27; types, 235-36
—endogenous, 27, 59, 62, 229-30
—Erythomatous, 77
—infantile
¤ cases, 283-84; etiology, 232; features, 231-32; types, 230-31
—infective, 35, 41, 42, 223ff
¤ flexura, 225; follicular, 224-25; post-traumatic, 224
—nummular, 43
¤ etiology, Pathogenesis, 234-35; treatment, 235
—seborrhoeic
¤ features, 231-32
—solar, 124-25
—Weeping
¤ case study, 274
Eczematides, 29
¤ see also Disseminated Eczema
Eczematoid infectious dermatitis
¤ see Dermatitis
Eczematous patient
¤ study of, 216-17
Elephantiasis, 80
¤ definition, 36
End bulbs of Krause
¤ see Sensory end-organs for cold
Endogenous Eczema(s)
¤ see Eczema
Epidemic Exfoliative Dermatitis
¤ see Dermatitis exploliative
Epidermic papule
¤ see Papule(s)
Epidermis, 12, 13, 19, 23-4, 72
¤ dendritic cells, 6; division of, 5; structure of, 4ff
Epidermodermal junction, 13, 24

Epidermolysis bullosa, 25, 30
Epithelial cells
◘ see cells
Epithelioma(s), 23, 30, 34, 37, 41, 42
◘ development of, 44
Epithelium, 14
◘ sequamous, stratified, 459; volar, 82
Erosions, 19, 32
Eruption(s), Drug, 28ff, 36
◘ development, 44; SOH, in, 27
—papular, 75
—urticarial, 159ff
Erythema, 32, 36
◘ caused by, 81, 289
—induratum, 25
—multiforme, 25, 28, 30, 35, 40, 42, 49, 58
◘ approach, 297-98; diagnosis, 292; drugs, 299; etiology, features (clinical); pathology, 291; prognosis, 291-92; repertory, 299-300
—Nosodum, 25, 29, 40, 43, 48, 293ff; course, 294; hallmark, diagonistic, 293; pathogenesis, 294; presentation clinical, 293-94; prognosis, 294; therapy, 294-95
—perinio
◘ see Chilblains
Erythomatous eczema
◘ see Eczema
—Macules
◘ see Macules
—rashes
◘ see Rashes
Erythrocyanosis
◘ and chilblains, 109
Erythroderma, 61
◘ meaning, 36
◘◘ see also Exfoliative dermatitis
—chronic, 65
—desquamativum (Leiner), 228
—Ichthyosiform congenita, 228
—Scarlatiniform, recurrent erythroderma, 229
Etiological stresses
◘ effects, 2
Exanthemata, 28, 32ff
◘ course of, 43; suppression: effect, 73; viral, 72
Exercise
◘ and sweating, 16
Excoriation (linear), 26, 32, 33
Excretion, 15-7
Exfoliative dermatitis
◘ see Dermatitis

FATTY ACIDS
◘ constituent of Sebum, 16
Female
◘ gonorrhoea in, 460-61
Filariasis, 36, 61
Fissure(s)
◘ examples, 33; repertory, 101-05
Fissure-in-ano, 33, 42
Flat warts (verruca plana)
◘ see Warts
Fluorescent antibody test, 423
Folliculitis, 43, 59, 65
◘ duration of, 43
—bacterial
◘ course, pathogenesis, presentation, clinical and prognosis, 490
—decalvans, 498
—fungal
◘ approach, course, pathogenesis, presentation, clinical 491
Formication
◘ see Crawling sensation
Fox-Fordyce's disease, 42
Frei's (intradermal) test, 61, 458
Friction
◘ and erythema, 81
Frost-bite, 34
◘ and immersion foot, 110-11
◘ repertory, 116-17

fungus affections
¤ (tropical countries), 43-4
Furuncle
¤ repertory, 413-18
Furunculosis, 31, 48, 65
¤ approach, 400-01 constitution, 399-400; cases, 408-12; environmental, 400; chronic, 68; etiology, 399; therapeutics, 401ff
Fusiform cells
¤ see Stratum Granulosum

GANGRENE, 48-79
General Medicine
¤ and Dermatology, 1
Germinal cells, basal
¤ see Basal germinal cells
Germinativum stratum
¤ see Stratum Germinativum
Giemsa's stain, 51, 52, 57
Glands, aprocrine, 10, 20
¤ distribution, 10
—Eccrine, 9-10, 20
¤ distribution, 9
—Sebaceous, 4, 7, 13ff, 20, 21, 25, 72
¤ and: disorders, dermatologica, puberty, 16; characteristics, 8-9, 16-7; structure, 9
—sweat, 7, 11ff, 22, 24, 25
¤ diseases of, 563ff; approach, 565-69; repertory, 569ff; stimulation of, 17-8; types, 9-10
Goitre
¤ case study, 284-85
Gold Chloride method, 6
Gonorrhoea, 77
¤ approach, 461ff; diagnosis, 461; features clinical, 459; in: female, 460-61; male, 459-60; newborn, 460; pathology, 459; repertory, 470ff
Gram's stain, 50, 52
Granuloma
¤ causes, 36-7; composition, 24; drugs, 37; infective, 36-7; Neoplastic, 37
—annulare, 35
—inguinale, 36, 42
—venereum, 61
¤ diagnosis, 456; features, clinical, 456; development, 44; incubation (period), 456; treatment, 456-57
Granulomata, 34, 52
Granulosum stratum
¤ see Stratum granulosum
Guttate Psoriasis, 318

HAHNEMANN
¤ Miasmatic theory, 72
¤ skin diseases classified
¤¤ under, 74ff
Hair, 10-3, 14, 21, 52, 53
¤ care of, 71; composition, 11-2; distribution, 10; growth, 11; types, 11
—follicles, 7, 8, 12ff, 21, 72
¤ characteristics, 11-3; root sheath, 12; segments, 11
—loss
¤ diseases associated with, 514ff; see also Alopecias
—shaft
¤ components, 12
Hard Chancre
¤ see Syphilis
Heat
¤ affections due to, 118-19
¤ sense of: importance, 27
¤ stress on, by Ayurveda, Galen, Hippocrates, 27
Hebra
¤ see Dermatitis exfoliative
Henoch-Schoenlein purpura
¤ see Purpura
Herpes, 181ff

¤ approach, 186ff; cases, 198ff; repertory, 204ff
—Circinatus, 75
—Progenitalis
¤ development, 44
—recurrent, 68
—Simplex, 30, 40, 41
¤ diagnosis, 183-84; features, clinical, 182-83; prognosis, 184
—Zoster, 26, 30, 33, 34, 38, 40ff, 75, 77, 184ff
¤ diagnosis, 185; features, clinical, 185; prognosis, 185-86
Herpes-Zoster like Lichen planus
¤ see Lichen planus
herpetic neuralgia, 27
Herpetic Whitlow, 530
Herpetiform, 38
Hidradenitis suppurativa, 42
Histochemical methods, 6
Histocytes, 7
Histological studies
¤ biopsy, 55-6; cytological examination, 56-7; histochemistry, 57; Tests: immunofluorescence, 57-8; Tissue stain, 55; Tzanck, 57
History of disease
¤ see Natural history of disease
Hodgkin's disease, 37, 72, 130
Holmes, Sherlock, 2, 219
Horny layer, 14
¤ water content in, 15
Human beings
¤ skin-keratinized
¤¤ waterproof epidermis, 14
Human Leucocyte
¤ Antigen (HL-A) system, 45-6
Human skin
¤ see Skin, human
Hunterian Chancre
¤ see Syphilis
Huxley's layer, 12
Hydroa aestivals, 48
Hyperaesthesia, 26, 27
Hyperchromatic nuclei, 24
Hyperhidrosis, 68, 563-64
¤ causes, prognosis, 564; treatment, 564-65
Hyper keratosis, 23, 24, 32
Hyperpigmentary macules, 28
Hyperplasia, 23, 37
Hypersensitivity, 46-8
¤ types, 48
Hypertrophy, 23, 36
Hypodermis, 4, 7, 12, 18
Hypopigmentation, 29
Hypothalamus
¤ heat-regulating centres in, 18

ICHTHYOSIS, 23, 32, 80
Ide eruptions, 43
Illiteracy
¤ and: diseases, contagious, 1-2; tropical countries, 2
Immersion foot
¤ see Frost-bite
Immunity
¤ definition, 44; mechanism, 44-5
—antibody mediated
¤ (humoral), 45
—cell mediated (T. cell), 45
Immunofluorescence
¤ (technique), 57-8
Immunoglobin (Ig)
¤ classification: IgA, 45; IgD, 45; IgE, 45; IgG, 45, 130; IgM, 45, 130
Impetigo Contagiosa, 30ff, 35, 41. 77, 78
¤ approach, 38ff; case, 395; diagnosis, 383; features, clinical, 381-82; histopathology, 382-83; prognosis, 383-84
Infantile Dermatitis
¤ see Dermatitis
—Eczema
Infection dorphacyngeal, 461
Infection gonococcal disseminated,

460-61
Infections
¤ and tropics, 1
Infectious eczematoid Dermatitis
¤ see Dermatitis
Infective Dermatitis
¤ see Dermatitis
—Eczema
¤ see Eczema
Inflammatory phimosis, 453
Ingrown Toe-nails, 530-31
Inhalants, 60
¤ and allergy tests, 60
Insect bites, 29ff
¤ frequency of, 44
Integument, 4, 8, 14, 22, 64, 68
¤ see also Skin, human
¤ agents (physical) affecting the, 81ff
Integumentary system
¤ anomalies, congential, 21-2
Intertrigo, 33, 40, 42, 68
¤ diagnosis, 341; drugs, 342ff; etiology, 340; features, clinical, 340-41; repertory, 346-48; treatment, 341-42
Intradermal tests, 59-60
Ions
¤ and skins, 19
Itching, 48, 49, 72
¤ causes, 26; result of, 540
—dermatoses, 540-41
Ito-Reenstierna test, 61; 454

JOINTS LESIONS, 429

KAHN TEST, 54
Kaposi's Varicelliform eruption, 32
Keloid, 30, 78
Keratin, 6
¤ constituent of sweat, 15
Keratinized
¤ epidermis, 14; structure, 11
Keratinocytes, 5, 6
Keratinous tissue, 52-3
Keratoderma(s), 23, 37, 43
Keratohyalin
¤ granules of, 5, 6, 20
Keratosis, 23, 37
Keratotic warts
¤ see Warts
Koebner phenomenon, 37
Koeim test, 61

LABORATORY AIDS
¤ and etiology, 50
Langerhan's cells, 6, 24
'Lanugo' hair, 10, 21
Leiner Erythoderma Desquamativum, 228
Leishmaniasis, 34, 37
Leishmania Vaccine test, 61
Lepromin test, 48, 61
Leprosy, 24, 28ff, 34, 36, 41, 43, 54, 77, 78
¤ anaesthesia in, 27; development, 44; diet in, 65; slit biopsy in, 51
Lesion(s)
¤ clinical: primary, 28-31, 37; secondary, 32-4, 56; erythomato-papular, 29; granulomatus, 31; in: bones, eyes, 49; of: bones, bursae, joints, muscles, tendons, 429; papulo-pustules, papulo-vesicular, 29; special: see Dermatological terms
Leucocyte(s), 45, 46
—counts, 27
Lewis (Sir), Thomas (1927), 46
Lichenoid
¤ description, 37; eruptions: types, 495-96
Lichen Myxoedematosus, 496
—Nitidus, 495
—plano-pilaris, 37, 494

—planus, 24, 29, 32, 37, 40ff, 58
¤ annular, 493; approach, 496-97; development, 44; diagnosis, 494; etiology, 492; features, clinical, 492-93; pathology, 492; prognosis, 496; variations, 493-94
Lichen Sclerosus et atrophicus, 24, 42
—scrofulosorum, 29, 37
—simplex chromicus, 75
spinulosus, 29, 37, 495
—striatus, 495
syphiliticus, 495
Lie detection
¤ basis, 16
Lipoma(s), 25, 30
Lunula
¤ definition, 13
L(upus) Erythematosus, 32, 35, 40, 41, 49, 58, 61, 109-10, 514
¤¤ cells, 56-7
L(upus) V(ulgaris), 34, 41ff
Lymphogranuloma
¤ development of, 44
—inguinale, 36, 42, 61
—venereum
¤ diagnosis, 458; features, clinical, 457-58; incubation, infection, 457; prognosis, 458
Lymphomas
¤ production of, 47

MACERATION, 23, 58, 68
¤ approach, description, 107; remedies, 108-09
Macular syphilids, 28, 425
Macule(s), 61
¤ causes, 28-9; definition, 28
—Erythematous, 28
—Pigmentary, 28-9
Maculo-papular syphilides, 425
Male
¤ gonorrhoea in, 459-60
Malpighian layer
¤ see Stratum Malpighii
Malpighian system
¤ see Melancocytes
Malpighee Stratum
¤ see Stratum Malpighii
Mantoux test
¤ see Tuberculin test
Mast cells, 45, 46
Mata
¤ see Smallpox
Medicine
¤ practice of, bases for, 3
Medulla
¤ see Hair shaft
Meibomian glands
¤ see Glands
Meissner's corpuscles, 7
Melanin (pigment), 5, 13, 20
¤ synthesis of, 15
Melancocytes, 5, 6, 13
¤ dendrites of, 5
Melanoma(s), 25, 56
—malignant
¤ development of, 44
Membrane, basement
¤ see Basal Lamina
Menicke's test, 54
Mental sweating
¤ see Cold sweating
Merkel's discs, 8
Mesenchymal cells
¤ see Cells
Miasm
¤ understanding of, 72ff
Microsporon, 480
Miliaria crystallina, 30
—rubra, 30
Milroy's disease, 25
Mitotic figures
¤ see Stratum Germinativum
Moisture
¤ stress on, by Ayurveda, Galen, Hippocrates, 27

Molluscum Contagiosum, 24
◘ approach, 489-90; diagnosis, 489; features, 489
Moniliasis, 42, 48
Mucous membrane(s)
◘ and skin, 14; lesions, 429
Mycological studies, 51-4
◘ material collection, 52; microscopic examination, 52-4; staining, 54
Mycosis fungoides, 30, 37
Myxoedematous skin
◘ see Skin

NAEVI, 25, 28ff, 38, 78
Nails 13-4, 21
◘ and: claws, hooves, 13
Nail colour changes
◘ banding, 528; splinter haemorrhages, 529-29
Nail diseases, 525ff
—dystrophy
◘ approach, 531; causes, 526ff
Nail splitting
◘ see Nail dystrophy
Napkin rash, 338ff
◘ diagnosis, 338-39; drugs, 339-40; prophylexis, 339; symptoms, 338-39; treatment, 339-40
Natural history of disease, 43-4
Necrobiosis, 48
◘ meaning, 25
Neoplastic ulcer, 33, 34
'Nettle rash'
◘ see Urticaria
Neuralgia, herpetic, 27
Neuritis, leprotic, 26
Neurodermatitis, 40ff, 75
◘ characteristics, 237; prognosis, treatment, 238
Neurofibromatosis, 29, 49, 62
Neuro-syphilis, 421, 430-31
Nodule(s), 61
◘ description, 29; examples, 29-30
Nummular eczema
◘ see Eczema

OCCUPATIONAL DERMATITIS
◘ see Dermatitis
Oedema, 19, 23ff, 31, 59
◘ angioneurotic, 164, 171-73
Oil, 69-70, 71
Onychomycosis
◘ see nail dystrophy and Tinea Unguium
Organs of Ruffini
◘ see sensory end-organs for heat

PAGET'S DISEASE
◘ see Epitheliomas
Palpable purpura
◘ see Purpura
Panniculitis
◘ subcutaneous tissue in (affected), 25
Papillary layer, 14
Papular eruptions
◘ see Eruption(s)
—syphilides, 425-26
—Urticaria, 31, 163ff
◘ diagnosis, etiology, prognosis, 164; treatment, 164-65
Papule(s), 29-30, 59, 61
◘ causes, description, 29
—epidermic
◘ description, 29
—in lines, 29
Papulous
◘ case study, 285-86
Parakeratosis, 23, 32
Paronychia, 107, 529-31
Paronychial inflammation
◘ Bacterial paronychia, 530; Candida paronychia, 529-30; herpetic whitlow, 530; ingrown toe-

nails, 530-31
Paronychial warts
¤ see Warts
Patch tests, 58-9
Patient
¤ bearing, clothing, 2; signs, symptoms, 72
Pediculoses, 41, 42
Pellagra, 32, 48
Pemphoid, 58
¤ course, 506; hallmarks, diagnositic, 505; pathogenesis, 506-07; presentation, clinical, 505-06; prognosis, variants, 506
Pemphigus, 30, 34, 41, 42, 57, 64
¤ approach, 507ff; diet, 65
—(of Hailey and Hailey), 23, 24, 33
—vegetans, 38
—vulgaris
¤ course, 504; hallmarks,
¤¤ diagnostic, 503, pathogenesis, 505; presentation, 503-04; prognosis, 504
Perioral dermatitis
¤ see Dermatitis
Perspiration, 8-9, 15, 17-8
¤ mechanism, 16
Petechial and Ecchymotic diseases, 297-300
Phagedaena, 42, 454
Phimosis, inflammatory, 453
Photodermatitis and contact Dermatitis, 218-19
Pigmentary macule
¤ see Macule
Pigmentary system
¤ see Melanocytes
Pigmentation, 48, 49
Pilonidal cyst
¤ see Cyst
Pilo-sebaceous, apparatus, 19, 24
Pimples
¤ repertory, 365ff
(Von) Pirquet, Vienne (1906)
¤ 'Allergy' coined, 46
Pituitary cachexia (Simmond's), 49
Pityriasis alba, 29
—capitis, 41
rubra pilaris, 23, 32, 36, 37
—rosea, 28, 32, 36, 42, 314
—versicolour, 32, 40ff
Pityrosporon ovale, 22
Plantar warts
¤ see Warts
Plastic planing
¤ see Cutaneous scars
Plexuses, 7, 17
Polyhedral cells, 5, 12
Porphyrinuria, 48, 54, 62
Portier and Richet (1902)
¤ Hypersensitivity
¤¤ concept introduced by, 46
Post-traumatic.infective eczema, 43, 224
Poverty
¤ and: countries, tropical; diseases, contagious, 2
Prausnitz-Kustner (passive transfer) reaction, 47
Pregnancy
¤ pruritus, 548-49
Pressure
¤ erythema caused by, 81
Prickle cell layer
¤ see Stratum Malpighii
Primary Chancre
¤ see Syphilis
Primary lesions
¤ see Lesions
Primary psora
¤ see Psora
Protein Keratin
¤ see Stratum Corneum
Prutritus, 74, 539ff
¤ causes, 540-41; discussion, 541-42; drugs, 549ff; treatment, 542-43; types, 543-44
—ani

◘ causes, 544-45; diagnosis, 545; etiology, 544-45; treatment, 545
—nocturnal, 557
—scrotum
◘ and penis, 547-48
—senile, 543
—summer, 543
—vulvae, 545ff
◘ diagnosis, 547; etiology, 546-47; prognosis, 547; treatment, 547
Psora, 72-3
Psoriasis, 7, 23, 24, 28, 29, 32, 35ff, 40ff, 74, 77, 526-27; approach, 320ff; cases, 328ff; development, 44; diagnosis, 318-19; pathology, 316; prognosis, 319-20; repertory, 336-37; see also Nail dystrophy
—Anthropathica, 317-18
—Flexural
—Guttate
—Pustular, 317
—Syphilitic, 319
Psoric miasm
◘ description, 73
Psychogenic dermatoses
◘ see Dermatoses
Puberty, 21
◘ and sebaceous glands, 16
Purpura, 25, 62, 302ff
◘ allergic, anaphylactoid, 304-05; approach, 305ff; treatment, 305
—ecchymosis
◘ repertory, 312-14
—Henoch-Schoenlein, 43, 48
—palpable
◘ course, 296; hallmarks, diagnostic, 295; pathogenesis, 296-97; presentation, clinical, 295-96; prognosis, 295
Pustular Psoriasis
◘ see Psoriasis
Pustule
◘ description, examples, 31
Pyoderma, 23, 41, 380ff
—chronic, 64
◘ diet in, 65
—gangrenosum
◘ development, 43
—vegetans, 24, 38

QUNCKE'S DISEASE

RADIATION
◘ way of heat loss, 17
Radio Dermatitis, 238
Radiological test, 62
Rash, drug, 31
◘ sense of heat (SOH) in, 27
Rash, Napkin
◘ see Napkin rash
Rashes, Erythematous, 289ff
◘ causes, 289-90
—syphilitic
◘ itching absent, 26
Raynaud's disease, 43, 49
Recurrent scarlatiniform Erythroderma
◘ see Erythroderma
Red cells
◘ extravasation of, 25
Regional differential diagnosis, 41-3
Remedies, anti-haemorrhagic, 308ff
Reticuloses, 25, 36, 37
Rhagades, 79
◘ repertory, 101-05
Richet (1902)
◘ 'anaphylaxis' coined, 46
Ringworm
◘ see Tinea
Ritter
◘ Dermatitis Exfoliative Neonatorum, 228
Roberts, 72
Rosacea (Acne Rosacea)
◘ see Acne

SABOURAUD'S MEDIUM, 53
Sarcoid, 24, 29, 30, 37
◘ histology of, 61
Sarcoidosis, 61, 62
Savill
◘ see Dermatitis
Scab
◘ see Crust
Scabies, 30, 31, 41, 42, 74
◘ alternate with asthma, 73; approach, 558-59; character, 44; complications, 558; features, clinical, 557-58; measures, preventive, 559; remedies, 559-62
Scale
◘ description, 32
Scaling
◘ causes, 32
Scar(s), 14, 31
◘ causes, description, 34
—cutaneous, 1
Schamberg's disease, 25
Schiff's stain, 54
Schoenlein purpura
◘ see Purpura
Scleroderma, 24, 25, 49
Scratch tests, 60
Scrofuloderma, 41, 42
Sebaceous Cyst
◘ see Cyst(s)
Sebaceous glands
◘ see Glands
Seborrhoea
◘ meaning of, 16
—corporis, 36
Seborrhocic conditions
◘ diet in, 65
—Dermatitis
◘ see Dermatitis
—eczema
◘ see Eczema
Sebum, 13
◘ constitutents, of, 16
Secondary Lesions
◘ see Lesions
Secondary psora
◘ see Psora
Secondary Syphilis
◘ see Syphilis
Sense of Heat (SOH)
◘ importance of, 27
Sensory
◘ end-organs for cold, heat, 18
◘ fibre, 7
Serological tests, 54
—for Syphilis, 423
Serotonim, 45, 46
Shelly test
◘ see Basophil degranulation Test
Skin, 52
◘ anatomy, 4ff; bacteriology, 22-3; embryology, 19-22; functions, 14ff; growth of, 19ff; pathology, 23ff; physiology, 14ff
—cancer, 29
◘ smears in, 57
—, cracks in
◘ approach, 96ff; cases, 106-07; remedies discussed, 96-101; repertory, 101-05; treatment, 95-6
—diathesis, 2, 9
disease(s), 46ff
◘ and dermal histology, 55ff; causes, characteristics, 1ff; diagnosis, 39-43; signs, 27ff; symptoms, 26; treatment, line of, 2-3
◘ see also Dermatoses
—grafting
◘ see scars, cutaneous
—, healthy
◘ aids to, 67ff
—, human
◘ characteristics, 4
—, macerated
◘ see Maceration
—, myxoedematous, 49

—temperature
◻ and blood flow, 17
Smallpox, 1, 29ff, 33
◻ course, limited, 43
Smears and stains, 50-1
Smegma glands
◻ see Glands
Soft chancre
◻ see Chancroid
Soft sore
◻ see Chancroid
Solar Dermatitis
◻ see Dermatitis
—Eczema
◻ see Eczema
—Urticaria, 125
Splinter haemorrhages
◻ see Nail colour changes
Squamous cell carcinoma
◻ see Epitheliomas
Staining, 54
Staphylococcus albus, 22, 23
Stinging, 26, 27
Stevens Johnson Syndrome
◻ Case study, 300-02
Stomatitis
◻ angular, 33, 41; approach, 396-98; drugs, 397-98
Stools test, 62
Stratum corneum, 6, 14, 15, 19, 20, 23, 32, 35, 37, 38
◻◻ desquamation, 22
—germinativum, 5, 6, 20, 24
—granulosum, 5, 6, 14, 20
—lucidum 5, 14, 20
—malpighii, 5, 6, 9, 12, 14, 20, 23, 24
Stresses, etiologica
◻ see Etiological stress
Subcutaneous layer
◻ see Hypodermis
—nodules, 74
—tissue, 23, 25
Sunburn
◻ treatment, 123
Sunlight, 15
◻ affections, 118; treatment, 119-22
Sunstroke
◻ affects, 122-23; treatment, 122-23
—acute
◻ treatment, 120-22
Superstitions
◻ and diseases, contagious, 1
Sweat, 15-6, 25
◻ constituents, 15; enzymes, 22; repertory, 569-71
—apparatus
◻ disorders of, 563ff
—glands
◻ see Glands
—partial
◻ repertory, 571-72
Sweating, 58
◻ and exercise, 16
Sycosis, 32, 41, 75, 497ff
◻ diagnosis, 498; etiology, 498; Prognosis, 498
—barbae, 31, 41
◻ approach, 499ff
—lupoides, 498
—nuchae, 41, 497
Syphilides, papular
◻ see Papular Syphilides
Syphilis, 25, 29, 30, 32ff, 36, 39, 43, 51, 61, 62, 75, 77
◻◻ approach, 433ff; benign, 41, 428-29; bone affection, 426, 429; bursae, 429; cardiovascular, 421; classification, 428ff; congenital, 431-33; course, 421; cutaneous, 428-29; diagnosis, 422-24, 432-33; drugs, 435-44; etiology, 419-20; features, clinical, 424-25; hair affection, 426; incubation, 424; infection, 420; joints affection, 426, 429; late (stage) 421, 428; latent, 427; liver, 429-30; mucous membrane, muscles, 429; nails

affection, ocular affection, 426; pathology, 421; relapse in, 427; repertory, 444ff; serological test, 54; signs, 421-32; syphilides, 425-26; tendons, 429; tests, 422ff; untreated, 420-21; visceral, 421, 429-30
—nodulo ulcerative, 33
—rupial, 33
Syphilitic chancre
◘ development, 44
—fissures, 33
—gumma
◘ development of, 44
Syringomyelia, 34
◘ anaesthesia in, 27
Systemic diseases
◘ see Diseases
—disorders
◘ and cutaneous lesions, 48-9

TENIA FAVOSA, 74, 76
Telangiectasia
◘ causes, description, 37
Telogen, 12, 13
◘ effluvium, 516-17
Temperament
◘ stress on, by Ayurveda, Galen, Hippocrates, 27
Tests
◘ see under respective names
Thermal sweating
◘ meaning, 15
T(hymus) Lymphocyte cells, 44-5
Tinea, 30, 42, 43, 53, 480ff
◘ approach, 486-88; types, 480ff
—barbae, 75
◘ types, 482-83
—capitis, 513-14
◘ case, 488-89; diagnosis, differential, 482; featues, clinical, 481-82
—circinata, 28, 35, 42
—corporis, 32
—cruris, 41, 42
◘ diagnosis, prognosis, 484
◘ diagnosis, differential, 483-84; features, clinical, 483; prognosis, 484
—(feet), 484-86
◘ diagnosis, 485; prognosis, 486
—(hands), 484-86
◘ diagnosis, 485; prognosis, 486
—pedis, 41
—unguium
◘ prognosis, 486
—Versicolor, 29, 32, 42, 54
—Vesicular, 75
Toad, skin
◘ glands, poisonous, 14
Toe-nail(s)
◘ arteriosclerotic changes of
◘ see Nail Dystrophy
◘ ingrown, 530-31
Tonfibrils
◘ see Cytoplasm
Tonofilaments
◘ see Cytoplasm
Toxic Erythemata, 292-93
Traumata, 13
◘ healing, 5
Treponema pallida agglutination (TPA) test, 423
—complement fixation (TPCA) test, 423
—immobilization (TPI) test, 423
—immune adherence (TPIA) test, 423
Treponema Pallidum, 51
Trophic ulcers, 33, 48
Tropical countries
◘ illiteracy, poverty in, 2
Tropical diseaes
◘ see Diseases
—Ulcers, 34
◘ development, 43
Tropics
◘ and infections, 1

Tubercular miasm, 73
Tuberculin test, 40, 61
Tuberous sclerosis, 49, 54
Tumour(s), 25
◘ description, 29; examples, 30
Tzanck test, 57

ULCERS, 19, 32
◘ causes, 33-4
Urine Analysis test, 62
Urticaria, 26, 31, 46, 48, 59, 62, 64, 75
◘ approach, 165ff; cases, 173ff; diagnosis, 162; etiology, 160-62; features, clinical, 160; pathology, 160; prognosis, 163; repertory, 177ff; sense of heat in, 27
Urticaria, Solar
◘ see Solar urticaria
Urticarial eruptions
◘ see Urticaria

VACCINATION, 77, 78, 80
Varicose dermatitis
◘ see Dermatitis
—Ulcer, 33, 34, 41, 43, 79
Vasculitis, neutrophilic type
◘ see Purpura
V.D.R.L. test, 422ff
Vegetations
◘ cause, 38
Vellus hair, 10, 11
Venereal Warts
◘ see Warts (condyloma acuminata)
Vernix caseosa, 20, 21
Vesicle, 31-33
◘ causes, description, 30
Viruses, 126ff
Visceral Syphilis, 421, 429-30
Vitiligo, 29, 38, 41, 54, 62, 79

WARTS, 23, 24, 29, 37, 44, 75
◘ approach, 132ff; cases, 134-36, 141ff; repertory, 154-59; treatment, 136-41, 152-54
—condyloma, acuminata, flat, 130ff
—paroenychial, plantar, verucca vulgaris, 128ff
Weal
◘ description, exmaple,s 31; reaction, 59
Whitlow
◘ case, 537-38
Wilson
◘ see Dermatitis
Wood's Lamp Examination, 54

XANTHOMATOSIS, 29, 48, 62

YAWS, 34, 36, 54

ZIEHL NEELSEN STAIN, 50, 51
Zosteriform
◘ description, example, 38